Clinical Immunology

Clinical Immunology

Edited by **Jim Wang**

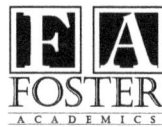

FA **FOSTER** ACADEMICS

New Jersey

Published by Foster Academics,
61 Van Reypen Street,
Jersey City, NJ 07306, USA
www.fosteracademics.com

Clinical Immunology
Edited by Jim Wang

International Standard Book Number: 978-1-63242-431-0 (Hardback)

Printed in the United States of America.

Contents

Preface

In my initial years as a student, I used to run to the library at every possible instance to grab a book and learn something new. Books were my primary source of knowledge and I would not have come such a long way without all that I learnt from them. Thus, when I was approached to edit this book; I became understandably nostalgic. It was an absolute honor to be considered worthy of guiding the current generation as well as those to come. I put all my knowledge and hard work into making this book most beneficial for its readers.

Immunology is the branch of medical science which deals with the study of the immune system and related issues. It generally studies the problems such as hypersensitivity, transplant rejection, autoimmune diseases, immune deficiency, etc. It has applications in wide variety of fields such as bacteriology, oncology, psychiatry, parasitology, and dermatology. Clinical immunology studies the problems caused by dysfunction of the immune system. This book is a compilation of chapters that discuss the most vital concepts and emerging trends in this field. It aims to shed light on some of the unexplored aspects of this subject and recent researches in this area. The studies collated in this book have been contributed by immunologists, researchers and veterans from across the globe. For all those who are interested in clinical immunology, this book will prove to be an essential guide.

I wish to thank my publisher for supporting me at every step. I would also like to thank all the authors who have contributed their researches in this book. I hope this book will be a valuable contribution to the progress of the field.

Editor

Recurrent Skin and Lung Infections in Autosomal Dominant Hyper IgE Syndrome with Transactivation Domain STAT3 Mutation

Chad J. Cooper, Sarmad Said, and German T. Hernandez

Department of Internal Medicine, Texas Tech University Health Sciences Center, 4800 Alberta Avenue, El Paso, TX 79905, USA

Correspondence should be addressed to Chad J. Cooper; chad.cooper@ttuhsc.edu

Academic Editors: M. Hummel, N. Kutukculer, and J. Litzman

Background. Hyper IgE is a rare systemic disease characterized by the clinical triad of high serum levels of IgE (>2000 IU/mL), eczema, and recurrent staphylococcal skin and lung infections. The presentation of hyper IgE syndrome is highly variable, which makes it easy to confuse the diagnosis with that of severe atopy or other rare immunodeficiency disorders. *Case Report.* A 23-year-old Hispanic presented with history of frequent respiratory and gastrointestinal infections as a child and multiple episodes of skin and lung infections (abscess) with *Staphylococcus aureus* throughout his adult life. He had multiple eczematous lesions and folliculitis over his entire body, oral/esophageal candidiasis, and retention of his primary teeth. The IgE was elevated (>5000 IU/mL). Genetic mutation analysis revealed a mutation affecting the transactivation domain of the STAT3 gene. *Conclusion.* The hallmark of hyper IgE syndrome is serum IgE of >2000 IU/mL. Hyper IgE syndrome is a genetic disorder that is either autosomal dominant or recessive. A definite diagnosis can be made with genetic mutation analysis, and in this case, it revealed a very rare finding of the transactivation domain STAT3 mutation. Hyper IgE syndrome is a challenge for clinicians in establishing a diagnosis in suspected cases.

1. Introduction

Hyper IgE is a rare systemic disease characterized by the clinical triad of high serum levels of IgE (>2000 IU/mL), eczema, and recurrent staphylococcal skin and lung infections [1]. It was first described as Job's syndrome in 1966, in patients suffering from recurrent sinopulmonary infections and cold skin abscesses due to *Staphylococcus aureus* [1]. The term was changed to hyper IgE syndrome, when an elevated level of IgE was discovered in these affected patients. There is no predilection for a certain gender or race. In recent years, the pathophysiology has been revealed through understanding the genetic components and consequences of the underlying condition. Hyper IgE syndrome is a complex immune deficiency with diverse clinical manifestations and heterogeneous genetic origins [2]. The presentation of hyper IgE syndrome is highly variability, which makes it easy to confuse the diagnosis with that of severe atopy or other rare immunodeficiency disorders.

The majority of patients with hyper IgE syndrome suffer from recurrent staphylococcal infections that predominantly involve the skin and lungs. Other features include abnormalities of the musculoskeletal system, hypermobility of the joints, prominent forehead, broad nasal bridge, macrocephaly, retention of primary teeth, and recurrent skin or respiratory infections [2]. Fungal infections, including mucocutaneous candidiasis and pulmonary aspergillosis, are also common. Patients with hyper IgE syndrome commonly have atopic dermatitis associated with very high levels of IgE and eosinophilia. But they do not have allergic manifestations, such as allergic rhinitis, asthma, urticaria, and anaphylaxis [3]. Hyper IgE syndrome has been associated with an increased risk of autoimmune diseases such as systemic lupus erythemathosus (SLE), dermatomyositis, and membranoproliferative glomerulonephritis [3]. These patients have an increased incidence of lymphoproliferative disorders such that non-Hodgkin and Hodgkin lymphomas have also been noted. Skeletal abnormalities include osteopenia, minimal trauma fractures, and scoliosis. Vascular abnormalities include middle-sized artery tortuosity and aneurysms, with infrequent clinical sequelae of myocardial infarction and subarachnoid hemorrhage.

The respiratory infections are most commonly caused by *Streptococcus pneumonia*, *Staphylococcus aureus*, or *Haemophilus influenzae* [4]. Pneumonias are usually complicated by lung abscesses, bronchopleural fistulas, bronchiectasis, and the formation of pneumatocele [4]. These bronchopulmonary lesions are predisposing factors for colonization by opportunistic microorganisms such as *Aspergillus fumigatus* and *Pseudomonas aeruginosa*. These pulmonary complications lead to the development of chronic respiratory insufficiency which is the main cause of mortality in hyper IgE syndrome [5]. Lung abscess with hemoptysis and cystic lung disease are other common causes of death in hyper IgE syndrome.

Characteristic oral and dental manifestations in hyper IgE syndrome include the delayed loss of primary teeth, abnormal development of permanent teeth, periodontitis, and severe dental caries with periapical abscess formation. Primary teeth usually fail to exfoliate, which may impair secondary dentition emergence [6]. The retention of primary teeth has been thought to be due to reduced resorption of the tooth roots that result in the failure of eruption of permanent teeth [7]. The extraction of primary teeth usually results in normal eruption of the permanent dentition. Other oral cavity abnormalities have also been described, including a high arched palate, central ridges, and fissures of the palate and deep grooves on the tongue and buccal mucosa with multiple fissures [8]. We present a classic case of a patient with autosomal dominant hyper IgE syndrome and the identification of a rare genetic mutation of the STAT3 gene.

2. Case Report

A 23-year-old Hispanic male presented to our care with a sore throat and odynophagia to liquid and solids for 3 days. He denied any fever, chills, nausea, vomiting, diarrhea, cough, or shortness of breath. He claimed that he had frequent respiratory and gastrointestinal infections when he was a child. On a previous hospital admission 2 years ago, he was discovered to have a lung abscesses (*Staphylococcus aureus*) and oral candidiasis. The computed tomography (CT) of the chest on the previous admission revealed a large consolidation involving the right lung and posterior segment of the left lower lobe with an air fluid level. These bilateral lung abscesses were drained and he was treated for aspiration pneumonia with clindamycin 300 mg PO four times a day for one month upon discharge. The CT of the chest (Figure 1) after drainage of the abscess revealed residual 6 cm thin walled cyst in the posterior aspect of the of left midlung field. Other past medical problems included recurrent *Staphylococcus aureus* skin infections. He had no family history of any immunodeficiency disorders. He admitted to smoking 1 pack of cigarettes per week for the last 9 years and social alcohol use. He denied any illicit drugs use.

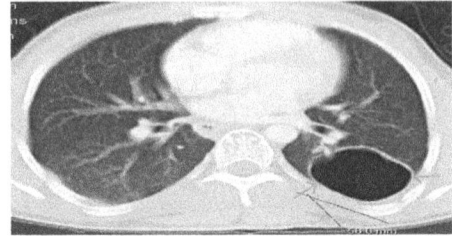

FIGURE 1: Chest CT: residual 6 cm thin walled cyst in the posterior aspect of the left midlung field (green arrows).

TABLE 1: Initial laboratory work-up.

White blood cell count	10.0×10^3 UL (4.5–11.0×10^3/UL)
Hemoglobin	12.4 g/dL (12.0–15.0 g/dL)
Hematocrit	37.0% (36.0–47.0%)
Platelet count	198×10^3/UL (150–450×10^3/UL)
Sodium	145 mmol/L (135–145 mmol/L)
Potassium	4.3 mmol/L (3.5–5.1 mmol/L)
Chloride	119 mmol/L (98–107 mmol/L)
CO_2	17 mmol/L (21–32 mmol/L)
Serum glucose	85 mg/dL (70–100 mg/dL)
BUN	25 mg/dL (7–22 mg/dL)
Creatinine	2.2 mg/dL (0.60–1.30 mg/dL)
Calcium	7.9 mmol/L (8.5–10.1 mmol/L)
Albumin	2.8 g/dL (3.4–5.0 g/dL)
Protein	5.9 g/dL (6.4–8.2 g/dL)
AST	29 IU/L (15–37 IU/L)
ALT	19 IU/L (12–78 IU/L)
Alkaline phosphatase	83 IU/L (50–136 IU/L)

Initial vital signs were significant for hypertension (blood pressure: 147/85), tachycardia (heart rate: 116), and tachypnea (respiratory rate: 25 breaths per minute). Physical examination revealed a cachectic individual with multiple eczematous lesions and folliculitis over his entire body. He had white lesions resembling thrush on his tongue, palate, and oropharynx. It was noted that he had retention of his primary teeth. Breath sounds were decreased bilaterally on auscultation. He was tachycardic but without murmurs. He had a decreased muscle mass of all four extremities. The initial lab work-up (Table 1) was only significant for acute renal insufficiency (BUN 25 mg/dL and creatinine 2.2. mg/dL), hypocalcemia (calcium 7.9 mmol/L), hypoalbuminemia (albumin 2.8 g/dL), and hypoproteinemia (7.9 mmol/L). The chest radiograph (Figure 2) on admission revealed a left lung cyst.

Our initial impression was oral/esophageal candidiasis and the possibility of an immunodeficiency disorder. For the treatment of oral/esophageal candidiasis, he was started on fluconazole 100 mg IV daily. The HIV test was negative. Other lab work-ups (Table 2) was ordered to rule out various immunodeficiency disorders. All the immunoglobulins (Ig) were within normal range except that IgE was very elevated (>5000 IU/mL). The normal value of IgE was <114 IU/mL. Genetic mutation analysis revealed a novel mutation affecting the transactivation domain of the STAT3 gene at exon 22. This

Recurrent Skin and Lung Infections in Autosomal Dominant Hyper IgE Syndrome...

3

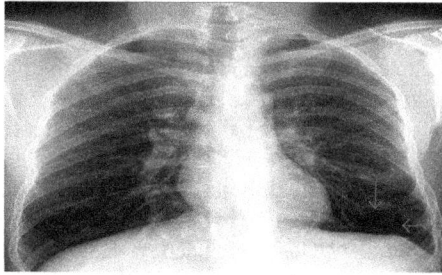

FIGURE 2: CXR: left lung cyst (red arrows).

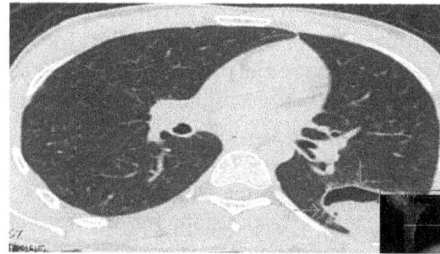

FIGURE 3: Chest CT: cavitation measuring 5.6 cm in the superior segment of the left lower lobe that contained soft tissue density (blue arrows).

TABLE 2: Other laboratory work-ups.

Complement 3 (C3)	113 mg/dL (74–148 mg/dL)
Complement 4 (C4)	35 mg/dL (14–39 mg/dL)
CH 50	52 U/mL (30–75 U/mL)
IgM	84 mg/dL (54–296 mg/dL)
IgD	9 mg/dL (<10 mg/dL)
IgE	>5000 IU/mL (<114 IU/mL)
IgA	158 mg/dL (50–400 mg/dL)
IgG	1480 mg/dL (600–1500 mg/dL)

provided a definite diagnosis of autosomal dominant hyper IgE syndrome which correlates with the clinical presentation. These results confirmed our suspicion of hyper IgE syndrome (Job's syndrome). No curative treatment is available for hyper IgE syndrome. We treated his multiple skin infections with mupirocin 2% ointment and started prophylactic treatment of recurrent skin and pulmonary infections with trimethoprim-sulfamethoxazole 160 mg tab every 12 hours to prevent recurrent staphylococcal infections.

Approximately one year after previous, he presented again with a productive cough with greenish sputum, fever, chills, generalized weakness, eczema, chest pain, and shortness of breath for 4 days. On the day of admission he had 3 bouts of hemoptysis. The CT of the chest (Figure 3) revealed the same cavitation measuring 5.6 cm in the superior segment of the left lower lobe (LLL) that contained soft tissue density that was suggestive of a mycetoma. A bronchoscopy was performed on this admission with findings of hemoptysis and cavitation in the LLL. The analysis of the bronchoalveolar lavage fluid did not reveal any pneumocystis or fundal organisms. He was discharged on amoxicillin-sulbactum 500 mg tab every 12 hours and itraconazole 200 mg tab every 12 hours. Even though the patient had recurrent infections typical of hyper IgE as a child, he never received an immunodeficiency investigation. Partly because hyper IgE is a rare disease that can have a variety of presentations and not all physicians may consider it in their differential diagnosis, another reason as stated by the patient was that he was treated for the infection and then either lost to follow up or went to another hospital once another infection recurred. This case demonstrates the chronic debilitating course of a patient with hyper IgE.

3. Discussion

The hallmark of hyper IgE syndrome is an increased concentration of immunoglobulin E (IgE) in the serum. A value of >2000 IU/mL has been considered the cutoff point in establishing a definitive diagnosis of the syndrome [9]. The diagnosis of hyper IgE syndrome is based on characteristic clinical phenotypes associated with increased serum levels of IgE and eosinophilia. In 93% of patients with hyper IgE syndrome will also exhibit peripheral eosinophilia [9]. Eosinophilia is common but does not always correlate with the serum IgE. In approximately 20% of cases, the IgE will normalize during adulthood [10]. Other immunoglobulins are frequently normal, although some may have low serum IgA or slightly low serum IgG. Hyper IgE syndrome is a genetic disorder that is either autosomal dominant or recessive. However, a definite diagnosis can be made with genetic mutation analysis. Autosomal dominant hyper IgE syndrome will have abnormalities in multiple systems, including skeletal/dental, connective tissue, and immune systems. Autosomal dominant hyper IgE syndrome manifests characteristics of coarse facies, skeletal/connective tissue abnormalities (pathological fracture, scoliosis, hyperextensibility, and retention of deciduous teeth), and pneumatocele after pulmonary staphylococcal infection [11].

The majority of autosomal dominant hyper IgE syndrome is sporadic mutations. The autosomal dominant hyper IgE syndrome is associated with a missense or in-frame deletions in the SH2 and DNA-binding domains in the STAT3 gene (Signal Transducer and Activator of Transcription 3) [12]. Woellner et al. found 18 novel mutations in STAT3 gene among a cohort of 100 patients with suspected hyper IgE syndrome [13]. It is deemed necessary to sequence the entire STAT3 gene to exclude possible mutations. Mutations could involve the exon or introns of the DNA-binding domain, SH2 domain, which are more common or the very rarely, and involve the transactivation domain or coiled-coil domain. Patients with the STAT 3 mutation have reduced numbers of interleukin (IL) 17 producing CD4 T cells. Those patients without the STAT3 mutation had a significant reduction of IFN-gamma producing CD4 T cells. Woellner et al. therefore suggest that Th-17 could also be used to distinguish hyper IgE syndrome patients with or without the STAT3 mutation [13]. IL-10 is one of the cytokines that are signaled through STAT3 gene. IL-10 plays an anti-inflammatory role that affects the extent of anti-/proinflammatory cytokine production and the regulation of monocytes [14]. It also inhibits the function of macrophages, suppresses inflammatory cytokines (IL-1, IL-6, IL-8, and TNF-alpha), and inhibits the function of antigen presenting cells (APC) [14].

Autosomal recessive hyper IgE syndrome is associated with a deficiency of tyrosine kinase 2 (TYK2). Tyrosine kinase 2 deficiency is responsible for the impairment of the innate and adaptive immune response due to defective cytokine signal transduction pathways which depend on interferon (IFN)-α, IL-6, IL-10, IL-12, and IL-23 [15]. Autosomal recessive hyper IgE syndrome displays abnormalities that are confined to the immune system. Autosomal recessive hyper IgE syndrome presents with severe viral infections, central nervous system involvement, and intracellular bacterial infections, but absence of pneumatocele and skeletal/connective tissue abnormalities [15]. Some cases of autosomal recessive hyper IgE syndrome will have a homozygous mutation of the cytokinesis gene, dedicator of cytokinesis 8 (DOCK8) that leads to a disruptive production of a protein involved in the regulation of actin skeleton [15]. Patients with autosomal recessive hyper IgE syndrome lack the connective tissue and skeletal manifestations, but an increased rate of viral infections (DOCK8 mutations) and intracellular bacteria (TYK2 mutations) [16]. Hematopoietic stem cell transplantation (HSCT) is not considered for hyper IgE syndrome but should be considered in DOCK8 deficiency [17].

The management of hyper IgE syndrome patients is difficult, mainly because the pathophysiology of the immunodeficiency is not completely understood. No curative treatment is available; however, prophylactic antibiotics, specific treatment depending on the involved organ system, and systemic antibiotics for infections have been suggested. Some authorities also recommend antifungal prophylaxis with itraconazole. A major goal of treatment is aggressive control of skin and sinopulmonary infections. Prophylactic antibiotic therapy with trimethoprim-sulfamethoxazole is recommended in patients with recurrent sinopulmonary and cutaneous infections to prevent Staphylococcal infections. The control of respiratory infections can help decrease the risk of parenchymal lung damage. The main therapeutic approach to hyper IgE syndrome is the prevention and management of infections. Empiric therapy of active respiratory infections with the introduction of antibiotics early on to cover such microorganisms as Staphylococcus aureus, Streptococcus pneumonia, and Haemophilus influenzae is recommended. Skin or lung abscesses may require surgical intervention.

There are a few studies in the current literature suggesting that intravenous immunoglobulin (IVIg) or hematopoietic cell transplantation (HCT) could be viable options in the treatment of hyper IgE. Wakim et al. reported no dramatic laboratory or clinical improvement with the use of IVIG in the treatment in patients with hyper IgE syndrome. IVIG does not provide a clear clinical benefit to help decrease IgE level [18]. Gennery et al. suggested that hematological and immunological reconstitution with donor bone marrow stem cells does not alter the disease process in hyper IgE

syndrome [19]. However, Mcdonald et al. reported on a child with autosomal recessive hyper IgE syndrome (ARHIES) with DOCK8 deficiency that underwent allogeneic hematopoietic cell transplantation (HCT) after myeloablative conditioning and demonstrated full donor chimerism early after transplant [20]. They suggested that HCT could be a viable therapy for these patients. Hematopoietic stem cell transplantation (HSCT) is not considered for hyper IgE syndrome but should be considered in DOCK8 deficiency. However, very few reports exist regarding the use of the IVIg or HCT for hyper IgE syndrome. Clearly more experience and further research are required to evaluate the clinical outcomes and future of these therapies.

Patients with the hyper IgE syndrome require interdisciplinary care by many specialists. Hyper IgE syndrome is a challenge for clinicians in establishing a diagnosis in suspected cases. Hyper IgE should be considered in the differential diagnosis when presented with a patient that exhibits clinical manifestations as mentioned above. Genetic mutation analysis provides a definitive diagnosis of hyper IgE syndrome. The case presented is very typical of STAT3 deficient autosomal dominant hyper IgE syndrome (ADHIES). The unique finding in this case is the very rare finding of the transactivation domain STAT3 mutation rather than the usual mutation of the SH2 or DNA-binding domain. There is no definitive therapy for hyper IgE syndrome. However, this case demonstrates a chronic debilitating course that requires further investigative research to develop a more effective therapy.

Conflict of Interests

All participated authors in this study declare no financial, professional, or personal conflict of interests.

Authors' Contribution

All authors were involved in paper preparation and literature review.

References

[1] L. Esposito, L. Poletti, C. Maspero et al., "Hyper-IgE syndrome: dental implications," Oral Surgery, Oral Medicine, Oral Pathology and Oral Radiology, vol. 114, no. 2, pp. 147–153, 2012.

[2] E. L. Rael, R. T. Marshall, and J. J. McClain, "The Hyper-IgE syndromes: lessons in nature, from bench to bedside," World Allergy Organization Journal, vol. 5, no. 7, pp. 79–87, 2012.

[3] Y. Minegishi, "Hyper-IgE syndrome," Current Opinion in Immunology, vol. 21, no. 5, pp. 487–492, 2009.

[4] S. Montella, M. Maglione, G. Giardino et al., "Hyper IgE syndrome presenting as chronic suppurative lung disease," Italian Journal of Pediatrics, vol. 38, article 45, 2012.

[5] Q. Zhang and H. C. Su, "Hyperimmunoglobulin e syndromes in pediatrics," Current Opinion in Pediatrics, vol. 23, no. 6, pp. 653–658, 2011.

[6] A. F. Freeman and S. M. Holland, "Clinical manifestations of hyper IgE syndromes," Disease Markers, vol. 29, no. 3-4, pp. 123–130, 2010.

[7] A. F. Freeman, D. L. Domingo, and S. M. Holland, "Hyper IgE (Job's) syndrome: a primary immune deficiency with oral manifestations," *Oral Diseases*, vol. 15, no. 1, pp. 2–7, 2009.

[8] P. F. K. Yong, A. F. Freeman, K. R. Engelhardt, S. Holland, J. M. Puck, and B. Grimbacher, "An update on the hyper IgE syndromes," *Arthritis Research & Therapy*, vol. 14, no. 6, p. 228, 2012.

[9] D. A. Koslovsky, V. A. Kostakis, A. N. Glied, R. D. Kelsch, and M. J. Wiltz, "An unusual lesion of the tongue in a 4-year-old with Job syndrome," *Journal of Oral and Maxillofacial Surgery*, vol. 71, no. 6, pp. 1042–1049, 2013.

[10] J. Heimall, A. Freeman, and S. M. Holland, "Pathogenesis of hyper IgE syndrome," *Clinical Reviews in Allergy and Immunology*, vol. 38, no. 1, pp. 32–38, 2010.

[11] J.-Y. Liu, Q. Li, T.-T. Chen, X. Guo, J. Ge, and L.-X. Yuan, "Destructive pulmonary staphylococcal infection in a boy with hyper-IgE syndrome: a novel mutation in the signal transducer and activator of transcription 3 (STAT3) gene (p.Y657S)," *European Journal of Pediatrics*, vol. 170, no. 5, pp. 661–666, 2011.

[12] P. Roxo, U. P. Menezes, S. Tucci Jr., M. F. Andrade, G. E. Barros Silva, and J. M. Lima Melo, "Renal abscess in hyper-IgE syndrome," *Urology*, vol. 81, no. 2, pp. 414–416, 2013.

[13] C. Woellner, E. M. Gertz, A. A. Schäffer et al., "Mutations in STAT3 and diagnostic guidelines for hyper-IgE syndrome," *The Journal of Allergy and Clinical Immunology*, vol. 125, no. 2, pp. 424.e8–432.e8, 2010.

[14] M. Giacomelli, N. Tamassia, D. Moratto et al., "SH2-domain mutations in STAT3 in hyper-IgE syndrome patients result in impairment of IL-10 function," *European Journal of Immunology*, vol. 41, no. 10, pp. 3075–3084, 2011.

[15] A. Szczawinska-Poplonyk, Z. Kycler, B. Pietrucha, E. Heropolitanska-Pliszka, A. Breborowicz, and K. Gerreth, "The hyperimmunoglobulin E syndrome—clinical manifestation diversity in primary immune deficiency," *Orphanet Journal of Rare Diseases*, vol. 6, no. 1, article 76, 2011.

[16] N. Rezaei and A. Aghamohammadi, "Hyper-IgE syndrome," *Journal of Postgraduate Medicine*, vol. 56, no. 2, pp. 63–64, 2010.

[17] P. Roxo Jr., L. A. G. M. Torres, U. P. Menezes, and J. M. L. Melo, "Lung function in hyper IgE syndrome," *Pediatric Pulmonology*, vol. 48, no. 1, pp. 81–84, 2013.

[18] M. Wakim, M. Alazard, A. Yajima, D. Speights, A. Saxon, and E. R. Stiehm, "High dose intravenous immunoglobulin in atopic dermatitis and hyper-IgE syndrome," *Annals of Allergy, Asthma and Immunology*, vol. 81, no. 2, pp. 153–158, 1998.

[19] A. R. Gennery, T. J. Flood, M. Abinun, and A. J. Cant, "Bone marrow transplantation does not correct the hyper IgE syndrome," *Bone Marrow Transplantation*, vol. 25, no. 12, pp. 1303–1305, 2000.

[20] D. R. Mcdonald, M. J. Massaad, A. Johnston et al., "Successful engraftment of donor marrow after allogeneic hematopoietic cell transplantation in autosomal-recessive hyper-IgE syndrome caused by dedicator of cytokinesis 8 deficiency," *Journal of Allergy and Clinical Immunology*, vol. 126, no. 6, pp. 1304.e3–1035.e3, 2010.

2

Persistent Lymphadenopathy due to IgG4-Related Disease

Benjamin Smith and Matthew B. Carroll

81st Medical Group Hospital, 301 Fisher Street, Keesler Air Force Base, MS 39534, USA

Correspondence should be addressed to Benjamin Smith, benjamin.smith.59@us.af.mil

Academic Editors: N. Martinez-Quiles, M. M. Nogueras, G. E. M. Reeves, and M. Trendelenburg

A 28-year-old healthy female presented to her primary care physician with lymphadenopathy, fatigue, malaise, and night sweats. Symptoms persisted despite conservative treatment and eventually the patient underwent multiple lymph node resections and a bone marrow biopsy before a diagnosis of IgG4-related disease (IgG4-RD) was made. IgG4-RD is a relatively new disorder first histopathologically recognized within the last decade. As the disease can affect a single organ or multiple organs, symptoms can vary greatly among patients. With symptoms ranging from mild, such as lower extremity edema, to severe, such as spinal cord compression, IgG4-RD must be considered in appropriate patients. Diagnostic criteria have been proposed based on organ involvement, serum IgG4 levels, and histopathological criteria. Diagnosis can be difficult to make with many studies suggesting different values for diagnostic criteria, such as the level of tissue IgG4+/IgG+ cell ratio to delineate IgG4-RD. Treatment consists of high dose glucocorticoids as a first line therapy with some patients choosing instead to simply undergo observation. This case illustrates the difficulty in diagnosis and the need for increased awareness among medical professionals.

1. Introduction

IgG4-RD is a relatively newly classified condition with unifying histopathologic features recognized only since the early 2000s [1]. The disorder is thought to mainly affect middle-aged to elderly men with a median age of onset of 58 years old [2, 3]. Exact incidence and prevalence are difficult to determine as many cases most likely go undiagnosed with limited awareness currently amongst medical professionals. Clinical findings vary by the organ system involved but many times are associated with tissue swelling or enlargement [1]. Due to the variety of clinical presentations, diagnosis can be delayed months to years and result in unnecessary tests and procedures.

2. Case Presentation

A 28-year-old female with no significant past medical history presented to her primary care physician with lymphadenopathy, night sweats, fatigue, and malaise. She was treated empirically and partially responded to a short course of glucocorticoids and an antibiotic. When initial laboratory workup was unrevealing for an obvious etiology and symptoms persisted, computed tomography (CT) of the neck and chest with contrast was performed that showed diffuse adenopathy (Figure 1) and hepatosplenomegaly. The patient was referred for lymph node resection that initially revealed only nonspecific B cell proliferation and did not support a specific etiology (Figure 2). With lymphoma a concern, she was referred to Hematology/Oncology for assessment. Hematology/Oncology evaluated the patient and performed a bone marrow biopsy which showed no cellular abnormalities consistent with lymphoma or leukemia. The patient's symptoms then stabilized for several months.

However, when her symptoms again worsened, she was referred to Infectious Disease who entertained a broad differential including Kikuchi's syndrome, Epstein-Barr virus (EBV), cytomegalovirus (CMV), toxoplasmosis, or human immunodeficiency virus (HIV) infection. Extensive serological testing was unrevealing and a second lymph node was removed, again without an obvious etiology. Rheumatology was then consulted and expanded the differential to include systemic lupus erythematosus, Sjögren's syndrome, Castleman's disease, autoimmune lymphoproliferative syndrome,

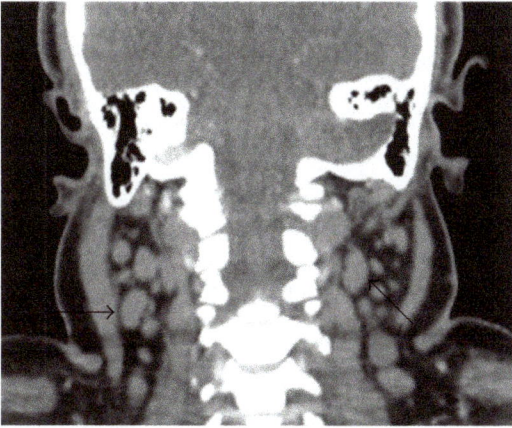

FIGURE 1: CT neck with contrast revealed diffuse cervical adenopathy (arrows demonstrate lymphadenopathy).

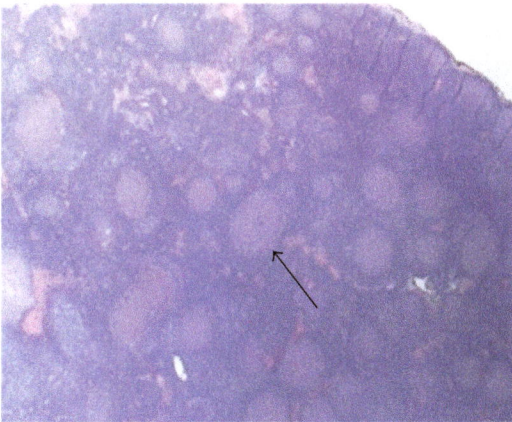

FIGURE 2: Hematoxylin and eosin stain of a resected lymph node, 2x magnification. This preparation shows nonspecific reactive follicular hyperplasia (arrow demonstrates secondary follicle with prominent germinal center).

and IgG4-related disease (IgG4-RD). Table 1 highlights the various serologic and tissue examinations performed as a part of the workup for this patient. An additional lymph node was removed and sent to Pathology for IgG4 staining (Figure 3) which, in combination with the patient's elevated serum IgG4 level of 206 mg/dL (normal 4–86 mg/dL), was very suspicious for IgG4-RD. Treatment modalities offered to the patient included a prolonged course of glucocorticoids or rituximab but she declined therapy as she and her spouse were attempting to conceive. The patient continues to attempt conception and therefore treatment has still not been initiated.

3. Diagnosis

The diagnosis of IgG4-RD can be difficult to make and misdiagnosis is common. One set of proposed diagnostic criteria as outlined in Table 2 calls for (1) organ enlargement, mass or nodular lesions, or organ dysfunction; (2) a serum

IgG4 concentration >135 mg/dL; (3) histopathological findings of >10 IgG4 cells/high powered field (HPF) with an IgG4+/IgG+ cell ratio >40%. Based on these criteria a diagnosis is "definite" in patients who fulfill criteria (1), (2), and (3), "possible" if criteria (1) and (2) are met, and "probable" in patients with criteria (1) and (3) satisfied. The situations in which these criteria prove most difficult to utilize are in those from whom tissue cannot safely be obtained or it is very difficult to biopsy the involved organ, such as in pancreatic disease. When the diagnosis is in question, further clarification can be sought using organ specific criteria for IgG4-RD, such as in autoimmune pancreatitis, Mikulicz's disease, and IgG4-related kidney disease. These additional organ-specific criteria greatly increase the specificity of the diagnostic criteria in applicable settings [2].

While the diagnostic criteria discussed earlier suggest an IgG4+/IgG+ cell ratio of >40%, other proposed diagnostic criteria recommend more stringent requirements such as a ratio of >50%. Others suggest that some cases of IgG4-RD may present with an even lower ratio such as >30% [1, 4]. A retrospective study performed by Masaki et al. looked at the various cutoffs and how this would alter the sensitivity and specificity of the diagnostic criteria, with results shown in Table 3.

Another aspect of the proposed diagnostic criteria state the serum IgG4 concentration should be >135 mg/dL. However, the serum IgG4 level can be misleading, with approximately 30% of patients with otherwise classic findings for this disease having normal serum IgG4 concentrations [1]. Conversely, the serum IgG4 level can be elevated in a variety of other unrelated conditions including primary sclerosing cholangitis, many forms of nonautoimmune pancreatitis, and atopic dermatitis. Even in the normal population, an elevated IgG4 level can be found in up to 5% of those tested [5].

Tissue biopsy and evaluation play a central role in diagnosis. Although IgG4-RD can manifest in nearly any organ system, it shares unique histologic findings regardless of location including dense lymphoplasmacytic infiltrate rich in IgG4-positive plasma cells, storiform fibrosis which is that of an irregularly whorled pattern, obliterative phlebitis, and an eosinophilic infiltrate [1, 6]. While the histology is characteristic, diagnosis requires specific immunohistochemical confirmation with IgG4 immunostaining. A finding of >10 IgG4 cells/HPF has benefits and shortcomings. In one study, setting the cutoff at >10 IgG4 cell/HPF provided 100% sensitivity but only 38.1% specificity [4]. Poor specificity has also been documented in various other studies that have revealed high numbers of IgG4 cells/HPF in other disease states, such as in cases of granulomatosis with polyangiitis [7].

Diagnosis can be difficult but the most important first step is a high clinical suspicion. This disease requires specific testing to be recognized and therefore must be sought out, not revealing itself on routine labs or biopsy. Furthermore, because of some shortcomings in the current diagnostic criteria, one must thoroughly consider other disorders in the differential diagnosis. In our case of unexplained generalized lymphadenopathy, fatigue, and night sweats, the differential

TABLE 1: Differential diagnosis with pertinent laboratory findings*.

Lymphoma	Bone marrow and lymph node biopsy performed HTLV-1+2 antibodies (nonreactive)
Castleman's disease	HHV-8 lymph node stains negative
Autoimmune Lymphoproliferative syndrome	Less than 1.5% double negative (CD4−CD8−) T-cell count on cytometry
Mycobacterial infection	AFB culture of lymph node (negative)
Systemic lupus erythematosus	ANA panel (1 : 160)
	Anti-dsDNA and anti-Sm antibodies (negative)
	Complement levels C3, C4 within normal range
Viral infections	EBV (nuclear Ag IgG positive, viral capsid IgG positive, viral capsid IgM negative), CMV (IgM negative, IgG negative), parvovirus B19 (IgM negative, IgG negative), Hepatitis (HBs Ag negative, HBc Ab negative, HBs Ab negative, HCV Ab negative)
Cat scratch disease	Bartonella panel (negative)
Sjögren's syndrome	SSA/SSB (negative)

* HTLV-1+2: human T-lymphotropic virus type I and II, HHV-8: human herpes virus 8; AFB: acid-fast bacilli, ANA: antinuclear antibodies, Anti-dsDNA: antidouble-stranded DNA, Anti-Sm: anti-Smith; EBV = Epstein-Barr virus, CMV: cytomegalovirus, HBs Ag = hepatitis B surface antigen, and HBc Ab: hepatitis B core antibody IgG, HBs Ab = hepatitis B surface antibody, HCV Ab: hepatitis C virus antibody, SSA: anti-Ro/SSA antibodies, and SSB: anti-La/SSB antibodies.

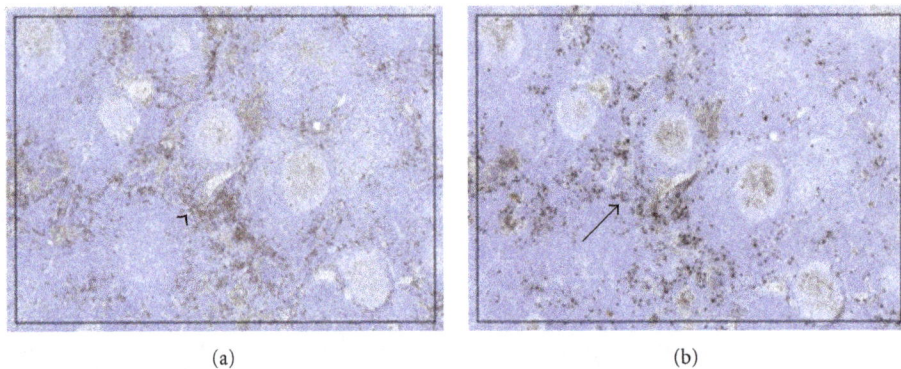

(a)   (b)

FIGURE 3: IgG (a) and IgG4 (b) stains, 4x magnification. These stains show an IgG4+/IgG+ cell ratio estimated at 30% (black arrow head: IgG staining, solid black arrow = IgG4 staining).

TABLE 2: Proposed comprehensive diagnostic criteria for IgG4-RD*.

(1) Organ enlargement, mass or nodular lesions, or organ dysfunction

(2) A serum IgG4 concentration >135 mg/dL

(3) Histopathological findings of >10 IgG4 cells/high powered field and an IgG4+/IgG+ cell ratio >40%

Definite = (1), Possible = (1) + (2), Probable = (1) + (3)

*Adapted from Umehara et al. [2].

TABLE 3: Specificity and sensitivity of IgG4+/IgG+ cell ratio for diagnosis of IgG4-RD*.

IgG4+/IgG+ Cell ratio	Sensitivity	Specificity
>30%	100%	71.4%
>40%	94.4%	85.7%
>50%	94.4%	95.2%

*Adapted from Masaki et al. [4].

4. Treatment

diagnosis included various infections (EBV, CMV, toxoplasmosis, HIV, and mycobacterium), lymphoma/leukemia, metastatic neoplasia, systemic lupus erythematous, Castleman's disease, autoimmune lymphoproliferative syndrome, and Sjögren's syndrome [8]. However, with a thorough evaluation to exclude alternative diagnoses, in the setting of our patient's elevated serum IgG level and significant staining for IgG4, her diagnosis was established.

Treatment strategies have not yet been validated by large randomized controlled trials. Recommendations are currently limited to case reports and consensus statements, with glucocorticoids considered first. Several glucocorticoid sparing regimens have also been suggested, with rituximab showing efficacy even in refractory disease [1, 6]. Treatment should include the input of the patient, as sometimes a watch-and-wait approach is sufficient depending on symptoms and organ involvement [1]. Regardless, patients should be monitored closely, because the disease process can progress and extensive fibrosis can occur making a treatment response less likely. Our patient chose a watch-and-wait approach as medication side effects were unacceptable to her and her husband as they were trying to conceive a child.

5. Conclusion

IgG4-RD is a new disease that has been present for many years but only better appreciated within the last decade. The currently proposed diagnostic criteria incorporate organ involvement, the serum IgG4 level, and tissue evaluation with IgG4+/IgG+ ratio and IgG4 cells/HPF. These criteria must be interpreted in the right clinical setting and diagnosis made only after a thorough consideration and exclusion of alternative diagnoses. Clinical features of the disease can be difficult to piece together given the wide variety of potential systems that can be involved and, therefore, the physician must have a high clinical suspicion. Treatment based on case reports and consensus consists mainly of glucocorticoids or similar agents that suppress lymphocytes. As the disease definition and our understanding of it continues to evolve, greater physician awareness is needed so that this diagnosis is not overlooked in future patients. Ongoing study of patient's with IgG4-RD will provide a better understanding of this disorder, how to best approach treatment, and potentially a more refined diagnostic scheme.

Acknowledgments

The authors would like to thank Dr. Geoffrey Sasaki for his help in obtaining and interpreting the histopathology provided in the figures of this paper. The views expressed in this material are those of the authors and do not reflect the official policy or position of the US Government, the Department of Defense, or the Department of the Air Force.

References

[1] J. H. Stone, Y. Zen, and V. Deshpande, "Mechanisms of disease: IgG4-related disease," *The New England Journal of Medicine*, vol. 366, no. 6, pp. 539–551, 2012.

[2] H. Umehara, K. Okazaki, Y. Masaki et al., "Comprehensive diagnostic criteria for IgG4-related disease (IgG4-RD), 2011," *Modern Rheumatology*, vol. 22, no. 1, pp. 21–30, 2012.

[3] H. Umehara, K. Okazaki, Y. Masaki, M. Kawano, M. Yamamoto, T. Saeki et al., "A novel clinical entity, IgG4-related disease (IgG4RD): general concept and details," *Modern Rheumatology*, vol. 22, no. 1, pp. 1–14, 2011.

[4] Y. Masaki, N. Kurose, M. Yamamoto et al., "Cutoff values of serum IgG4 and histopathological IgG4+ plasma cells for diagnosis of patients with IgG4-related disease," *International Journal of Rheumatology*, vol. 2012, Article ID 580814, 5 pages, 2012.

[5] J. H. Ryu, R. Horie, H. Sekiguchi, T. Peikert, and E. S. Yi, "Spectrum of disorders associated with elevated serum IgG4 levels encountered in clinical practice," *International Journal of Rheumatology*, vol. 2012, Article ID 232960, 6 pages, 2012.

[6] M. N. Carruthers, J. H. Stone, and A. Khosroshahi, "The latest on IgG4-RD: a rapidly emerging disease," *Current Opinion in Rheumatology*, vol. 24, no. 1, pp. 60–69, 2012.

[7] S. Y. Chang, K. Keogh, J. E. Lewis, J. H. Ryu, and E. S. Yi, "Increased IgG4-positive plasma cells in granulomatosis with polyangiitis: a diagnostic pitfall of IgG4-related disease," *International Journal of Rheumatology*, vol. 2012, Article ID 121702, 6 pages, 2012.

[8] G. S. Kerr, A. Aggarwal, and S. McDonald-Pinkett, "A woman with rheumatoid arthritis, Sjögren's syndrome, leg ulcer, and significant weight loss," *Arthritis Care & Research*, vol. 64, no. 5, pp. 785–792, 2012.

Does the Maternal Serum IgG Level during Pregnancy in Primary Antibody Deficiency Influence the IgG Level in the Newborn?

Vasantha Nagendran,[1,2] **Noel Emmanuel,**[3] **and Amolak S. Bansal**[1]

[1]*Epsom and St Helier University Hospitals NHS Trust, Carshalton, Surrey SM5 1AA, UK*
[2]*St Georges University of London, London SW17 0RE, UK*
[3]*St George's University Hospitals NHS Foundation Trust, Tooting, London SW17 0QT, UK*

Correspondence should be addressed to Vasantha Nagendran; nagendran@doctors.org.uk

Academic Editor: Alessandro Plebani

Purpose. To find out if the serum IgG level in the newborn baby was affected by low maternal serum IgG during pregnancy in two newly diagnosed primary antibody deficient patients. *Method.* Infant cord blood IgG level was compared with maternal IgG level in 2 mothers with newly diagnosed primary antibody deficiency, who declined replacement IgG treatment during pregnancy. *Results.* Both mothers delivered healthy babies with normal IgG levels at birth. *Conclusions.* The normal IgG levels and sound health in these 2 babies in spite of low maternal IgG throughout pregnancy raise interesting discussion points about maternofoetal immunoglobulin transport mechanisms in primary antibody deficiency.

1. Introduction

It is conventional wisdom that the foetus and neonate depend on transplacental transfer of IgG antibodies from the mother for immune protection, until maturation of their own humoral immunity. IgG is the only immunoglobulin class that is significantly transferred across the human placental barrier. The crossing of IgG from the mother to foetus occurs throughout pregnancy via endosomes within the syncytiotrophoblasts of the placenta, through a pH dependent mechanism involving FcRn receptors, with a possible role for other IgG Fc receptors, yet to be fully elucidated. The transfer is influenced by the maternal IgG and specific antibody concentrations, IgG subclass, gestational age, placental integrity, and the nature of the antigen, being more intense for thymic dependent antigens [1].

IgG transport to the foetus begins mainly in the second trimester of pregnancy and is maximal in the third trimester. IgG1 subclass is transported most efficiently and IgG2 least efficiently, and transfer of pneumococcal antibodies appears to be serotype specific and IgG subclass dependent [2, 3].

Common variable immunodeficiency (CVID) and hyper IgM syndrome (HIGM) which was previously included under the umbrella of CVID are heterogeneous primary antibody deficiency states characterised by low IgG and impaired antibody responses. Management of both of these conditions involves replenishing the IgG deficiency and monitoring and treating infections, autoimmune diseases, and other complications. Immunoglobulin replacement therapy (RIT) may be administered by intravenous (IVIg) or subcutaneous (SCIg) routes.

If pregnant mothers with CVID or HIGM had no RIT, placental transfer of IgG may be reduced, causing a deficiency of protective antibodies to defend the foetus from intrauterine infections. This lack of passive immunity may also increase the risk of infection in the child's first few months of life, until its immune system matures.

There are presently no published protocols on the management of CVID or HIGM patients during pregnancy. CVID mothers receiving intravenous immunoglobulin (IVIg) therapy are believed to transfer exogenous IgG through the placenta in similar patterns as endogenous immunoglobulins,

TABLE 1: Summary of serum/cord blood total IgG and specific IgG levels against pneumococcal polysaccharides, *H. influenzae* b, and tetanus toxoid in patients and their babies.

Test (units)	Patient 1	Baby of patient 1	Transfer ratio	Patient 2	Baby of patient 2	Transfer ratio
IgG (g/L)	2.5*	5.5**	2.20	4.3*	9.2**	2.14
Pneumococcal antibody ug/mL (protective level >20 ug/mL)	2.0	2.0	1.0	8.0	Insufficient sample	—
H. influenzae antibody ug/mL (protective level >0.15 ug/mL)	0.90	0.03	0.033	0.10	Insufficient sample	—
Tetanus antibody u/mL (protective level >0.01 u/mL)	0.31	0.43	1.39	0.24	Insufficient sample	—

*Normal range of serum IgG for adults: 6.0–16.0 g/L.
**Normal range of cord blood IgG: 5.2–18.0 g/L.

and therefore mothers are advised to continue regular RIT (by intravenous or subcutaneous route) and encouraged to breast-feed their babies [4–8].

The management of CVID or HIGM that is *first* diagnosed during pregnancy is more complicated and has *not* hitherto been addressed in the literature. We report our experience of 2 women in this situation who declined replacement immunoglobulin therapy during their pregnancy.

2. Case Reports

2.1. Patient 1. A 40-year-old woman pregnant with her second child was seen for recurrent upper respiratory tract infections. She had suffered a series of colds and bouts of productive cough after the birth of her first child, born by Caesarian delivery at term, 3 years earlier. At 20 years of age, she had required 6 months of oral prednisolone therapy for low platelets.

Blood tests at 9 weeks of gestation confirmed a total IgG of 2.5 g/L (normal 6.0–16.0), IgM of 1.22 g/L (0.5–1.9), and IgA of <0.056 g/L (normal 0.8–2.8). There was no paraprotein on immunoelectrophoresis. Her B cell count was normal at 0.17 × 109/mL and she had normal numbers of CD4 and CD8 T cells.

She was advised to start immunoglobulin therapy for CVID, but, in spite of detailed discussions with medical staff on several occasions, she was reluctant to do this until after she had delivered the child by elective Caesarian delivery. The patient remained well during pregnancy and had only minor upper respiratory tract infections, not requiring antibiotic therapy.

A healthy female baby weighing 3150 gm was born at term and cord blood analysis detailed in Table 1 showed a total IgG 5.5 g/L (cord blood normal range: 5.2–18.0 g/L), IgA <0.18 g/L, and IgM <0.23 g/L. IgG subclasses showed IgG1 4.07 g/L, IgG2 0.13 g/L, IgG3 0.51 g/L, and IgG4 <0.083 g/L. Pneumococcal Abs at 2 μg/mL and Hib Abs at 0.03 μg/mL were sub-therapeutic according to accepted values [9–11], but the level was satisfactory for tetanus toxoid at 0.43 IU/mL [12, 13]. Numbers of CD19 B cells and CD4 T cells were normal but CD8 T cells were slightly reduced. The child was breast-fed

and remained well in infancy. Repeat serum immunoglobulin assessment at one year of age showed normal levels.

The patient's Caesarian scar became infected and required antibiotics. She commenced regular IVIg therapy 2 months later following detailed investigations for specific antibody production after vaccination. CT scan of the chest showed mild bronchiectasis but pulmonary function tests were essentially normal. Approximately 6 years from delivery, she was relatively free of infections but had a relapse of idiopathic thrombocytopenia (ITP) and also developed autoimmune haemolytic anemia (AIHA).

2.2. Patient 2. A 38-year-old lady was investigated for suspected parvovirus infection in the first trimester of her second pregnancy as 4 children in the nursery where she worked were thought to have "slapped cheek" virus infection. Her results showed previous exposure and immunity (IgG antibody to parvovirus, but no IgM antibody). However, her serum immunoglobulins IgG was found to be low. She had been previously well with no significant sinus, ear, chest, or gastrointestinal infections. Her first pregnancy was uneventful, and she had delivered a healthy baby boy.

Our initial investigations in the first trimester confirmed low total IgG 4.3 g/L (normal: 6.0–16.0), low IgA 0.56 (normal: 0.8–2.8), and high IgM 8.32 g/L (normal: 0.5–1.9). The immunoelectrophoresis did not detect any paraprotein to account for this profile. Serum IgG subclass measurements showed low IgG 1 (3.07 g/L) and normal IgG2, IgG3, and IgG4. The pneumococcal antibodies and *Haemophilus* antibodies were low, and tetanus antibodies were normal. There was lymphopenia with low T and B cell counts and low CD4 and CD8 subset counts. The B cell proportion was high (35%) with slight decrease in T cell proportion (54%) and normal CD4-CD8 ratio. CVID classification is as follows: Warnatz Class = 1a, Piqueras Class = MB1, and EuroClass = SmB (−) Tr(norm)21(low). The autoantibody screen, RF, ANCA, TPO, and ACA (IgG) were negative, but ACA IgM was slightly elevated at 13.1.MPLU/mL (normal: 0–9.8).

She was well in herself and very reluctant to embark on any further investigations (for the high IgM) or new treatments, so we arranged to monitor her for infections and check serum immunoglobulins during her pregnancy. Although she remained well, repeat serum IgG in the third trimester was lower (3.6 g/L), IgM remained elevated at 8.16 g/L, and IgA was 0.57 g/L. The lymphopenia noted in the first trimester had reverted to normal. We discussed that maternofoetal transfer of immunoglobulins occurred in the third trimester of pregnancy and strongly advised immunoglobulin replacement. After a detailed discussion of the pros and cons with medical staff, she made an informed decision to consider this only *after* the birth of her baby. She had a full term normal delivery of a healthy female baby weighing 3570 grams and cord blood analysis showed a total IgG 9.2 g/L (cord blood normal range: 5.2–18.0 g/L), IgA <0.18 g/L, and IgM <0.23 g/L. There was insufficient sample to measure IgG subclasses and specific antibodies.

Mother breast-fed her baby, from birth. She postponed her postpartum clinic visit but confirmed that she and her baby were in good health. Blood tests arranged through her general practitioner 10 months after the birth showed low IgG (5.2 g/L), low IgA (0.7), and elevated IgM (10.5 g/L) in the mother, who confirmed her good health but declined further investigations for HIGM. The baby was infection-free and thriving, and her serum immunoglobulins at 10 months were normal (IgG 5.07 g/L, IgM 0.38 g/L, and IgA 0.18 g/L). Mother has moved away from our area and has not attended for follow-ups.

3. Discussion

We present two women discovered to have low IgG during their second pregnancy. The first had experienced chest infections over the preceding three years and had previous treatment for presumed idiopathic thrombocytopenia. The second patient had no history of infections. Both mothers had informed discussions with the consultant immunologists about RIT. The importance of maternofoetal immunoglobulin transfer to protect the foetus and the newborn baby and the potential of blood products (including IVIg) to transmit hitherto unidentified infections (e.g., prions) were discussed. Both mothers opted to defer RIT until after they delivered their babies. In spite of low maternal IgG levels, both delivered healthy babies with normal cord blood total IgG. Patient 1 commenced RIT 2 months after delivery. Patient 2 chose to defer RIT, as she was symptom-free and her serum IgG was 5.2 g/L 10 months postpartum (compared to 3.6 g/L in the third trimester).

The cord/maternal IgG ratios noted in our antibody deficient women were within the 0.75 to 2.86 range reported in healthy women [14]. It is interesting that the ratios were similar in both mother/baby pairs despite significantly different total maternal IgG levels, and the transfer ratio was slightly higher in patient 1 who had lower levels of maternal IgG, confirming an active transfer process to maintain foetal IgG levels.

Specific IgG transfer ratios could only be calculated for patient 1 due to insufficient sample in newborn 2. Here, the transfer ratios of specific IgG antibodies to tetanus and pneumococcal capsular polysaccharides were preserved, but the transfer ratio was significantly reduced for *Haemophilus influenzae* b (Hib).

Importantly both of our babies remained well and infection-free after birth, with normal serum immunoglobulins, and neither appears to have suffered infection with either Hib or *S. pneumoniae*.

Our findings raise interesting questions about physiological mechanisms that may operate to maintain normal foetal IgG levels when maternal levels are low. Observations that neonatal cord blood antibody level is higher than maternal levels date back to several decades but were disregarded or attributed to measurement error. In 1966, a study from Scripps Clinic, California, using more "advanced methods" concluded that cord blood IgG was significantly higher than in the mother and attributed this to active placental transport [15]. In 1968, a Finnish study found significantly higher titres of IgG antibodies in full-term cord sera compared to maternal titres, in 7 out of 12 antibodies studied [16]. Other studies showed that low maternal values did *not* necessarily predict equally low levels in cord blood; in fact, they tended to exceed the maternal level [17]. An inverse relationship between maternal and foetal levels of IgG antibodies to herpes simplex, tetanus toxoid, streptolysin O, and *S. pneumoniae* was reported in 1996 [18].

We speculate that an "upregulation" of FcRn and other IgG Fc receptors in the endosome of the syncytiotrophoblast may help increase the transport of IgG from mother to foetus, when maternal IgG is low. This may explain why both of our patients delivered babies with normal IgG and high IgG transfer ratios, in spite of low IgG levels in their mothers.

Although high transfer ratios were achieved without IgG replacement therapy in our two patients, IgG level in newborn of patient 1 is considered low and could have been raised if the mother had received IVIg therapy during pregnancy, and this may have also improved her Hib level, affording optimal protection for the newborn.

The recent worldwide interest in maternal immunisation is aimed at protecting the newborn in the first few months of life (before primary immunisation becomes effective), and the basis of this is the demonstration of a strong positive correlation between maternal and infant specific antibody responses to vaccine-preventable infections such as pertussis, tetanus, *Haemophilus*, and *pneumococcus* [19]. Mothers with primary antibody deficiency states (e.g., CVID and HIGM) are unable to respond effectively to immunisations and must therefore rely on immunoglobulin infusions (IVIg or SCIg) to boost their levels of specific antibodies. In a detailed study of two mothers with IVIg treated CVID and their newborns, it was demonstrated that cord blood IgG levels were greater than maternal IgG; subclasses IgG1, IgG3, and IgG4 were preferentially transferred compared with IgG2; anti-protein (tetanus) IgG antibodies were equivalent to or higher than maternal levels with good transfer of polysaccharide (Hib) IgG antibodies; and anti-*Streptococcus pneumoniae* avidity indices were similar between mothers and their neonates [6].

Therefore, in primary antibody deficiency states, the potential benefit of immunoglobulin therapy to both the pregnant mother and the baby cannot be overemphasised.

4. Conclusion

Women with hypogammaglobulinemia can deliver healthy infants with normal IgG levels, but careful monitoring of both mother and baby is important. Further research is required to fully understand transplacental transfer of protective IgG antibodies in the presence of low maternal serum IgG levels.

Conflict of Interests

The authors declare that there is no conflict of interests regarding the publication of this paper.

Acknowledgments

The authors thank all members of staff who were involved in the care of patient 1 and patient 2 in the Department of Clinical Immunology, St Helier Hospital, and the Maternity Units at St Helier Hospital and East Surrey Hospital, Surrey, UK.

References

[1] P. Palmeira, C. Quinello, A. L. Silveira-Lessa, C. A. Zago, and M. Carneiro-Sampaio, "IgG placental transfer in healthy and pathological pregnancies," *Clinical and Developmental Immunology*, vol. 2012, Article ID 985646, 13 pages, 2012.

[2] N. E. Simister, "Placental transport of immunoglobulin G," *Vaccine*, vol. 21, no. 24, pp. 3365–3369, 2003.

[3] B. T. Costa Carvalho, M. M. Carneiro-Sampaio, D. Solé, C. Naspitz, L. E. Leiva, and R. U. Sorensen, "Transplacental transmission of serotype-specific pneumococcal antibodies in a Brazilian population," *Clinical and Diagnostic Laboratory Immunology*, vol. 6, no. 1, pp. 50–54, 1999.

[4] F. M. Schaffer and J. A. Newton, "Intravenous gamma globulin administration to common variable immunodeficient women during pregnancy: case report and review of the literature," *Journal of Perinatology*, vol. 14, no. 2, pp. 114–117, 1994.

[5] H. Osada, Y. Morikawa, T. Nishiwaki, and S. Sekiya, "Intravenous immunoglobulin replacement therapy for common variable immunodeficiency during pregnancy," *Archives of Gynecology and Obstetrics*, vol. 258, no. 3, pp. 155–159, 1996.

[6] P. Palmeira, B. T. Costa-Carvalho, C. Arslanian, G. N. Pontes, A. T. Nagao, and M. M. S. Carneiro-Sampaio, "Transfer of antibodies across the placenta and in breast milk from mothers on intravenous immunoglobulin," *Pediatric Allergy and Immunology*, vol. 20, no. 6, pp. 528–535, 2009.

[7] A. Gardulf, E. Anderson, M. Lindqvist, S. Hansen, and R. Gustafson, "Rapid subcutaneous IgG replacement therapy at home for pregnant immunodeficient women," *Journal of Clinical Immunology*, vol. 21, no. 2, pp. 150–154, 2001.

[8] N. Vitoratos, P. Bakas, H. Kalampani, and G. Creatsas, "Maternal common variable immunodeficiency and pregnancy," *Journal of Obstetrics & Gynaecology*, vol. 19, no. 6, pp. 654–655, 1999.

[9] T. Cherian, "WHO expert consultation on serotype composition of pneumococcal conjugate vaccines for use in resource-poor developing countries, 26-27 October 2006, Geneva," *Vaccine*, vol. 25, no. 36, pp. 6557–6564, 2007.

[10] World Health Organization, "Recommendation for the production and control of pneumococcal conjugate vaccines," WHO Technical Report Series 927, 2005.

[11] H. Kayhty, H. Peltola, V. Karanko, and P. H. Makela, "The protective level of serum antibodies to the capsular polysaccharide of *Haemophilus influenzae* type b," *The Journal of Infectious Diseases*, vol. 147, no. 6, pp. 1100–1101, 1983.

[12] R. Booy, S. J. M. Aitken, S. Taylor et al., "Immunogenicity of combined diphtheria, tetanus, and pertussis vaccine given at 2, 3, and 4 months versus 3, 5, and 9 months of age," *The Lancet*, vol. 339, no. 8792, pp. 507–510, 1992.

[13] J. W. Smith, "Diptheria and tetanus toxoids," *British Medical Bulletin*, vol. 25, no. 2, pp. 177–182, 1969.

[14] A. P. Machado, G. Gonçalves, H. Barros, and M. S. Nascimento, "Mother-child transmission of immunoglobulins G," *Acta Medica Portuguesa*, vol. 8, no. 2, pp. 81–85, 1995.

[15] P. F. Kohler and R. S. Farr, "Elevation of cord over maternal IgG immunoglobulin: evidence for an active placental IgG transport," *Nature*, vol. 210, no. 5040, pp. 1070–1071, 1966.

[16] P. Toivanen, R. Mäntyjärvi, and T. Hirvonen, "Maternal antibodies in human foetal sera at different stages of gestation," *Immunology*, vol. 15, no. 3, pp. 395–403, 1968.

[17] R. Mäntyjärvi, T. Hirvonen, and P. Toivanen, "Maternal antibodies in human neonatal sera," *Immunology*, vol. 18, no. 3, pp. 449–451, 1970.

[18] M. I. de Moraes-Pinto, A. C. M. Almeida, G. Kenj et al., "Placental transfer and maternally acquired neonatal IgG immunity in human immunodeficiency virus infection," *The Journal of Infectious Diseases*, vol. 173, no. 5, pp. 1077–1084, 1996.

[19] C. Jones, L. Pollock, S. M. Barnett, A. Battersby, and B. Kampmann, "Specific antibodies against vaccine-preventable infections: a mother–infant cohort study," *BMJ Open*, vol. 3, no. 4, Article ID e002473, 2013.

Behcet's Disease with Intracardiac Thrombus Presenting with Fever of Unknown Etiology

**Sajal Ajmani,[1] Durga Prasanna Misra,[1] Deep Chandh Raja,[2]
Namita Mohindra,[3] and Vikas Agarwal[1]**

[1]*Department of Clinical Immunology, Sanjay Gandhi Postgraduate Institute of Medical Sciences, Lucknow 226014, India*
[2]*Department of Cardiology, Sanjay Gandhi Postgraduate Institute of Medical Sciences, Lucknow 226014, India*
[3]*Department of Radiodiagnosis, Sanjay Gandhi Postgraduate Institute of Medical Sciences, Lucknow 226014, India*

Correspondence should be addressed to Sajal Ajmani; sajalajmani@gmail.com

Academic Editor: Alessandro Plebani

A young male was referred to us for evaluation of fever of unknown origin (FUO). He had history of recurrent painful oral ulcers for one year and moderate to high grade fever, pustulopapular rash, and recurrent genital ulcers for 6 months and hemoptysis for 3 days. He was detected to have intracardiac thrombi and pulmonary arterial thrombosis along with underlying Behcet's disease (BD). Patient responded to high dose prednisolone (1 mg/Kg/day) along with monthly parenteral cyclophosphamide therapy. This case highlights the fact that BD is an important cause for pulmonary artery vasculitis with intracardiac thrombus formation, and such patients can present with FUO.

1. Introduction

Behcet's disease (BD) is a multisystem inflammatory disease. There is no definitive laboratory test to confirm BD; hence diagnosis is based on clinical features. A number of diagnostic criteria have been proposed for BD. The 1990 International Study Group (ISG) criteria [1] mandate the presence of oral ulcers along with two of the following: recurrent genital ulceration, eye lesion (anterior or posterior uveitis), skin lesions (erythema nodosum, pseudofolliculitis, papulopustular lesions, and acneiform nodules), and positive pathergy test. The International Criteria for Behcet's Disease (ICBD) [2] have a higher sensitivity and provide a weighted score to the various manifestations of BD. Ocular lesions, oral aphthosis, and genital aphthosis are each assigned 2 points, while skin lesions, central nervous system involvement, and vascular manifestations score 1 point each. The pathergy test, when used, scores 1 point. A score of at least 4 points is classified as BD.

Despite the multisystem involvement, cardiac pathology is unusual. Pancarditis, acute myocardial infarction, conduction system disturbances, and valvular disease have all been described [3]. Intracardiac thrombus formation is very uncommon. We present a case of a young male who was referred to us as fever of unknown origin (FUO) and was subsequently diagnosed to have BD with pulmonary artery vasculitis and intracardiac thrombus.

2. Case Presentation

A 36-year-old male was referred to us for evaluation of FUO. He had history of recurrent painful oral ulcers, 4 episodes in the past 1 year, each time lasting for around 2 months. For the past 6 months, he complained of daily high grade fever, with chills and rigors, documented to be around 39.4–40°C. In addition to fever, recurrent crops of erythematous papulopustular rash over the abdomen, forearm, and thigh and recurrent genital ulcers on the scrotum and shaft of penis were reported for last 6 months. For the past month, he had right lower chest pain, worse on coughing, associated with shortness of breath which had progressed over the month to the extent that he had shortness of breath even on day-to-day activities. He had history of streaky hemoptysis for the past 3 days. He also had history of significant weight loss, night

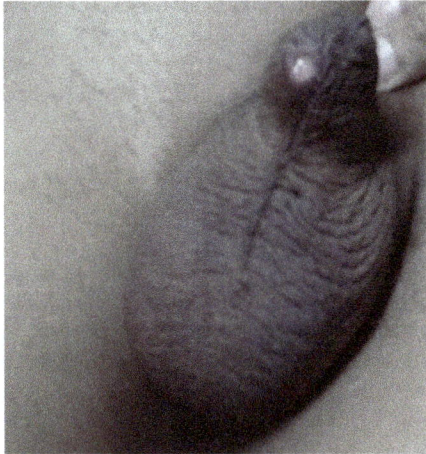

FIGURE 1: Ulcer in the ventral surface of the shaft of the penis.

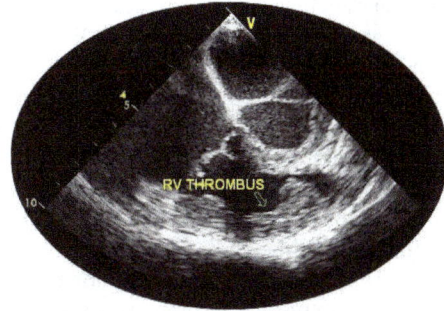

FIGURE 2: Transoesophageal Echocardiographic (TOE) image at midoesophagus (short axis) showing the right ventricular (RV) thrombus (arrow mark) along the free wall of RV, extending from just below tricuspid valve to the right ventricular outflow beneath the pulmonary valve.

sweats, and loss of appetite. There was no history of joint pain, abdominal pain, diarrhea or blood mixed stools, lymph node enlargement, recent onset hypertension, oliguria, hematuria, edema over feet or periorbital edema, altered sensorium, headache, stroke, and thrombosis in the past. There was no family history of stroke in young or deep venous thrombosis to suggest a hypercoagulable state. He was in a stable monogamous relationship for a number of years. He had not received blood transfusions in the past or ever abused intravenous drugs. There was no history of contact with tuberculosis. He had received multiple courses of broad spectrum antibiotics elsewhere without any relief. On examination pulse rate was 90/min, blood pressure was 126/70 mm Hg in the right upper limb, and respiratory rate was 22/min. General physical examination revealed severe pallor, oral ulcers over tongue and cheek, small, 0.5×0.5 cm with clean base. A genital ulcer (Figure 1) measuring 2×2 cm was present over the penile shaft ventral surface with erythematous border and showing signs of healing with healthy granulation tissue at the base. There were hyperpigmented macules over back and abdomen, suggestive of healed rash. Rest of the general physical and systemic examinations were unremarkable.

Hematological investigations revealed a normocytic anemia (hemoglobin 8.7 g/dL), total leucocyte count was 10,200/mm^3 (neutrophils 72%, lymphocytes 28%), platelet count was 327000/mm^3, normal renal (blood urea 16 mg/dL, serum creatinine 1 mg/dL) and liver function tests (bilirubin 0.5 mg/dL, aspartate aminotransferase 37 U/L, alanine aminotransferase 28 U/L, alkaline phosphatase 155 U/L, serum protein 6.7 g/dL, and serum albumin 3.6 g/dL). He had markedly elevated acute phase reactants (ESR by Westergren's method 70 mm/hr, C-reactive protein 9.25 mg/dL, normal <0.6 mg/dL). Computed tomography (CT) of chest and abdomen revealed minimal effusion in right pleural cavity and mild hepatosplenomegaly and thickening of the distal ileum and caecum. Serology for HBsAg, anti-HCV, and HIV-ELISA were negative. Three blood cultures did not grow any microorganisms. Two-dimensional transthoracic and transesophageal echocardiography (Figure 2) revealed a thrombus

in right ventricle with broad base and extending from the tricuspid valve to the pulmonary valve. Mantoux (10 TU) and pathergy tests were negative. CT pulmonary angiography was done in view of hemoptysis and revealed multiple peripheral pulmonary artery thrombi.

Our patient fulfilled both ISG and ICBD criteria (orogenital ulcers, skin lesions, and vascular manifestations—hence scoring 6 points, fulfilling ICBD criteria for the classification of BD) and hence was diagnosed as having BD. Mild pleural effusion [4] and bowel thickening akin to Crohn's disease [5] have been well described in BD and hence were attributed to the primary disease. In view of the fact that he had been extensively evaluated prior to presenting to us and no cause of fever was identified in spite of multiple prior hospital visits and admissions, he was labeled as FUO, subsequently identified to be due to cardiac and pulmonary artery thrombi [6]. He was started on colchicine, 1 mg/kg of prednisolone, and aspirin and given 1st dose of cyclophosphamide (he has been planned for 6 doses of monthly cyclophosphamide, 750 mg/m^2). With therapy, all his symptoms improved in a week and he was discharged in stable condition. He was asymptomatic when contacted over the phone a month later and was due for the second dose of cyclophosphamide.

3. Discussion

Although it was possible to suspect BD from the first instance itself due to presence of oral and genital ulcers, fever is considered to be an uncommon manifestation of BD. A study in 500 patients of BD reported that 22% of patients reported a history of febrile episodes. The presence of fever was found to be strongly associated with vascular, neurological, or joint involvement [5]. In our patient, subsequent investigation revealed presence of intracardiac and pulmonary artery thrombi which were the cause of fever.

Intracardiac thrombosis in BD is rare. A review of literature done in 2000 [7] reported only 24 cases in literature till then. Intracardiac thrombus can occur not only in adults, but also in children with BD [8]. It is a serious complication with poor prognosis and often occurs in association with pulmonary artery aneurysm (42%), pulmonary thromboembolism (52%), and venous thrombosis (56%). At the time of detection of intracardiac thrombus, fever, hemoptysis, dyspnea, and cough are the predominant symptoms (seen in 52%, 48%, 44%, and 20% of patients, resp.). Young men (usually third decade) are most often affected, and the right heart is the most frequent site of involvement. Because intracardiac thrombus is tightly attached to the endocardium or myocardium, thromboembolism from the cardiac cavity seems to be relatively uncommon. The pulmonary abnormalities have been seen to resolve in some cases after administration of immunosuppressive treatment rather than anticoagulation [9–11]. It is, therefore, likely that the pulmonary vascular involvement is a result of in situ inflammation rather than embolization. Patients of BD with intracardiac thrombus usually have prominent constitutional symptoms such as fever, due to which it is difficult to differentiate it from infective endocarditis and atrial myxoma. The pathologic mechanism of thrombus formation in BD is believed to be endothelial cell ischemia or disruption leading to platelet aggregation [12]. Decreased release of antithrombotic tissue plasminogen activator from blood vessels has also been reported [13].

Treatment of intracardiac thrombus is unclear. Some patients have been treated surgically with removal of thrombus. In the small number of cases published in literature, patients treated with medical therapy tend to do better than those treated surgically [14]. Most patients have been treated with colchicine and steroids. Some have been treated with cyclophosphamide in addition and have shown good response. Anticoagulation in patients with cardiac thrombus is controversial since these have a low chance of thromboembolism and a high risk of bleeding in presence of pulmonary artery aneurysm, which can be life threatening. Often, resolution of the thrombus has been seen with just immunosuppression with or without antiplatelet agent [7]. Our patient responded to treatment with steroids, cyclophosphamide, and aspirin without anticoagulation.

In conclusion, BD should be kept in differential diagnosis in a young male with intracardiac thrombus. Such patients usually have marked constitutional symptoms and can present with FUO. It is also important to look for vascular, neurological, and joint involvement in patients with BD if they have fever. A keen clinical acumen is essential to diagnose these patients in a timely manner and institute life-saving immunosuppression at the earliest.

Conflict of Interests

The authors declare that there is no conflict of interests regarding the publication of this paper.

References

[1] International Study Group for Behçet's Disease, "Criteria for diagnosis of Behçet's disease," *The Lancet*, vol. 335, no. 8697, pp. 1078–1080, 1990.

[2] F. Davatchi, S. Assaad-Khalil, K. T. Calamia et al., "The international criteria for Behcet's disease (ICBD): a collaborative study of 27 countries on the sensitivity and specificity of the new criteria," *Journal of the European Academy of Dermatology and Venereology*, vol. 28, no. 3, pp. 338–347, 2014.

[3] M. Ozkan, O. Emel, M. Ozdemir et al., "M-mode, 2-D and Doppler echocardiographic study in 65 patients with Behcet's syndrome," *European Heart Journal*, vol. 13, no. 5, pp. 638–641, 1992.

[4] F. Erkan, E. Kıyan, and A. Tunacı, "Pulmonary complications of Behçet's disease," *Clinics in Chest Medicine*, vol. 23, no. 2, pp. 493–503, 2002.

[5] E. Seyahi, H. Karaaslan, S. Ugurlu, and H. Yazici, "Fever in Behcet's syndrome," *Clinical and Experimental Rheumatology*, vol. 31, no. 3, supplement 77, pp. S64–S67, 2013.

[6] G. E. Thwaites, "Pyrexia of unknown origin," *Acute Medicine*, vol. 4, no. 1, pp. 10–14, 2005.

[7] N. Mogulkoc, M. I. Burgess, and P. W. Bishop, "Intracardiac thrombus in Behcet's disease: a systematic review," *Chest*, vol. 118, no. 2, pp. 479–487, 2000.

[8] B. Krupa, R. Cimaz, S. Ozen, M. Fischbach, P. Cochat, and I. Koné-Paut, "Pediatric Behçet's disease and thromboses," *The Journal of Rheumatology*, vol. 38, no. 2, pp. 387–390, 2011.

[9] S. Demirelli, H. Degirmenci, S. Inci, and A. Arisoy, "Cardiac manifestations in Behcet's disease," *Intractable & Rare Diseases Research*, vol. 4, no. 2, pp. 70–75, 2015.

[10] E. Seyahi and H. Yazici, "Behçet's syndrome: pulmonary vascular disease," *Current Opinion in Rheumatology*, vol. 27, no. 1, pp. 18–23, 2015.

[11] G. Geri, B. Wechsler, L. Thi Huong du et al., "Spectrum of cardiac lesions in Behcet disease: a series of 52 patients and review of the literature," *Medicine*, vol. 91, no. 1, pp. 25–34, 2012.

[12] N. Butta, I. Fernández-Bello, F. López-Longo, and V. Jiménez-Yuste, "Endothelial dysfunction and altered coagulation as mediators of thromboembolism in Behçet disease," *Seminars in Thrombosis & Hemostasis*, 2015.

[13] S. Yurdakul, N. Hekim, T. Soysal et al., "Fibrinolytic activity and d-dimer levels in Behçet's syndrome," *Clinical and Experimental Rheumatology*, vol. 23, no. 4, supplement 38, pp. S53–S58, 2005.

[14] Y.-L. Zhu, Q.-J. Wu, L.-L. Guo et al., "The clinical characteristics and outcome of intracardiac thrombus and aortic valvular involvement in Behcet's disease: an analysis of 20 cases," *Clinical and Experimental Rheumatology*, vol. 30, supplement 72, pp. S40–S45, 2012.

Systemic Sarcoidosis Presenting with Headache and Stroke-Like Episodes

J. Campbell,[1] R. Kee,[1] D. Bhattacharya,[2] P. Flynn,[2] M. McCarron,[3] and A. Fulton[1]

[1]Department of Neurology, Royal Victoria Hospital, Belfast BT12 6BA, UK
[2]Department of Neuroradiology, Royal Victoria Hospital, Belfast BT12 6BA, UK
[3]Neurology Centre, Altnagelvin Area Hospital, Londonderry BT47 6SB, UK

Correspondence should be addressed to J. Campbell; jcampbell@talk21.com

Academic Editor: Takahisa Gono

Sarcoidosis is a multisystem granulomatous disorder. Neurological manifestations as a presenting symptom are relatively rare. A 26-year-old male presented with a five-week history of headache suggestive of raised intracranial pressure. He subsequently developed transient episodes of mild right-sided hemiparesis and numbness. Magnetic resonance imaging (MRI) of brain revealed widespread inflammatory white matter lesions, an ischaemic focus in the left corona radiata, and widespread microhaemorrhages consistent with a more diffuse vasculopathy. Serum angiotensin-converting enzyme (ACE) level was normal. Lumbar puncture revealed an elevated opening pressure (36 cmH$_2$O) and inflammatory cerebrospinal fluid (CSF). Computerised tomography (CT) of chest, abdomen, and pelvis revealed widespread lymphadenopathy and biopsy of axillary lymph nodes revealed the presence of noncaseating granulomata in keeping with systemic sarcoidosis. The patient responded well to corticosteroids. This case highlights the importance of considering sarcoidosis to be a rare but potentially treatable cause of stroke in younger patients.

1. Introduction

Sarcoidosis is a multisystem granulomatous disorder characterised by noncaseating granulomata. The respiratory system is one of the most commonly involved sites and patients may present with cough and dyspnoea [1].

The nervous system is affected in approximately 5% of patients with sarcoidosis [2]. The neurological manifestations can be diverse but most commonly include cranial neuropathies (particularly involving the facial or optic nerves) [2, 3]. Other less frequent presentations include meningoencephalitis, hydrocephalus, intracranial mass lesions, psychiatric symptoms, spinal cord disease, peripheral nerve involvement, or even myopathy [4–7].

Despite pathological evidence of granulomatous involvement of cerebral blood vessels in neurosarcoidosis [8], stroke or transient ischaemic episodes are reported only very rarely. We report a case of an unusual presentation of systemic sarcoidosis with headache and stroke-like symptoms.

2. Case Report

A 26-year-old right-handed male was admitted to a district general hospital with a five-week history of gradual onset, dull, and global headache that was worse when supine and exacerbated by valsalva manoeuvres. There was associated nausea and frequent early morning vomiting. He also complained of prominent lethargy and approximately 5 kg of weight loss in the preceding four months.

He denied visual disturbance or other focal neurological symptoms at presentation. There was no history of febrile illness or recent travel. Soon after admission he experienced several transient episodes of sudden onset right upper limb weakness and numbness lasting up to 15 minutes without impairment of consciousness.

His past medical history was notable for an episode of right-sided uveitis six years prior to this presentation. He also had a history of well-controlled childhood epilepsy.

Approximately eighteen months prior to his current admission he was discovered to have renal impairment

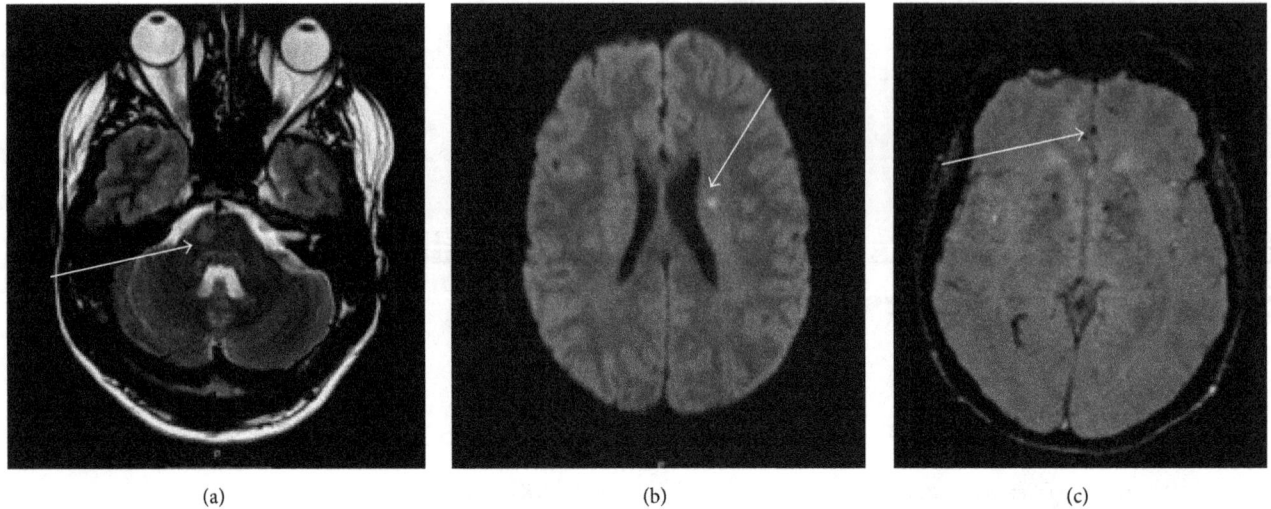

(a)   (b)   (c)

FIGURE 1: MRI scan of brain. MRI of brain. Axial T2-weighted image showing T2 hyperintense lesion within the right pons (arrow) (a). Axial DWI (B1000) demonstrates restricted diffusion within the left centrum semiovale (arrow) (b). Gradient recalled ECHO T2 susceptibility weighted imaging showing diffuse hypointense lesions suggestive of microhaemorrhages (arrow) (c).

(urea 14.8 mmol/L and creatinine 226 umol/L) after a routine check-up revealed hypertension. He underwent renal biopsy that was consistent with interstitial nephritis and which was attributed to sodium valproate that he had been taking for treatment of epilepsy. The sodium valproate was switched to levetiracetam and he was started on prednisolone and lisinopril. Renal function subsequently stabilised, blood pressure normalised, and the prednisolone was gradually weaned over the following 18 months and had been stopped several weeks prior to this admission.

Medications on this admission were levetiracetam 2500 mg daily, omeprazole 20 mg daily, and lisinopril 2.5 mg daily.

3. Examination

On examination chest was clear on auscultation. There was no hepatosplenomegaly. On neurological examination tone, power, and coordination were normal. Reflexes were symmetrically brisk; however both plantar responses were flexor. Visual acuity was 6/6 in both eyes. On fundoscopy there was blurring of the optic disc margins bilaterally as well as absent spontaneous venous pulsations in both eyes. Blood pressure was 150/107. Systemic examination revealed the presence of diffuse, nontender cervical and axillary lymphadenopathy. There were no visible skin lesions. The remainder of the examination was normal.

Initial investigations included a mild normocytic anaemia (Hb 11.6 g/dL). Serum white cell count, erythrocyte sedimentation rate, C-reactive protein, liver function tests, and serum electrolytes (including calcium) were normal. Blood urea was 7.1 mmol/L; creatinine was 282 umol/L.

Other laboratory tests including tests for human immunodeficiency virus, VDRL, double stranded DNA, anti-nuclear antibodies, anti-neutrophil cytoplasmic antibodies, serum angiotensin-converting enzyme, antibodies to extractable nuclear antigens, anti-Ro, anti-La, anti-Sm, anti-RNP, anti-Scl, and anti-Jo1 as well as tuberculosis quantiferon and mantoux testing were normal or negative. Serology for herpes simplex virus, cytomegalovirus, Epstein-Barr virus, and varicella virus was negative. Chest radiograph was normal on admission.

CT brain on admission was normal. Cerebrospinal fluid analysis revealed an opening pressure of 36 cmH$_2$O. CSF protein was 0.74 g/L and glucose was 2.9 mmol/L (no paired serum was sent for analysis). There were 9 lymphocytes/μL and 72 erythrocytes/μL. CSF was sterile. Oligoclonal bands were not detected.

MRI brain showed multiple small T2-weighted hyperintense lesions predominantly within the subcortical white matter throughout both cerebral hemispheres and also within the right pons. Microhaemorrhages were also observed on susceptibility weighted imaging (SWI) and an area of restricted diffusion was observed in the left centrum semiovale on diffusion weighted MRI consistent with a small acute infarct (Figure 1).

Repeat MRI imaging upon transfer to a tertiary neurology unit revealed further linear areas of T2 hyperintensity with postcontrast T1 enhancement extending from the periventricular regions into the centrum semiovale bilaterally.

A differential diagnosis of cerebral vasculitis, a neoplastic process, or granulomatous disease was considered. CT of chest, abdomen, and pelvis revealed multiple lymph nodes in both axillae measuring up to 14 mm, as well as mediastinal and left para-aortic lymphadenopathy (Figure 2).

The patient underwent excision of one of the axillary lymph nodes, which revealed the presence of noncaseating granulomata in keeping with sarcoidosis (Figure 3). The original kidney biopsy was subsequently reviewed but did not contain evidence of granulomata.

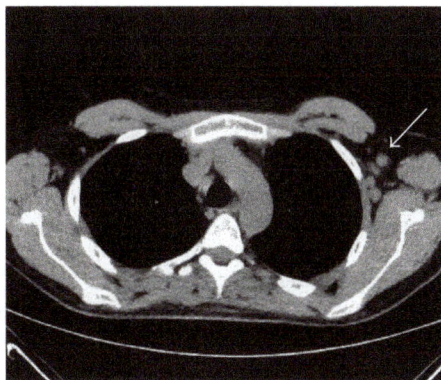

FIGURE 2: CT scan of thorax. CT of chest showing enlarged axillary nodes (arrow).

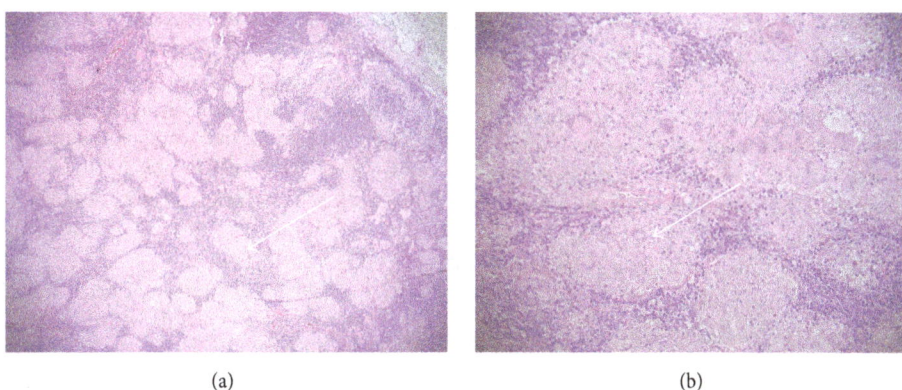

(a)   (b)

FIGURE 3: Axillary lymph node biopsy showing noncaseating granulomata (arrow) at ×50 magnification (a) and noncaseating granulomata (arrow) at ×200 magnification (b).

4. Treatment and Outcome

The patient was treated with one gram of intravenous methylprednisolone for three days followed by 60 mg daily of oral prednisolone with rapid clinical improvement. Renal function improved to baseline following commencement of steroids. Repeat lumbar puncture one month following introduction of steroids revealed opening pressure of 19 cmH$_2$O, protein 0.29 g/L, glucose 4.6 mmol, 2 lymphocytes/μL, and 72 erythrocytes/μL. Oligoclonal bands remained negative. At 12-month follow-up, the patient was well with no relapse of symptoms. He was maintained on 5 mg of prednisolone daily.

5. Discussion

Sarcoidosis is a systemic granulomatous disorder most commonly presenting between the ages of 20 and 40 years and is particularly prevalent among African Americans and Northern Europeans [9, 10]. The diagnosis of sarcoidosis most often relies on identifying systemic manifestations of the condition and obtaining histological demonstration of noncaseating granulomata on biopsy of affected tissue. Histologically, a central collection of macrophages is seen to exist with an oligoclonal T-cell population situated peripherally [11].

About 30–60% of patients with sarcoidosis develop granulomatous uveitis at some point in the course of the disease [12] but this can precede the systemic manifestations by up to eleven years [13]. Renal involvement may appear as interstitial nephritis and long-term treatment is often required to prevent progression to end stage renal failure [14].

Neurosarcoidosis is known to affect a minority of patients with sarcoidosis. The neurological features of sarcoidosis can be diverse and where neurological symptoms are the sole manifestation of the condition it can be particularly challenging to make a definitive diagnosis [15]. To further the investigation of suspected neurosarcoidosis, investigation with CSF analysis and measurement of CSF ACE levels are often undertaken. Both have limited sensitivity and specificity in the diagnosis of neurosarcoidosis [16]. Although tissue diagnosis remains the gold standard, it is invasive and not always feasible. MRI therefore remains an important investigation. The most common MRI findings in neurosarcoidosis include cranial nerve involvement, enhancing and nonenhancing parenchymal lesions, dural thickening, and leptomeningeal enhancement. Occasionally intracranial mass lesions are seen [17].

Our case is of interest for several reasons. The interval between the initial manifestations of sarcoidosis (presumed to be anterior uveitis) and subsequent symptoms was significant (over six years). The episode of acute onset right-sided weakness was shown to be related to an area of diffusion restriction on MRI. Focal ischaemic change in conjunction with MRI evidence of more diffuse microhaemorrhages was felt consistent with a vasculopathy. The neurovascular complications of neurosarcoidosis are extremely rare.

Although granulomatous involvement of cerebral blood vessels is described in neurosarcoidosis [8], stroke or transient ischaemic episodes are only rarely reported and such case reports largely precede the routine use of MRI [18–20]. Only isolated case reports exist of ischaemic stroke in the context of neurosarcoidosis confirmed on diffusion weighted MRI [21, 22]. Haemorrhagic manifestations of neurosarcoidosis are also reported but are a rare presentation [23–26]. Vascular complications of this nature are felt to result from a small-vessel vasculopathy, usually due to the destruction of elastic lumen by inflammatory cells and subsequent luminal occlusion. Acute necrotizing vasculopathy has also been observed [27].

The optimum treatment of neurosarcoidosis is unclear. Corticosteroids are generally considered the first-line treatment; however high doses may be required and relapse can occur during drug taper [28]. A number of agents including methotrexate, chloroquine, azathioprine, mycophenolate mofetil, cyclophosphamide, and infliximab can be used as second-line or steroid sparing agents [29–32]. Due to the rarity of neurosarcoidosis, large scale randomized controlled trial evidence is lacking.

6. Conclusion

We report a case of biopsy proven systemic sarcoidosis presenting with neurological features of raised intracranial pressure and transient neurological deficits, which were felt to be of vascular origin. Serial MRI over a short period showed significant change both revealing an area of restriction diffusion indicative of ischaemia and showing evidence of cerebral microhaemorrhages on susceptibility weighted imaging sequences as a result of small-vessel granulomatous vasculopathy.

In retrospect, the past medical history of anterior uveitis and interstitial nephritis is felt to be in keeping with systemic sarcoidosis and serves to highlight the considerable variation that can be seen in the natural history of this condition.

This case highlights that neurosarcoidosis should be considered a potentially treatable cause of otherwise unexplained vasculopathy or stroke, particularly in the context of other atypical neurological features or salient past medical history.

Conflict of Interests

The authors declare that there is no conflict of interests regarding the publication of this paper.

References

[1] R. P. Baughman, E. E. Lower, and R. M. du Bois, "Sarcoidosis," *The Lancet*, vol. 361, no. 9363, pp. 1111–1118, 2003.

[2] T. M. Burns, "Neurosarcoidosis," *Archives of Neurology*, vol. 60, no. 8, pp. 1166–1168, 2003.

[3] J. P. Zajicek, N. J. Scolding, O. Foster et al., "Central nervous system sarcoidosis—diagnosis and management," *QJM: Monthly Journal of the Association of Physicians*, vol. 92, no. 2, pp. 103–117, 1999.

[4] B. J. Stern, A. Krumholz, C. Johns, P. Scott, and J. Nissim, "Sarcoidosis and its neurological manifestations," *Archives of Neurology*, vol. 42, no. 9, pp. 909–917, 1985.

[5] J. L. Sponsler, M. A. Werz, R. Maciunas, and M. Cohen, "Neurosarcoidosis presenting with simple partial seizures and solitary enhancing mass: case reports and review of the literature," *Epilepsy and Behavior*, vol. 6, no. 4, pp. 623–630, 2005.

[6] F. Fayad, F. Lioté, F. Berenbaum, P. Orcel, and T. Bardin, "Muscle involvement in sarcoidosis: a retrospective and followup studies," *Journal of Rheumatology*, vol. 33, no. 1, pp. 98–103, 2006.

[7] L. Wang and Y. Li, "Longitudinal ultra-extensive transverse myelitis as a manifestation of neurosarcoidosis," *Journal of the Neurological Sciences*, vol. 355, no. 1-2, pp. 64–67, 2015.

[8] A. B. Herring and H. Urich, "Sarcoidosis of the central nervous system," *Journal of the Neurological Sciences*, vol. 9, no. 3, pp. 405–422, 1969.

[9] B. A. Rybicki, M. Major, J. Popovich Jr., M. J. Maliarik, and M. C. Iannuzzi, "Racial differences in sarcoidosis incidence: a 5-year study in a health maintenance organization," *American Journal of Epidemiology*, vol. 145, no. 3, pp. 234–241, 1997.

[10] J. M. Reich, "A critical analysis of sarcoidosis incidence assessment," *Multidisciplinary Respiratory Medicine*, vol. 8, no. 1, article 57, 2013.

[11] D. R. Moller, "Cells and cytokines involved in the pathogenesis of sarcoidosis," *Sarcoidosis Vasculitis and Diffuse Lung Disease*, vol. 16, no. 1, pp. 24–31, 1999.

[12] H. Takase, K. Shimizu, Y. Yamada, A. Hanada, H. Takahashi, and M. Mochizuki, "Validation of international criteria for the diagnosis of ocular sarcoidosis proposed by the first international workshop on ocular sarcoidosis," *Japanese Journal of Ophthalmology*, vol. 54, no. 6, pp. 529–536, 2010.

[13] G. Rizzato, M. Angi, P. Fraioli, L. Montemurro, E. Pilotto, and A. Tommasini, "Uveitis as a presenting feature of chronic sarcoidosis," *European Respiratory Journal*, vol. 9, no. 6, pp. 1201–1205, 1996.

[14] R. Rajakariar, E. J. Sharples, M. J. Raftery, M. Sheaff, and M. M. Yaqoob, "Sarcoid tubulo-interstitial nephritis: long-term outcome and response to corticosteroid therapy," *Kidney International*, vol. 70, no. 1, pp. 165–169, 2006.

[15] V. Oksanen, "Neurosarcoidosis: clinical presentations and course in 50 patients," *Acta Neurologica Scandinavica*, vol. 73, no. 3, pp. 283–290, 1986.

[16] S. J. Borucki, B. V. Nguyen, T. Ladoulis Ch., and R. R. McKendall, "Cerbrospinal fluid immunoglobulin abnormalities in neurosarcoidosis," *Archives of Neurology*, vol. 46, no. 3, pp. 270–273, 1989.

[17] D. H. Miller, B. E. Kendall, S. Barter et al., "Magnetic resonance imaging in central nervous system sarcoidosis," *Neurology*, vol. 38, no. 3, pp. 378–383, 1988.

[18] M. M. Brown, A. J. Thompson, J. A. Wedzicha, and M. Swash, "Sarcoidosis presenting with stroke," *Stroke*, vol. 20, no. 3, pp. 400–405, 1989.

[19] A. M. Corse and B. J. Stern, "Neurosarcoidosis and stroke," *Stroke*, vol. 21, no. 1, pp. 152–153, 1990.

[20] A. Michotte, P. Dequenne, D. Jacobovitz, and J. Hildebrand, "Focal neurological deficit with sudden onset as the first manifestation of sarcoidosis: a case report with MRI follow-up," *European Neurology*, vol. 31, no. 6, pp. 376–379, 1991.

[21] M. H. Hodge, R. L. Williams, and M. B. Fukui, "Neurosarcoidosis presenting as acute infarction on diffusion-weighted MR imaging: summary of radiologic findings," *American Journal of Neuroradiology*, vol. 28, no. 1, pp. 84–86, 2007.

[22] I. González-Aramburu, E. Ruiz-Pérez, J. Gómez-Román, R. Quirce, D. Larrosa, and J. Pascual, "Sarcoidosis presenting as transient ischemic attack status," *Journal of Stroke and Cerebrovascular Diseases*, vol. 21, no. 6, pp. 515–517, 2012.

[23] J.-P. Ferroir, A. Khalil, V. Gounant, and B. Milleron, "Brain and medullar neurosarcoidosis, complicated by stroke with local vasculitis," *Revue Neurologique*, vol. 165, no. 6-7, pp. 596–600, 2009.

[24] J. P. O'Dwyer, B. A. Al-Moyeed, M. A. Farrell et al., "Neurosarcoidosis-related intracranial haemorrhage: three new cases and a systematic review of the literature," *European Journal of Neurology*, vol. 20, no. 1, pp. 71–78, 2013.

[25] G. K. Dakdouki, Z. A. Kanafani, G. Ishak, M. Hourani, and S. S. Kanj, "Intracerebral bleeding in a patient with neurosarcoidosis while on corticosteroid therapy," *Southern Medical Journal*, vol. 98, no. 4, pp. 492–494, 2005.

[26] K. Berek, S. Kiechl, J. Willeit, G. Birbamer, G. Vogl, and E. Schmutzhard, "Subarachnoid hemorrhage as presenting feature of isolated neurosarcoidosis," *The Clinical Investigator*, vol. 71, no. 1, pp. 54–56, 1993.

[27] E. Reske-Nielsen and A. Harmsen, "Periangiitis and panangiitis as a manifestation of sarcoidosis of the brain: report of a case," *The Journal of Nervous and Mental Disease*, vol. 135, pp. 399–412, 1962.

[28] J.-L. Dumas, D. Valeyre, C. Chapelon-Abric et al., "Central nervous system sarcoidosis: follow-up at MR imaging during steroid therapy," *Radiology*, vol. 214, no. 2, pp. 411–420, 2000.

[29] O. P. Sharma, "Effectiveness of chloroquine and hydroxychloroquine in treating selected patients with sarcoidosis with neurological involvement," *Archives of Neurology*, vol. 55, no. 9, pp. 1248–1254, 1998.

[30] B. J. Stern, S. A. Schonfeld, C. Sewell, A. Krumholz, P. Scott, and G. Belendiuk, "The treatment of neurosarcoidosis with cyclosporine," *Archives of Neurology*, vol. 49, no. 10, pp. 1065–1072, 1992.

[31] D. J. Kouba, D. Mimouni, A. Rencic, and H. C. Nousari, "Mycophenolate mofetil may serve as a steroid-sparing agent for sarcoidosis," *British Journal of Dermatology*, vol. 148, no. 1, pp. 147–148, 2003.

[32] M. Sollberger, F. Fluri, T. Baumann et al., "Successful treatment of steroid-refractory neurosarcoidosis with infliximab," *Journal of Neurology*, vol. 251, no. 6, pp. 760–761, 2004.

Successful Desensitization of a Patient with Rituximab Hypersensitivity

Pinar Ataca,[1] Erden Atilla,[1] Resat Kendir,[2] Sevim Bavbek,[2] and Muhit Ozcan[1]

[1]*Department of Hematology, Ankara University, Cebeci, 06590 Ankara, Turkey*
[2]*Department of Pulmonary Medicine, Immunology and Allergy Clinic, Ankara University, Cebeci, 06590 Ankara, Turkey*

Correspondence should be addressed to Pinar Ataca; pinar@ataca.tk

Academic Editor: Ahmad M. Mansour

Rituximab is a monoclonal antibody which targets CD20 in B cells that is used for the treatment of CD20 positive oncologic and hematologic malignances. Rituximab causes hypersensitivity reactions during infusions. The delay of treatment or loss of a highly efficient drug can be prevented by rapid drug desensitization method in patients who are allergic to rituximab. We report a low grade B cell non-Hodgkin lymphoma patient with rituximab hypersensitivity successfully treated with rapid drug desensitization. In experienced centers, drug desensitization is a novel modality to break through in case of hypersensitivity that should be considered.

1. Introduction

Monoclonal antibody research has entered a new era in targeting of specific proteins associated with disease pathogenesis [1]. However, hypersensitivity reactions to monoclonal antibodies limit their practicality [2]; these reactions have been reported following initial or repeated exposures [1]. Most of these reactions involve nonimmune cytokine releases that occur during the intravenous administration of the agent. IgE-related type I hypersensitivity reactions may also occur [3]. IgE-related mast cell activation promotes the release of histamine, leukotrienes, prostaglandins, proteases, and proteoglycans, which mediate early-type hypersensitivity reactions that can be accompanied by urticaria, shock, or even death [2].

If a patient develops hypersensitivity to a mandatory agent, drug desensitization should be applied. Desensitization is a treatment method that enables patients, who have previously experienced hypersensitivity reactions, to be treated with the culprit drug [1]. Desensitization is the rapid signal attenuation in response to stimulation on the other hand reduction in response to a drug after repeated administration defined as tolerance. Desensitization is effective for IgE-dependent or IgE-independent hypersensitivity

reactions [4] but is contraindicated in patients with a history of Stevens-Johnson syndrome, toxic epidermal necrolysis, serum sickness, or hemolytic anemia [5].

Rituximab is a chimeric mouse-human anti-CD20 monoclonal antibody that is effective in non-Hodgkin's lymphoma (NHL), chronic lymphocytic lymphoma (CLL), rheumatoid arthritis, Wegener's granulomatosis, and microscopic polyangiitis [6]. In the rituximab prescription insert, the infusion-related reactions due to massive cytokine release are described as urticaria, hypotension, angioedema, hypoxia, bronchospasm, pulmonary infiltrates, acute respiratory distress syndrome, myocardial infarction, ventricular fibrillation, cardiogenic shock, anaphylactoid events, and death within 30–120 minutes of infusion [6]. The occurrence of an infusion reaction in NHL is reported to be 77% [6]. However, 5% to 10% of the reactions to rituximab are considered as immediate type I hypersensitivity [3]. Studies demonstrated that the prolongation of treatment should be managed by rapid drug desensitization in patients who are allergic to rituximab [7, 8]. Rapid desensitization allows safe readministration of a medication after certain types of immediate hypersensitivity. However, desensitization protocols for monoclonal agents are followed in few centers, and most researchers are unaware of the involved methods. Therefore,

TABLE 1: Rituximab desensitization protocol.

Step	Solution	Rate (mL/h)	Time (min)	Dose	Total dose
1	1	2.0	15	0.015	
2	1	5.0	15	0.037	
3	1	10.0	15	0.075	
4	1	20.0	15	0.150	0.277
5	2	5.0	15	0.375	
6	2	10.0	15	0.750	
7	2	20.0	15	1.500	
8	2	40.0	15	3.000	5.625 (1–8: 5.902) 750–5.902: 744 mg will be given in next steps
9	3	10.0	15		
10	3	20.0	15		
11	3	40.0	15		
12	3	75.0	240		

Solution 1: 250 mL, 5% dextrose, /0.8 mL rituximab (0.03 mg/mL: 1 : 100 of total dose, 250 mL/7.5 mg).
Solution 2: 250 mL, 5% dextrose, /7.5 mL rituximab (0.30 mg/mL: 1 : 10 of total dose, 250 mL/75 mg).
Solution 3: 250 mL, 5% dextrose, /74.4 mL rituximab.
Premedication: 20 minutes before pheniramine 45.5 mg IV, prednisolone 100 mg IV, and famotidine 20 mg IV.

we present a patient with NHL who was treated successfully with rituximab in our center despite having a history of severe rituximab related adverse reaction.

2. Case Presentation

A 54-year-old male was admitted to the gastroenterology clinic with epigastric pain, weight loss of 6 kg, night sweats, and high fever that started a month prior to admission. He reported no severe allergic reactions in medical history; however, he described flushing and flu-like symptoms during gardening. In his physical examination, we detected nonmobile pathologically lymphadenopathies in bilateral cervical, axillary and inguinal regions, and splenomegaly. His routine laboratory results were as follows: lactate dehydrogenase: 133 U/L, Beta2 microglobulin: 4.246 mg/dL, leucocytes: 5.6×10^9/L, erythrocytes: 3.92×10^{12}/L, platelets: 137×10^9/L, and hemoglobin: 12.6 g/dL. In his cervical and inguinal ultrasonography and thoracoabdominal computed tomography (CT) scan, bilateral axillary, mediastinal, hilar, paraceliac, peripancreatic, portal hepatogastric, and inguinal pathological lymphadenopathies were detected. His right axillary region lymph node biopsy and bone marrow biopsy results indicated low-grade B cell (follicular) NHL. We diagnosed him with Stage 4 disease and prescribed 6 cycles of an R-CHOP (rituximab 375 mg/m^2, cyclophosphamide 750 mg/m^2, adriamycin 50 mg/m^2, vincristine 1.4 mg/m^2 (max: 2 mg), and prednisone 100 mg/day) protocol. Prior to the first dose of rituximab, 45.5 mg of pheniramine (intravenous) and 500 mg of acetaminophen (peroral) were administered. The patient developed flushing within 5 minutes following administration. The infusion was then interrupted, and 45.5 mg of pheniramine was administered. The infusion

was slowly restarted. Ten minutes following readministration, generalized urticaria, dyspnea, and nausea developed. His physical examination revealed the following: 38.2°C body temperature, arterial blood pressure of 100/60 mmHg (initial arterial blood pressure of 120/80 mmHg), arterial O_2 saturation: 92%, 120 beats/min tachycardia, and bilateral rhonchi with no stridor or pharynx edema. The infusion was stopped and the reaction was treated with the administration of 100 mg methylprednisolone and pheniramine. The tryptase level was 24.60 μg/L (n: <11 μg/L) at four hours after the hypersensitivity reaction. Next day, the patient received CHOP only protocol (no rituximab) uneventfully. We referred the patient to the Immunology and Allergy Clinic to continue rituximab treatment.

In the Immunology and Allergy Clinic, his reaction was defined as Grade 3 according to the Brown Classification, which indicates a severe systemic hypersensitivity reaction [9]. A 12-step rapid drug desensitization protocol was planned for the patient. He was premedicated with H1 and H2 blockers with systemic steroids and was desensitized by an experienced allergist and nurses according to established protocols (Table 1). The rituximab dosage was not decreased throughout the following cycles. The basal tryptase level was 8.89 μg/L. At the twelfth step of the protocol, he developed urticaria in his face and body; thus, desensitization was interrupted and treatment was administered. The infusion was restarted without adverse effects. He had a positive skin prick test result for rituximab before second course. During further cycles, the same dose rituximab was administered with minimal urticaria in his face and body so desensitization protocols were completed with increased premedications. The patient is followed by complete response after 6 cycles of R-CHOP; the bone marrow involvement was disappeared.

The patient's desensitization protocol is currently ongoing during maintenance therapy.

3. Discussion

Rituximab is a chimeric monoclonal antibody, changed the natural history of some catastrophic disorders, directed to the CD20 molecule and currently used in treatment of lymphoproliferative diseases and several rheumatologic disorders. Intentionally, rituximab is one of the most frequent causes of acute infusion reactions due to massive cytokine release [10]. Clinical manifestations of IgE-related and non-IgE related infusion reactions overlap; rash, hypotension, nausea, tachycardia, and shortness of breath have been described in both reactions [3]. The severity of infusion reactions is associated with high tumor burden or advanced disease which usually occurs after the first administration of rituximab [11]. Although our patient had high tumor burden, elevated tryptase levels, positive skin test supported the hypersensitivity reaction rather than infusion reaction.

Monoclonal antibodies have increasingly been used in routine practice; thus, hypersensitivity reactions are becoming increasingly more common. Recent studies reported the presence of serum anti-drug antibodies in pretreated patients [10]. Anti-drug antibodies are mostly IgG and IgE which shows the adaptive immune response to the drug [12]. Castells et al. reported 413 cases of desensitization in 98 patients for reactions to carboplatin, cisplatin, oxaliplatin, paclitaxel, liposomal doxorubicin, doxorubicin, and rituximab. A twelve-step rituximab desensitization protocol was performed seven times in three of the 98 patients. Two of these patients were diagnosed with lymphoma and one was diagnosed with polymyositis. Two patients with lymphoma had rashes and pruritus, while the third patient experienced syncope. Similar to our case, the infusion rate was decreased; however, there were no changes in the hypersensitivity reactions. Regression due to the reduction of the infusion rate could indicate immune-related or non-IgE-related hypersensitivity reactions [4].

The same researchers performed another study of 23 patients with 105 cases of desensitization. A total of 14 patients with no prior monoclonal antibody exposure developed (primarily) intermediate-grade hypersensitivity to rituximab. Eleven of the 14 patients had a reaction during the first administration that was similar to our case, while 1 patient experienced a reaction during his third administration, 1 patient during her fourth administration, and another patient during repeated administrations. None of the patients in the study exhibited skin prick test positivity with rituximab; however, 6 of the 9 tested patients had intradermal skin test positivity [3]. To prevent false-negative results, skin tests should be administered two weeks after a reaction; however, if the waiting period would interrupt the patient's treatment, the desensitization protocol should be performed first [13]. We desensitized the patient prior to the skin test; however, before second course the skin test was positive. The increase in the tryptase level in our patient indicates a hypersensitivity reaction due to IgE. In rapid drug desensitization protocols, the drug is administered in small increments [1]. The goal of this method is to decrease the mast cell and basophil response to the drug [14]. Rapid drug desensitization precipitates transient unresponsiveness; thus, the patient should be desensitized again during each exposure [2].

Using rapid drug desensitization protocols, it is possible to continue monoclonal antibody administration after hypersensitivity reactions. As a result, early hypersensitivity reactions to rituximab can be managed in appropriately trained centers via rapid drug desensitization to enable rituximab continuation with transient tolerance. By this, an important drug, rituximab, which is opening a new era in management of hematological malignancies, can be prevented from early cessation.

Conflict of Interests

The authors declare that there is no conflict of interests regarding the publication of this paper.

References

[1] D. I. Hong, L. Bankova, K. N. Cahill, T. Kyin, and M. C. Castells, "Allergy to monoclonal antibodies: cutting-edge desensitization methods for cutting-edge therapies," *Expert Review of Clinical Immunology*, vol. 8, no. 1, pp. 43–54, 2012.

[2] M. Castells, M. D. C. Sancho-Serra, and M. Simarro, "Hypersensitivity to antineoplastic agents: mechanisms and treatment with rapid desensitization," *Cancer Immunology, Immunotherapy*, vol. 61, pp. 1575–1584, 2012.

[3] P. J. Brennan, T. Rodriguez Bouza, F. I. Hsu, D. E. Sloane, and M. C. Castells, "Hypersensitivity reactions to mAbs: 105 desensitizations in 23 patients, from evaluation to treatment," *Journal of Allergy and Clinical Immunology*, vol. 124, no. 6, pp. 1259–1266, 2009.

[4] M. C. Castells, N. M. Tennant, D. E. Sloane et al., "Hypersensitivity reactions to chemotherapy: outcomes and safety of rapid desensitization in 413 cases," *Journal of Allergy and Clinical Immunology*, vol. 122, no. 3, pp. 574–580, 2008.

[5] J. A. Meyerhardt, A. S. LaCasce, M. C. Castells, and H. Burstein, "Infusion reactions to therapeutic monoclonal antibodies used for cancer therapy," http://www.uptodate.com/contents/infusionreactions-to-therapeutic-monoclonalantibodies-used-for-cancertherapy.

[6] Rituxan (package insert), South San Francisco, Calif, USA: Biogen Idec and Genentech, 2013.

[7] S. G. A. Brown, "Clinical features and severity grading of anaphylaxis," *Journal of Allergy and Clinical Immunology*, vol. 114, no. 2, pp. 371–376, 2004.

[8] P. J. Brennan, T. Rodriguez Bouza, F. I. Hsu, D. E. Sloane, and M. C. Castells, "Hypersensitivityreaction to mAb: 105 desensitizations in 23 patients, from evaluation to treatment," *Journal of Allergy and Clinical Immunology*, vol. 124, pp. 1259–1266, 2009.

[9] P. J. Bugelski, R. Achuthanandam, R. J. Capocasale, G. Treacy, and E. Bouman-Thio, "Monoclonal antibody-induced cytokine-release syndrome," *Expert Review of Clinical Immunology*, vol. 5, no. 5, pp. 499–521, 2009.

[10] E. Schmidt, K. Hennig, C. Mengede, D. Zillikens, and A. Kromminga, "Immunogenicity of rituximab in patients with severe pemphigus," *Clinical Immunology*, vol. 132, no. 3, pp. 334–341, 2009.

[11] H. S. Kulkarni and P. M. Kasi, "Rituximab and cytokine release syndrome," *Case Reports in Oncology*, vol. 5, no. 1, pp. 134–141, 2012.

[12] A. Vultaggio, E. Maggi, and A. Matucci, "Immediate adverse reactions to biological: from pathogenic mechanisms to prophylactic management," *Current Opinion in Allergy and Clinical Immunology*, vol. 11, no. 3, pp. 262–268, 2011.

[13] P. Lieberman and M. Castells, "Desensitization to chemotherapeutic agents," *The Journal of Allergy and Clinical Immunology*, vol. 2, no. 1, pp. 116–117, 2014.

[14] A. Liu, L. Fanning, H. Chong et al., "Desensitization regimens for drug allergy: state of the art in the 21st century," *Clinical & Experimental Allergy*, vol. 41, no. 12, pp. 1679–1689, 2011.

Fever of Unknown Origin: An Unusual Presentation of Kikuchi-Fujimoto Disease

Piyush Ranjan,[1] **Manish Soneja,**[1] **Nellai Krishnan Subramonian,**[2] **Vivek Kumar,**[2] **Shuvadeep Ganguly,**[2] **Tarun Kumar,**[3] **and Geetika Singh**[3]

[1]Department of Medicine, All India Institute of Medical Sciences, New Delhi 110029, India
[2]All India Institute of Medical Sciences, New Delhi 110029, India
[3]Department of Pathology, All India Institute of Medical Sciences, New Delhi 110029, India

Correspondence should be addressed to Manish Soneja; manishsoneja@gmail.com

Academic Editor: Alessandro Plebani

Kikuchi-Fujimoto disease is a rare, benign, and self-limiting condition that mostly affects young females. Cervical lymphadenopathy with fever is the most common presentation of the disease. It may have unusual presentations that can lead to diagnostic dilemma and delay in diagnosis. We report a case of a 25-year-old female who presented with relapsing fever and cervical lymphadenopathy. Because of atypical presentation, there was a delay in diagnosis and increase in morbidity. High index of suspicion with collaboration between clinicians and pathologists is essential for early and accurate diagnosis of the disease.

1. Introduction

Fever of unknown origin (FUO) represents a condition in which the cause of fever remains elusive even after extensive investigations. Infection is the most common cause of FUO, whereas, connective tissue disorders and neoplasms are the other leading causes among adults [1, 2]. Despite considerable development in the imaging and serological and immunohistopathological modalities, the task of diagnosis is often difficult and cannot be achieved in up to 50% of the cases [3]. The diagnosis of FUO becomes even more difficult and often gets delayed when the cause is a rare disease. Kikuchi-Fujimoto disease (KFD) is a rare but important cause of FUO affecting mostly young population. We present an interesting case of FUO in which the diagnosis was delayed due to atypical presentation leading to unnecessary invasive investigations.

2. Case Report

A 25-year-old female presented with the complaint of episodes of high grade fever and cervical lymphadenopathy requiring multiple hospitalizations. The patient developed low grade fever with headache three months before for which she was initially prescribed NSAIDS on outpatient basis. Subsequently, she was admitted in an outside hospital for further investigation and management. Her routine hemogram, urine and blood cultures, chest X-ray, and ultrasound of the abdomen were normal. No significant lymphadenopathy was noted. She responded to conservative management and was discharged after defervescence in 4-day time.

After three weeks, she noticed 3-4 small nodular swellings in the neck. She developed high grade fever and headache, following which she was admitted in the hospital. At the time of admission, she had stable vitals and four enlarged, firm, and discrete lymph nodes in the posterior triangle of the neck. There were no meningeal signs. Her routine hemogram showed leukopenia (TLC-3200/μL). Other investigations including urine and blood cultures, a contrast enhanced computed tomography (CECT) of the chest and abdomen along with lumbar puncture, and CSF examination were noncontributory. She was given symptomatic and supportive treatment and the fever subsided and the lymph nodes regressed. She was discharged in two-week time.

After two weeks, she was again hospitalized with high grade fever and headache. Clinical examination revealed

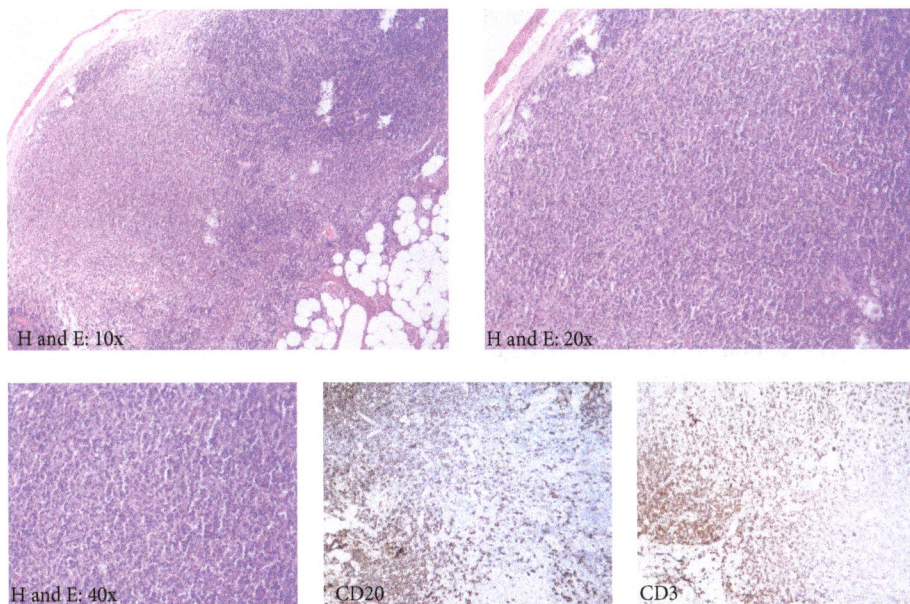

FIGURE 1: Photomicrophotograph of lymph node biopsy shows paracortical necrosis, histiocytes, apoptotic bodies, and nuclear dust (karyorrhexis). CD3 and CD20 immunostains demonstrate the reactive population of lymphoid cells including both B cells (CD20 immunopositive) and T cells (CD3 immunopositive).

multiple, enlarged, firm, enlargement of cervical and axillary lymph nodes of size about two centimeters. She was again subjected to extensive investigations including lumbar puncture and CSF examination, all of which were noncontributory except for mild anaemia, leukopenia, and raised ESR (70 mm in first hour). Immunological tests like ANA and RF were within normal limits. CECT of chest and abdomen was done and revealed enlarged axillary and cervical lymphadenopathy. Excision biopsy of cervical lymph nodes and histopathological examination was done and revealed multiple well circumscribed areas of necrosis with histiocytes and marked karyorrhexis (Figure 1). These features were suggestive of KFD. To exclude the differential diagnosis of infective aetiology stains for acid fast bacilli and fungus were performed which were negative. The patient was given symptomatic and supportive treatment and was discharged in afebrile condition in one week. She is asymptomatic at 4 months follow-up.

3. Discussion

The patient had certain unusual presentation that caused delay in the diagnosis and increase in morbidity. Usually fever is of low to moderate grade and self-limiting in KFD; our case had high grade fever. Cervical lymphadenopathy appeared late in the course and disappeared after first episode of the febrile illness. This probably delayed the decision to do lymph node biopsy. Our case showed early recurrence which is rare in the disease.

KFD is a benign condition of unknown cause that usually presents with lymphadenopathy and fever. It mostly affects younger population with female preponderance. Although more prevalent in Southeast Asia, it is described in different parts of the world including the United States [4].

The etiopathogenesis of KFD is unknown. Current knowledge suggests that it may be due to the excessive immune response of histiocytes to an infectious agent. Many viruses like Epstein Barr virus, human herpes virus, human immunodeficiency virus, parvovirus B19, and paramyxoviruses have been implicated in its pathogenesis [5, 6].

Fever is an important symptom which is present in almost half of the patients [1]. Fever is usually of low grade and persists for weeks. Sometimes, excessive fatigue and joint pains may be present [7]. Lymphadenopathy is present in almost all cases. They are multiple and usually involve cervical group. However other groups like axillary, mediastinal, and inguinal lymph nodes may also be involved. These are usually multiple and moderately enlarged and are typically firm, discrete, and nontender [4]. Other uncommon findings are rash, arthritis, and hepatosplenomegaly that are present in less than 10% of the cases. Complete blood count is usually normal; however cytopenias of various degrees may be present [8]. Immunological antibodies like ANA and RF are usually negative.

The diagnosis of KFD is delayed and, at times, missed mostly because of its rarity and self-limiting course. Lymph node biopsy is the cornerstone of the diagnosis. Histopathological findings of KFD may simulate with that of SLE and lymphoma posing difficulty in diagnosis. There are certain reports where the case was misdiagnosed as lymphoma and cytotoxic drugs were started [4].

The disease has a benign self-limiting course and usually symptomatic and supportive treatment is sufficient. In severe cases with persistent symptoms, high dose steroids are beneficial. In about 10% of the cases, early as well as delayed recurrences have been described [9]. There are reports of the development of SLE in the cases of KFD. Very rarely, death has also been reported [10].

Prolonged pyrexia, lymphadenopathy with noncontributory haematological and biochemical investigations, and sterile cultures of urine and blood usually raise the possibility of relatively common conditions like lymphoma, tuberculosis, SLE, HIV infection, and myeloid tumour. However, KFD is also an important differential in similar settings. High index of suspicion and careful histopathological examination are essential for early and accurate diagnosis. Delayed diagnosis leads to unnecessary investigations and inappropriate aggressive treatment.

This case report shares two important messages. Firstly, KFD can have atypical presentation in the form of high grade fever and late appearance of cervical lymphadenopathy causing delay in the diagnosis. Secondly, there should be low threshold for tissue biopsy as a diagnostic modality in such cases.

Consent

The authors have obtained the written informed consent from the patient for publication of this case report and the images included.

Conflict of Interests

The authors declare that there is no conflict of interests regarding the publication of this paper.

References

[1] X.-J. Ma, A.-X. Wang, G.-H. Deng, and R.-Y. Sheng, "A clinical review of 449 cases with fever of unknown origin," *Zhonghua Nei Ke Za Zhi*, vol. 43, no. 9, pp. 682–685, 2004.

[2] R. H. Hassan, A. E. Fouda, and S. M. Kandil, "Fever of unknown origin in children: a 6 year-experience in a Tertiary Pediatric Egyptian hospital," *International Journal of Health Sciences (Qassim)*, vol. 8, pp. 13–19, 2014.

[3] C. P. Bleeker-Rovers, F. J. Vos, E. M. H. A. de Kleijn et al., "A prospective multicenter study on fever of unknown origin: the yield of a structured diagnostic protocol," *Medicine (Baltimore)*, vol. 86, no. 1, pp. 26–38, 2007.

[4] R. F. Dorfman and G. J. Berry, "Kikuchi's histiocytic necrotizing lymphadenitis: an analysis of 108 cases with emphasis on differential diagnosis," *Seminars in Diagnostic Pathology*, vol. 5, no. 4, pp. 329–345, 1988.

[5] M. Imamura, H. Ueno, A. Matsuura et al., "An ultrastructural study of subacute necrotizing lymphadenitis," *The American Journal of Pathology*, vol. 107, no. 3, pp. 292–299, 1982.

[6] F. G. N. Rosado, Y. W. Tang, R. P. Hasserjian, C. M. McClain, B. Wang, and C. A. Mosse, "Kikuchi-Fujimoto lymphadenitis: role of parvovirus B-19, Epstein-Barr virus, human herpesvirus 6, and human herpesvirus 8," *Human Pathology*, vol. 44, no. 2, pp. 255–259, 2013.

[7] X. Bosch and A. Guilabert, "Kikuchi-Fujimoto disease," *Medicina Clinica*, vol. 123, no. 12, pp. 471–476, 2004.

[8] Y. Kucukardali, E. Solmazgul, E. Kunter, O. Oncul, S. Yildirim, and M. Kaplan, "Kikuchi-Fujimoto disease: analysis of 244 cases," *Clinical Rheumatology*, vol. 26, no. 1, pp. 50–54, 2007.

[9] J. Y. Song, J. Lee, D. W. Park et al., "Clinical outcome and predictive factors of recurrence among patients with Kikuchi's disease," *International Journal of Infectious Diseases*, vol. 13, no. 3, pp. 322–326, 2009.

[10] T. Kampitak, "Fatal Kikuchi-Fujimoto disease associated with SLE and hemophagocytic syndrome: a case report," *Clinical Rheumatology*, vol. 27, no. 8, pp. 1073–1075, 2008.

8

A Precocious Cerebellar Ataxia and Frequent Fever Episodes in a 16-Month-Old Infant Revealing Ataxia-Telangiectasia Syndrome

Luigi Nespoli,[1] **Annapia Verri,**[2] **Silvia Tajè,**[1] **Francesco Paolo Pellegrini,**[1] **and Maddalena Marinoni**[1]

[1] *Pediatrics Unit, Department of Clinical and Experimental Medicine, University of Insubria, 21100 Varese, Italy*
[2] *Neurological Institute C. Mondino Foundation IRCCS, 27100 Pavia, Italy*

Correspondence should be addressed to Annapia Verri; annapia.verri@mondino.it

Academic Editors: N. Martinez-Quiles and N. Tulek

Ataxia-telangiectasia (AT) is the most frequent progressive cerebellar ataxia in infancy and childhood. Immunodeficiency which includes both cellular and humoral arms has variable severity. Since the clinical presentation is extremely variable, a high clinical suspicion will allow an early diagnosis. Serum alpha-fetoprotein is elevated in 80–85% of patients and therefore could be used as a screening tool. Here, we present a case of a 5-year-old female infant who was admitted to our department at the age of 16 months because of gait disorders and febrile episodes that had begun at 5 months after the cessation of breastfeeding. Serum alfa-fetoprotein level was elevated. Other investigations showed leukocytopenia with lymphopenia, reduced IgG$_2$ and IgA levels, and low titers of specific postimmunization antibodies against tetanus toxoid and Haemophilus B polysaccharide. Peripheral lymphocytes subsets showed reduction of T cells with a marked predominance of T cells with a memory phenotype and a corresponding reduction of naïve T cells; NK cells were very increased (41%) with normal activity. The characterization of the ATM gene mutations revealed 2 specific mutations (c.5692C > T/c.7630-2A > C) compatible with AT diagnosis. It was concluded that AT syndrome should be considered in children with precocious signs of cerebellar ataxia and recurrent fever episodes.

1. Introduction

Ataxia-telangectasia (AT) is a complex multisystem disorder characterized by progressive neurological impairment, variable immunodeficiency, and oculocutaneous telangiectasia [1]. AT is a member of chromosomal breakage syndromes caused by a mutation in the ataxia-telangiectasia mutated (ATM) gene [2, 3]. The immunodeficiency is of variable severity in relation to the specific ATM mutation and is associated with sinopulmonary infections, radiation hypersensitivity, and increased incidence of malignancy [3, 4]. Cells from patients show increased sensitivity to ionizing radiation, defective DNA repair, and frequent chromosomal abnormalities [5, 6].

Gait instability with or without recurrent infection is the earliest symptom and oculocutaneous teleangiectasias will appear later [7]. The complete phenotype occurs over a number of years, usually within the school age [8, 9]. An easy and reliable marker in case of suspected AT is the elevated serum level of alpha-fetoprotein which is present in 80–85% of the affected patients [1]. An early diagnosis is possible today by using the molecular approach which will identify the specific ATM mutations and by measuring the ATM protein levels and the ATM kinase activity [3, 4]. AT is transmitted as an autosomal recessive disorder, and its incidence is about 1 per 40.000 live births in the USA, but the frequency varies considerably from country to country [3, 10].

2. Case Report

Our patient is a 5-year-old girl who presented to our outpatient service at the age of 16 months with a history of repeated episodes of fever (lasting 3-4 days) of unknown origin sometimes associated with upper respiratory tract infections and oral candidiasis. The episodes subsided without antibiotics and responded to acetaminophen treatment. The infant was not introduced to daycare and she was cared for at home by

TABLE 1: Lymphocyte subsets. A low count of CD3$^+$ cells and of CD4$^+$ and CD8$^+$ T cells with an increase of CD16/CD56$^+$ cells (NK cells) and a normal number of B cells (CD19$^+$) was found in our patient.

Lymphocyte subsets	Absolute number ($\times 10^9$/L)	Reference values (5th–95th centiles)
Total lymphocyte	1776	2180–8270
CD3$^+$	578	1460–5440
CD4$^+$	340	1020–3060
CD8$^+$	185	570–2230
CD16/CD56$^+$	1458	309–1135
CD19$^+$	710	300–774
CD4/CD8$^+$	1.8	1–2.2

TABLE 2: Immunoglobulin levels. A reduction of IgG, IgA and IgG$_2$ subset was found at diagnosis.

Immunoglobulin levels	Absolute number (mg/dL-UI/mL)	Reference values (5th–95th centiles)
IgG	88	264–1509
IgA	<4	17–178
IgM	187	48–337
IgE	<0.1	≤20
IgG$_2$	13	30–170

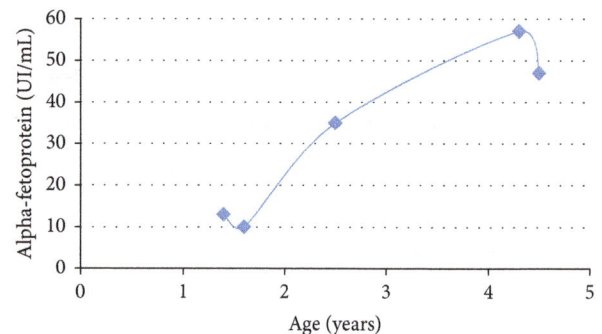

FIGURE 2: Alpha-fetoprotein trend.

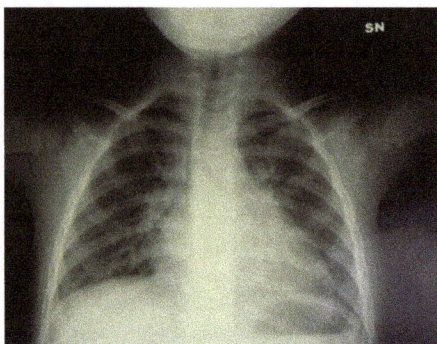

FIGURE 1: Chest X-ray: the chest X-ray showed reinforcement of the bronchial tree shadows, no bronchiectasis, and a markedly reduced thymic image.

her grandmother. She began walking just a few weeks before our visit. Her development was within the normal limits. Her parents are from Albania and are nonconsanguineous. Family history was noninformative. She was the first child of the family; the gestational period was normal as well as the birth parameters. Her previous medical history was positive for an exanthema subitum at the age of 8 months. Clinical examination was within the normal range: lymph nodes and intravelic tonsils were present; neurologic examination at that time revealed minimal hypotonia and a gait instability with slightly enlarged basis.

The first blood count showed a leukocyte number at the lower normal limits, microcytic anemia (the mother carries a beta-thalassemia trait), IgG below the lower limits for the age, IgA being absent, and IgM in the normal range. The chest X-ray did show a markedly reduced thymic image (Figure 1).

Our first hypothesis was a combined immunodeficiency; therefore, we performed more in-depth immunological investigations, but in the meantime the patient presented high fever and severe, nonbloody diarrhoea and was hospitalized.

At the admission, her general status was not compromised; she was present, conscious, and reacting to environmental stimuli. Weight was 10.100 kg (50th centile), length was 76.5 cm (50th centile), head circumference was 45 cm (25th centile), hearth rate was 180/min while crying, respiratory rate was 40/min, and ear temperature was 39.2°C;

hyperemia was found in the oropharynx and tonsils were visible and covered by grayish exudate with rare rales on the chest; clinical examination of the abdomen and the heart was normal.

Neurological examination revealed ataxic deambulation with frequent falls, forced right deviation, and left rotation of the head with left preferred look and oculomotor apraxia suggestive for cerebellar ataxia. Brain MRI was programmed for the following week and subsequently was normal.

Further laboratory investigations were carried out which showed border line levels of alpha-fetoprotein (13 ng/mL, n.v. < 10 ng/mL). The levels of this protein increased progressively over the years reaching 58 ng/mL when the patient was 4.5 years old (Figure 2). The complete blood count was in the normal range, but after 2 days leucopenia was present (6.820–3.280 WBC/cmm). The absolute number of circulating lymphocytes was below the normal range (Table 1). IgG, IgA, and IgM levels were unchanged as compared to the previous testing (Table 2). Isohemagglutinins, IgM natural antibodies against blood group specific antigens, were absent since the infant carried AB blood group. Postimmunization antibodies against tetanus toxoid and HiB conjugated polysaccharide were present at low levels. Cytofluorimetric analysis showed a low count of CD3$^+$ cells and of CD4$^+$ and CD8$^+$ T cells with a marked predominance of T-memory cells (CD45RO) and a reduction of naïve T cells (CD45RA), an increase of CD16$^+$/CD56$^+$ cells (NK cells), and a normal number of B cells, CD19$^+$ (Table 1 and Figure 3).

A karyotype test was performed that showed a normal female karyotype with t(7; 14)(p13; q11.2) in 3 metaphases, and t(4; 14)(q13.2; q13) t(5; 6)(p15.3; q23.3) del (7q11.23) in 1 metaphase, respectively.

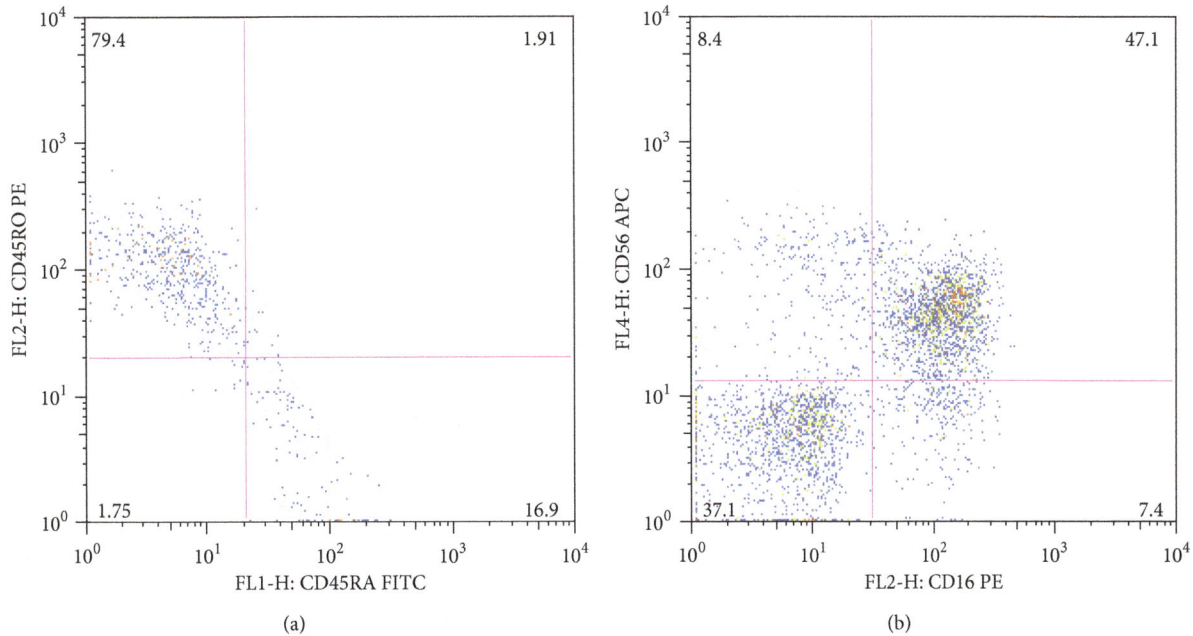

FIGURE 3: Cytofluorimetric CD45RA/CD45RO ratio (a) and CD16/CD56 $^+$ population (b). Note the reduced number of naïve T cells (CD45RA) versus peripheral T cells (CD45RO) (17% versus 80%, resp.) and the prevalent NK population (47.1%).

A blood sample was sent to the laboratory for the DNA molecular study of the ATM gene mutations which revealed 2 specific mutations (c.5692C > T/c.7630-2A > C) compatible with AT diagnosis (mother: c.5692C > T mutation; father: c.7630-2A > C on intron 53).

The child began replacement therapy with i.v. IgG every 21 days to maintain the serum IgG levels within the normal range. This treatment caused a reduction of episodes of fever and infections.

She progressively presented ataxic deambulation with frequent falls, forced right deviation, and left rotation of the head, with left preferred look and motor apraxia. Over a 2-year period, she developed deep gait instability and a difficult feeding due to supervening dysphagia that improved since the 3rd year of life with physiotherapy and exercises. She developed regular relational and cognitive skills and actually she is attending the kindergarten regularly, can eat without problems, walk safely, and drive a tricycle.

As expected, oculocutaneous telangiectasias became apparent when she was 3 years old. At 4.6 years of age she presented with enlargement of the spleen at the clinical examination which was repeatedly confirmed by the abdominal ultrasound. This fact made us suspect the appearance of a lymphoma. Virological research did document the presence of EBV-DNA (135.000 number of copies/mL) in blood which decreased to 15800 copies/mL after 3 weeks. IgM-specific antibodies were never present in the serum, whereas specific IgG antibodies were detectable but were from the transfused IgG. CMV or other viral DNAs were persistently negative. At the same time, an increase in the IgM serum levels (200 → 700 → 370 mg/dL) range was observed (Figure 4) which persisted for several weeks while the spleen size is in reduction but still not within the physiological range.

3. Discussion

Patients affected by AT typically present early onset gait disturbances which evolve in typically cerebellar ataxia [1, 7]. The observation of our patient deserves to be taken into account because it shows how careful clinical history together with clinical examination enables us to issue a diagnostic suspicion that today, thanks to molecular studies, can be easily confirmed or denied.

A firm diagnosis has positive effects on the choice of treatment by the doctors and on the procreative planning for the parents [3]. Our patient today has a younger, healthy sister.

Our infant had a history of recurrent fevers seemingly trivial, typical of children of this age, which were associated with an uncertain gait, common in an infant who had just started walking at the age of 15 months. Some peculiarities have led to the diagnosis: febrile episodes were initiated at cessation of breastfeeding at 5-6 months of age which is associated with transient infant hypogammaglobulinemia that had lasted too long in our infant (16-17 months of age when first tested) and was associated with the deficiency of IgA [9]. In addition, history of oral candidiasis is itself an indication of a deficiency of T lymphocytes [11, 12]. The thymic hypoplasia (Figure 1) in association with the low number of circulating lymphocytes further pointed to the diagnosis of combined immunodeficiency [11, 12]. The gait instability suggestive of cerebellar ataxia prompted us to the diagnosis of AT which was further supported by the simultaneous increase in alpha-fetoprotein (13 ng/mL) (Figure 3) [1]. The severity of the immunodeficiency associated with AT is correlated with the reduction of circulating naïve T-cell numbers as observed in our patient [13]. ATM is critically important

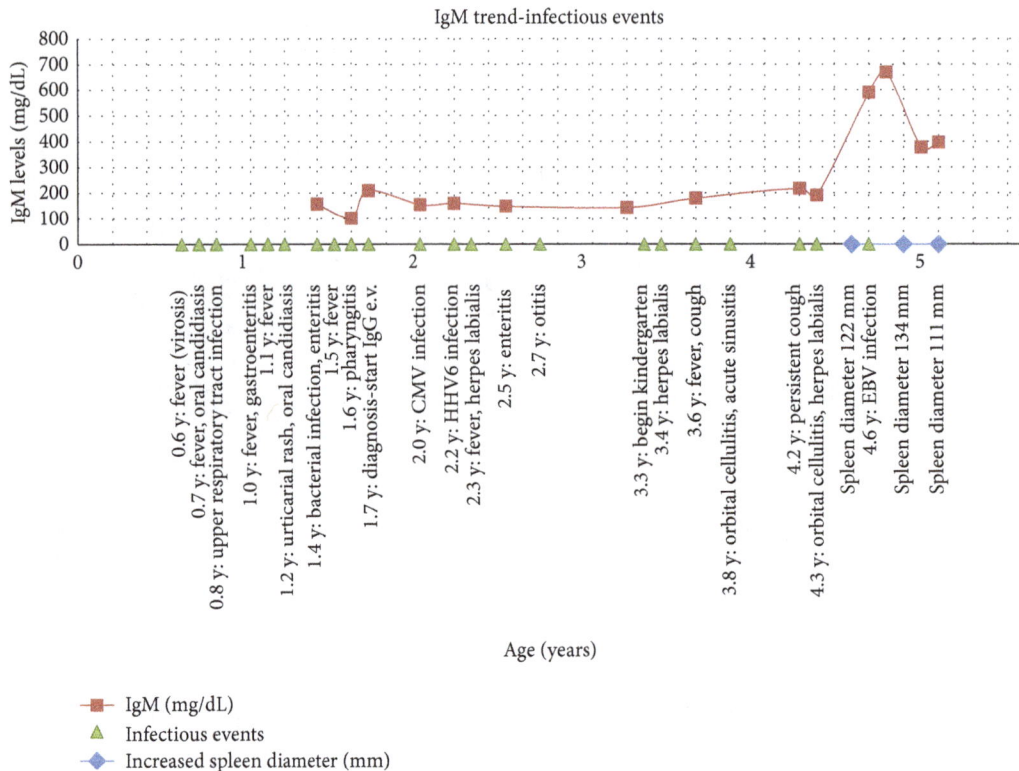

FIGURE 4: IgM levels according to history infections. Note the increasing levels of IgM simultaneously to EBV-DNA copies and spleen enlargement.

for the lymphocyte development that relies on double-strand break repair [14, 15] such as V(D)J recombination [16] and class switch recombination of immunoglobulin genes [17, 18].

In our child, as a result of infection with EBV, we observed both an increase in splenic volume and total IgM without, however, the rise of IgM antibodies specific for EBV (Figure 4). Low levels of total IgG and of specific postimmunization IgG antibodies document their defective synthesis in our child. The important reduction of the circulating viral DNA in the child as well as the healing of the previous exanthema subitum, sustained by HHV-6, in our patient demonstrates that the NK cell function is very effective and capable of containing the infections. The increased percentage of circulating NK cells may reflect their increased activity (Figure 3). Even the early onset AT patients referred to in the literature were associated with severe hypogammaglobulinemia and had been diagnosed with isolated severe hypogammaglobulinemia [4, 19]. The precocious introduction of i.v. IgG treatment has allowed our little girl to attend kindergarten without severe infections and to regularly follow the physiotherapeutic treatment. She is now able to speak in an understandable way and to communicate with other children and adults, as well as to walk and ride a tricycle. In fact, to date there is no codified and accepted treatment for neurological manifestations of AT [20], but there are many lines of evidence in other conditions associated with neurological suffering that early therapeutic intervention is able to create new synaptic network in the brain [21].

4. Conclusion

AT syndrome should be considered in children with precocious signs of cerebellar ataxia especially if associated with the evidence of defective immune function. A reflection on our case allows us to state that although the diagnostic hypothesis should always start from the clinical observation and the patient history, the possibility of a genetic investigation that is offered to us today is essential for therapeutic intervention to be ready, focused, and motivated.

References

[1] R. A. Gatti, S. Becker-Catania, H. H. Chun et al., "The pathogenesis of ataxia-telangiectasia: learning from a Rosetta stone," *Clinical Reviews in Allergy and Immunology*, vol. 20, no. 1, pp. 87–108, 2001.

[2] G. Rotman and Y. Shiloh, "ATM: from gene to function," *Human Molecular Genetics*, vol. 7, no. 10, pp. 1555–1563, 1998.

[3] H. H. Chun and R. A. Gatti, "Ataxia-telangiectasia, an evolving phenotype," *DNA Repair*, vol. 3, no. 8-9, pp. 1187–1196, 2004.

[4] E. R. Staples, E. M. McDermott, A. Reiman et al., "Immunodeficiency in ataxia telangiectasia is correlated strongly with the presence of two null mutations in the ataxia telangiectasia mutated gene," *Clinical and Experimental Immunology*, vol. 153, no. 2, pp. 214–220, 2008.

[5] P. J. McKinnon, "Ataxia-telangiectasia: an inherited disorder of ionizing-radiation sensitivity in man," *Human Genetics*, vol. 75, no. 3, pp. 197–208, 1987.

[6] A. M. Taylor, D. G. Harnden, C. F. Arlett et al., "Ataxia telangiectasia: a human mutation with abnormal radiation sensitivity," *Nature*, vol. 258, no. 5534, pp. 427–429, 1975.

[7] V. Leuzzi, R. Elli, A. Antonelli et al., "Neurological and cytogenetic study in early-onset ataxia-telangiectasia patients," *European Journal of Pediatrics*, vol. 152, no. 7, pp. 609–612, 1993.

[8] A. Nissenkorn, Y. Banet Levi, D. Vilozni et al., "Neurologic presentation in children with ataxia-telangiectasia: is small head circumference a hallmark of the disease?" *Journal of Pediatrics*, vol. 159, no. 3, pp. 466–471, 2011.

[9] S. Perreault, G. Bernard, A. Lortie, F. Le Deist, and H. Decaluwe, "Ataxia-telangiectasia presenting with a novel immunodeficiency," *Pediatric Neurology*, vol. 46, no. 5, pp. 322–324, 2012.

[10] M. Swift, D. Morrell, E. Cromartie, A. R. Chamberlin, M. H. Skolnick, and D. T. Bishop, "The incidence and gene frequency of Ataxia-telangiectasia in the United States," *American Journal of Human Genetics*, vol. 39, no. 5, pp. 573–583, 1986.

[11] S. M. Holland and J. A. Bellanti, "Immunodeficiency disorders," in *Immunology IV. Clinical Applications in Health and Disease*, J. A. Bellanti, Ed., pp. 429–457, I Care Press, Bethesda, Md, USA, 2012.

[12] L. D. Notarangelo, "Primary immunodeficiencies," *The Journal of Allergy and Clinical Immunology*, vol. 125, supplement 2, no. 2, pp. S182–S194, 2009.

[13] G. J. Driessen, H. Ijspeert, C. M. R. Weemaes et al., "Antibody deficiency in patient with ataxia teleangiectasia is caused by disturbed B- and T-cell homeostasis and reduced immune repertoire diversity," *The Journal of Allergy and Clinical Immunology*, vol. 131, no. 5, pp. 1367–1375, 2013.

[14] B.-B. S. Zhou and S. J. Elledge, "The DNA damage response: putting checkpoints in perspective," *Nature*, vol. 408, no. 6811, pp. 433–439, 2000.

[15] Y. Xu, "DNA damage: a trigger of innate immunity but a requirement for adaptive immune homeostasis," *Nature Reviews Immunology*, vol. 6, no. 4, pp. 261–270, 2006.

[16] A. L. Bredemeyer, G. G. Sharma, C.-Y. Huang et al., "ATM stabilizes DNA double-strand-break complexes during V(D)J recombination," *Nature*, vol. 442, no. 7101, pp. 466–470, 2006.

[17] B. Reina-San-Martin, H. T. Chen, A. Nussenzweig, and M. C. Nussenzweig, "ATM is required for efficient recombination between immunoglobulin switch regions," *Journal of Experimental Medicine*, vol. 200, no. 9, pp. 1103–1110, 2004.

[18] J. M. Lumsden, T. McCarty, L. K. Petiniot et al., "Immunoglobulin class switch recombination is impaired in Atm-deficient mice," *Journal of Experimental Medicine*, vol. 200, no. 9, pp. 1111–1121, 2004.

[19] A. Stray-Pedersen, I. S. Aaberge, A. Früh, and T. G. Abrahamsen, "Pneumococcal conjugate vaccine followed by pneumococcal polysaccharide vaccine; immunogenicity in patients with ataxia-telangiectasia," *Clinical and Experimental Immunology*, vol. 140, no. 3, pp. 507–516, 2005.

[20] S. Buoni, R. Zannolli, L. Sorrentino, and A. Fois, "Betamethasone and improvement of neurological symptoms in ataxia-telangiectasia," *Archives of Neurology*, vol. 63, no. 10, pp. 1479–1482, 2006.

[21] M. Hadders-Algra, "Early brain damage and the development of motor behavior in children: clues for therapeutic intervention?" *Neural Plasticity*, vol. 8, no. 1-2, pp. 31–49, 2001.

Lepra Reaction with Lucio Phenomenon Mimicking Cutaneous Vasculitis

Durga Prasanna Misra,[1] **Jyoti Ranjan Parida,**[1] **Abhra Chandra Chowdhury,**[1]
Krushna Chandra Pani,[2] **Niraj Kumari,**[2] **Narendra Krishnani,**[2] **and Vikas Agarwal**[1]

[1]*Department of Clinical Immunology, Sanjay Gandhi Postgraduate Institute of Medical Sciences, Lucknow 226014, India*
[2]*Department of Pathology, Sanjay Gandhi Postgraduate Institute of Medical Sciences, Lucknow 226014, India*

Correspondence should be addressed to Durga Prasanna Misra; durgapmisra@gmail.com

Academic Editor: Rajni Rani

Leprosy is a disease typically found in the tropics. Patients with leprosy can have varying presentation with constitutional symptoms, joint pains, skin nodules, and rarely a vasculitis-like picture with skin ulcers and neuropathy. We present a young lady who presented with the rare manifestation of skin infarcts mimicking cutaneous vasculitis, diagnosed on histopathology to have Lucio phenomenon on a background of lepromatous leprosy. With increasing migration and widespread use of biologic response modifiers, clinicians all over the world need to be aware of various presentations of leprosy as well as needing to keep an open mind while considering the differential diagnoses of vasculitis.

1. Introduction

Leprosy refers to systemic infection caused by *Mycobacterium leprae*, or less commonly *Mycobacterium lepromatosis*. Only the former has been reported from India. Although endemic to the tropics, it is increasingly being found in developed countries outside of the tropical regions [1, 2], predominantly due to activation of latent infection in the context of immunosuppression with biologic response modifiers. This serves as a reminder of the global importance of this problem at a time when boundaries are shrinking [3] and widespread use of biologics is becoming the norm rather than the exception in the treatment of many immune-mediated diseases, including ankylosing spondylitis and rheumatoid arthritis.

Patients with leprosy can present with symptoms varying from constitutional to arthralgias and arthritis, mononeuritis multiplex, or frank lepra reactions [4, 5]. These can mimic a wide variety of common conditions including rheumatoid arthritis, lupus, and vasculitis [6]. We present a young lady who presented with large cutaneous infarcts that on the first impression were vasculitic but were subsequently proven to be due to Lucio phenomenon in the context of lepromatous leprosy.

2. Case Presentation

A 20-year-old lady presented with history of multiple nodular skin lesions, which were erythematous and were associated with stinging pain, 1-2 cm in size over both the upper and lower limbs and face for the past 1 year. This was associated with a low grade fever, on and off, responsive to antipyretic agents, for the same duration. She had history of pain in both knees at the onset of illness, for a period of 3 months, not associated with swelling, early morning stiffness, or pain in other joints, which was worse during the times she had fever. She had no dryness of eyes or mouth, tingling or numbness of extremities, shortness of breath, cough, chest pain, nasal or ear discharge, epistaxis, hearing loss, abdominal pain, weight loss, diarrhea, or dysuria. She had no foot drop or redness of eyes. She was investigated and found to have anemia (hemoglobin (Hb) 9.9 g%), normal total leucocyte count ((TLC) 6200/mm^3), differential leucocyte count ((DLC) neutrophils 50%, lymphocytes 46%) and platelet count ((Plt), 261000/mm^3), elevated erythrocyte sedimentation rate ((ESR), 36 mm/hour), and positive rheumatoid factor (RF) in serum by ELISA (26.11 IU, reference 0–15 IU). With this, she was thought to have rheumatoid arthritis

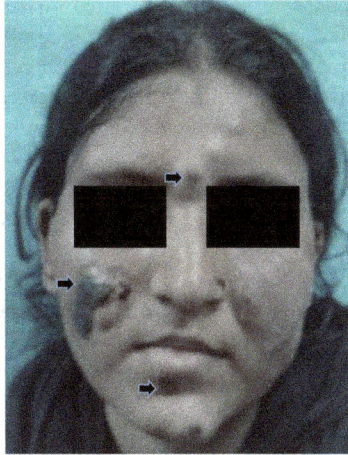

FIGURE 1: Image of face showing papulonodular lesions over the left cheek and necrotic skin infarct with irregular borders over the right cheek, chin, and forehead (black arrows).

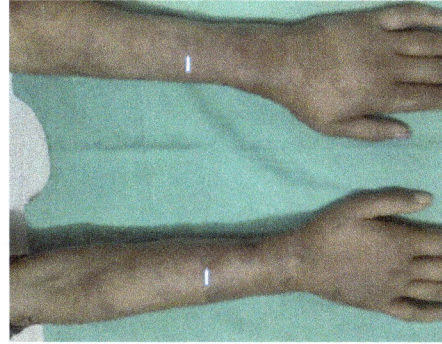

FIGURE 2: Picture of forearms and hands showing papulonodular infiltrating erythematous lesions over the forearms and dorsum of hands (white arrows).

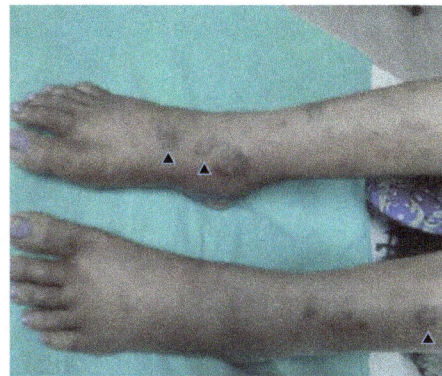

FIGURE 3: Picture of legs showing papules and nodules on dorsum of legs, necrotic lesions with irregular borders over lower leg and feet, and dorsal tenosynovitis of both feet (black arrowheads).

and started on methotrexate 5 mg/week, hydroxychloroquine sulfate 200 mg daily, and methylprednisolone 4 mg daily. Subsequently, the skin lesion, fever, and joint pains subsided.

Three months later, while on the above-mentioned medications, the fever and skin lesions recurred and were of a similar nature and distribution as before. She now consulted a dermatologist who investigated and detected a persisting anemia (Hb 10.4 g%), mild leukocytosis (TLC 11230/mm^3, DLC showing neutrophils 69%, lymphocytes 23%), normal platelet count (295000/mm^3), and ESR elevation of 99 mm/hr. On the basis of her symptoms, she was diagnosed to have type II lepra reaction (erythema nodosum leprosum (ENL)) and started on prednisolone 60 mg/day and antileprotic therapy with rifampicin 600 mg/month, clofazimine 300 mg/month and 50 mg/day, dapsone 100 mg/day, and ofloxacin. There was a transient relief of symptoms, but these again recurred. As a consequence she visited multiple physicians over the next 4 months without avail, while continuing the same antileprotic drugs.

A week prior to presenting to us, she developed additional similar skin lesions over the trunk, along with blackish discolouration over the skin lesions on the face, legs, and dorsum of feet. 2 days prior to presentation, she developed pain and swelling of dorsa of both feet and ankles. Review of her past history and family history were insignificant for any diagnoses of leprosy.

Examination revealed a temperature of 98°F, pulse rate of 98/minute with symmetry of all peripheral pulses, and blood pressure of 110/80 mm Hg in the right upper limb. There was mild pallor. She had multiple elevated plaque to nodule-like tender rashes, 1–3 cm in diameter, over arms, trunk, and upper and lower limbs (Figures 1, 2, and 3). The rashes over the face and both legs were necrotic, with black discolouration of the surface but no discharge or ulceration. She had bilateral axillary lymph nodes in the central group, 1 × 1 cm in size, discrete, nontender, and freely mobile. Musculoskeletal exam revealed extensor tenosynovitis over both feet (Figure 3); neurologic exam revealed thickening of both common peroneal and right ulnar nerves; however

there was no tenderness or sensory impairment. There was an anaesthetic patch of 7 cm × 6 cm size with loss of sweating and appendages over the back. Systemic examination was otherwise unremarkable. Investigations revealed Hb 12.6 g%, microcytic and normochromic, TLC 16300/mm^3, DLC showing neutrophils 80%, lymphocytes 15%, platelet count 463000/mm^3, serum creatinine 0.8 mg%, serum alanine aminotransferase 28 U/L, serum bilirubin 0.7 mg%, serum lactate dehydrogenase mildly elevated (471 mg%, normal less than 450), and normal serum creatinine (0.8 mg%). Chest radiograph and urine examination were normal.

Such a clinical picture was consistent with Lucio phenomenon; however it was unusual for the same to occur so many months after starting antileprotic therapy. Also the cutaneous infarcts had occurred in spite of being on high dose steroids and antileprotic therapy for the past 4 months. There was no histologic evidence of leprosy until now, and medicines had been started based on a clinical diagnosis. So other differential diagnoses were considered, namely, cutaneous polyarteritis nodosa (fever, skin nodules, and skin infarcts with elevated ESR, neutrophilic leukocytosis, and thrombocytosis), cutaneous T-cell lymphoma (fever, subacute onset of skin rash, and poor response to steroids) and lupus profundus (fever with tender nodular skin rash affecting trunk and face; odd was skin infarcts).

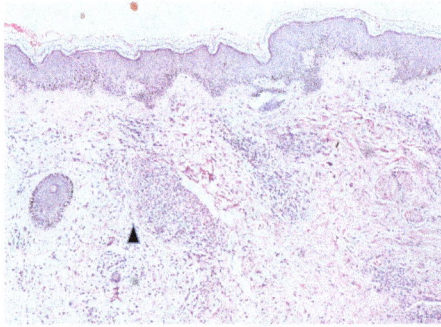

FIGURE 4: Skin biopsy from leg (hematoxylin and eosin stain, 20X magnification) showing largely unremarkable epidermis. Dermis shows collection of foamy histiocytes (black arrowhead).

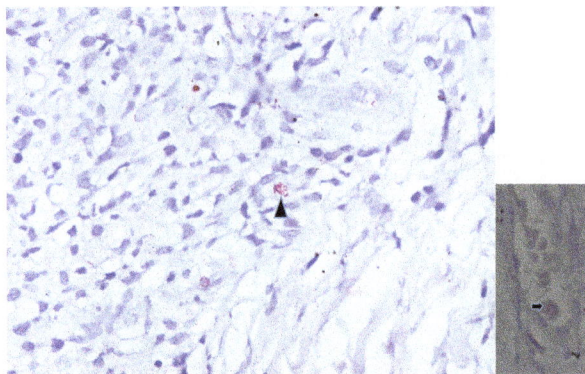

FIGURE 5: Magnified view of dermis showing foam cells with collection of lepra bacilli (globi) (black arrowhead) (Wade-Fite stain, 100X magnification); inset shows infiltration of capillary wall with lepra bacilli (black arrow) suggestive of Lucio phenomenon.

A skin biopsy was done to facilitate differential diagnosis. It showed unremarkable epidermis, foam cells with numerous lepra bacilli in dermis, and dermal capillaries showing vasculitis with neutrophilic infiltrate and damage to capillary wall with invading lepra bacilli (on Wade-Fite stain) (Figures 4 and 5), consistent with lepromatous leprosy with Lucio phenomenon. She was continued on prednisolone at 45 mg/day, with planned taper after 6 weeks, and rifampicin, clofazimine, and dapsone at the doses she was previously on (planned to be given for 24 months as per World Health Organisation recommendation for treating multibacillary leprosy). In addition, thalidomide was added at a dose of 100 mg daily to help with the lepra reaction. On OPD follow-up after 5 months, she was on prednisolone 10 mg/5 mg alternate day and continuing thalidomide 100 mg/day with antileprotic therapy as before. Her skin lesions and skin infarcts had healed and tenosynovitis and fever had resolved. ESR had normalized (13 mm/hour).

3. Discussion

Immunologic reactions in the context of leprosy can be of two types. Type I lepra reaction occurs on a background of tuberculoid leprosy, where cell-mediated immunity is robust, and is characterized by inflammation occurring inside existing skin lesions as well as appearance of new nodules and skin infiltrates. Type II lepra reaction, called ENL, occurs in lepromatous or borderline spectra, where cell-mediated immunity is weak and bacillary load is usually high. A rare form of lepra reaction is Lucio phenomenon, which manifests as tender nodules with ulceration, bulla formation, and necrotic areas [7–11]. Our patient had lepromatous leprosy with Lucio phenomenon.

What was odd in our patient for Lucio phenomenon was the onset of skin infarcts 4 months after starting antileprotic therapy. Lucio phenomenon is usually the presenting feature that heralds a diagnosis of leprosy [8, 12]. Also, the presence of cutaneous infarcts in the absence of blistering or ulcerating lesions is distinctly unusual for Lucio phenomenon (Magaña et al. reported a similar finding in only 3 out of 12 patients with Lucio phenomenon) [8]. Hence we considered differential diagnoses of cutaneous vasculitis or necrotising erythema nodosum. The skin biopsy was conclusively in favour of Lucio phenomenon occurring on a background of lepromatous leprosy and helped guide subsequent appropriate therapy, namely, continuing antileprotic therapy and prednisolone as well as addition of stronger immunosuppression with thalidomide. Our patient made a good recovery with this regimen.

Leprosy mimicking vasculitis has been rarely reported [9, 13–15]. Often the picture is complicated by the presence of autoantibodies as rheumatoid factor, antinuclear antibodies, and antineutrophil cytoplasmic antibodies. The pathology in Lucio phenomenon shows foam cells with lepra bacilli demonstrable inside them, as well as a cutaneous vasculitis involving medium and small-sized vessels [11]. Lucio phenomenon per se is common in Mexico and has only been rarely reported from India [16–20].

It is important for the clinician to differentiate leprosy from other presentations of cutaneous vasculitis, as the former is eminently curable with antibiotics and prudent use of immunosuppressive agents. A general principle is to always keep infectious etiologies in the differential diagnosis of vasculitis, as the treatment for the two is dramatically different and inappropriate immunosuppression alone can be disastrous in the context of infection. Leprosy is gaining attention as a global health problem due to reactivation of latent, previously undiagnosed cases even in the western world due to use of strong immunosuppressive regimens for a variety of diseases [1, 2]. When in doubt, a skin biopsy often helps to get the final diagnosis.

Conflict of Interests

The authors declare that there is no conflict of interests regarding the publication of this paper.

References

[1] D. M. Scollard, M. P. Joyce, and T. P. Gillis, "Development of leprosy and type 1 leprosy reactions after treatment with infliximab: a report of 2 cases," Clinical Infectious Diseases, vol. 43, no. 2, pp. e19–e22, 2006.

[2] E. M. Oberstein, O. Kromo, and E. C. Tozman, "Type I reaction of Hansen's disease with exposure to adalimumab: a case report," *Arthritis Care & Research*, vol. 59, no. 7, pp. 1040–1043, 2008.

[3] A. Soni, R. Manhas, L. John, L. Whittam, and L. Williamson, "Tropical rheumatology in a UK district general hospital: a case report of leprosy presenting as acute vasculitis," *Rheumatology*, vol. 49, no. 4, pp. 826–828, 2010.

[4] S. Chauhan, A. Wakhlu, and V. Agarwal, "Arthritis in leprosy," *Rheumatology*, vol. 49, no. 12, pp. 2237–2242, 2010.

[5] S. Prasad, R. Misra, A. Aggarwal et al., "Leprosy revealed in a rheumatology clinic: a case series," *International Journal of Rheumatic Diseases*, vol. 16, no. 2, pp. 129–133, 2013.

[6] S. Salvi and A. Chopra, "Leprosy in a rheumatology setting: a challenging mimic to expose," *Clinical Rheumatology*, vol. 32, no. 10, pp. 1557–1563, 2013.

[7] J. P. Bernadat, J. F. Faucher, and M. Huerre, "Diffuse lepromatous leprosy disclosed by cutaneous vasculitis. The Lucio phenomenon," *Annales de Dermatologie et de Vénéréologie*, vol. 123, no. 1, pp. 21–23, 1996.

[8] M. Magaña, J. Fernández-Díez, and M. L. Magaña, "Lucio's phenomenon is a necrotizing panvasculitis: mostly a medium-sized granulomatous arteritis," *The American Journal of Dermatopathology*, vol. 30, no. 6, pp. 555–560, 2008.

[9] L. S. Guedes-Barbosa, E. V. Batista, D. C. Martins, L. Neder, N. Crepaldi, and E. V. Martins, "Necrotizing cutaneous vasculitis in multibacillary leprosy disease (lucio's phenomenon)," *Journal of Clinical Rheumatology*, vol. 14, no. 1, pp. 57–59, 2008.

[10] S. Sarita, K. Muhammed, R. Najeeba et al., "A study on histological features of lepra reactions in patients attending the Dermatology Department of the Government Medical College, Calicut, Kerala, India," *Leprosy Review*, vol. 84, no. 1, pp. 51–64, 2013.

[11] P. F. Curi, J. S. Villaroel, N. Migliore et al., "Lucio's phenomenon: report of five cases," *Clinical Rheumatology*, 2014.

[12] L. Fogagnolo, E. M. de Souza, M. L. Cintra, and P. E. N. F. Velho, "Vasculonecrotic reactions in leprosy," *The Brazilian Journal of Infectious Diseases*, vol. 11, no. 3, pp. 378–382, 2007.

[13] S. Chauhan, S. D'Cruz, H. Mohan, R. Singh, J. Ram, and A. Sachdev, "Type II lepra reaction: an unusual presentation," *Dermatology Online Journal*, vol. 12, no. 1, article 18, 2006.

[14] L. Sampaio, L. Silva, G. Terroso et al., "Hansen' s disease mimicking a systemic vasculitis," *Acta Reumatologica Portuguesa*, vol. 36, no. 1, pp. 61–64, 2011.

[15] T. Camps-García, I. P.-D. Pedro, I. M. Gómez, D. Narankiewicz, M. Ayala-Gutierrez, and A. Sanz-Trelles, "Clinical images: cutaneous necrotizing vasculitis in a patient with lepromatous leprosy," *Arthritis and Rheumatism*, vol. 63, no. 11, article 3639, 2011.

[16] V. Saoji and A. Salodkar, "Lucio leprosy with lucio phenomenon," *Indian Journal of Leprosy*, vol. 73, no. 3, pp. 267–272, 2001.

[17] C. Kaur, G. P. Thami, and H. Mohan, "Lucio phenomenon and Lucio leprosy," *Clinical and Experimental Dermatology*, vol. 30, no. 5, pp. 525–527, 2005.

[18] R. Kumari, D. M. Thappa, and D. Basu, "A fatal case of Lucio phenomenon from India," *Dermatology Online Journal*, vol. 14, no. 2, article 10, 2008.

[19] P. S. S. Ranugha, L. Chandrashekar, R. Kumari, D. M. Thappa, and B. Badhe, "Is it lucio phenomenon or necrotic erythema nodosum leprosum?" *Indian Journal of Dermatology*, vol. 58, no. 2, article 160, 2013.

[20] V. V. Pai, S. Athanikar, K. N. Naveen, T. Sori, and R. Rao, "Lucio phenomenon," *Cutis*, vol. 93, no. 2, pp. E12–E14, 2014.

10

Effective Treatment of Rheumatoid Arthritis-Associated Interstitial Lung Disease by B-Cell Targeted Therapy with Rituximab

Wolfgang Hartung,[1] Judith Maier,[2] Michael Pfeifer,[3] and Martin Fleck[1,2]

[1] Department of Rheumatology and Clinical Immunology, Asklepios Clinic, 93077 Bad Abbach, Germany
[2] Department of Internal Medicine I, University of Regensburg, 93042 Regensburg, Germany
[3] Department of Pulmonology and Internal Medicine II, University of Regensburg, 93042 Regensburg, Germany

Correspondence should be addressed to Wolfgang Hartung, w.hartung@asklepios.com

Academic Editors: N. Kutukculer, T. Manigold, and A. Plebani

Rheumatoid arthritis- (RA-) associated interstitial lung disease (RA-ILD) is the extra-articular complication with most adverse impact on the quality of life and survival in RA patients. However, treatment options are limited and controlled studies are lacking. Here, we present the case of a 66-year-old patient suffering from severe RA-ILD, which has been successfully treated with Rituximab (RTX). After failure of conventional DMARD therapy, our patient showed sustained improvement of clinical pulmonary parameters as well as joint inflammation following B-cell depletion with RTX. The six-minute-walk test improved from 380 meters to 536 meters and the forced vital capacity from 2.49 liters to 3.49. The disease activity score could be reduced from 7.7 to 2.8. Therefore, RTX might be considered as an alternative treatment for RA-ILD in patients not responding to conventional DMARD therapy.

Rheumatoid arthritis-associated interstitial lung disease (RA-ILD) is RA's extra-articular complication with most adverse impact on quality of life and survival. However, treatment options are limited and controlled studies are lacking. We report a 66-year-old man suffering from severe RA-ILD. Treatment with methotrexate as well as cyclophosophamide failed to improve the respiratory function. Surprisingly, we noticed a fast and sustained improvement with rituximab. Thus we consider rituximab as an alternative treatment strategy for DMARD-resistant RA-ILD.

A now 66-year-old Caucasian was diagnosed with idiopathic pulmonary fibrosis (IPF) due to persistent dry coughing and dyspnea concomitant with impaired functional capacity of the lung and typical radiographic findings two years ago. A few months later, the initial respiratory symptoms were followed by polysynovitis associated with high systemic inflammatory activity. With regard to the clinical symptoms and presence of high titers of rheumatoid factor (Rf) as well as anticyclic citrullinated peptide (CCP) antibodies, the diagnosis of RA was established. Consequently,

treatment with NSAIDs, prednisolone and a course of leflunomide for half a year has been initiated in a community hospital without substantial improvement. Therefore, the patient presented to our outpatient clinic with persistent polysynovitis and severe systemic inflammatory response (DAS28: 7.47; CRP: 77 mg/L).

In light of the previous findings in combination with HRCT (Figure 1) we diagnosed RA-ILD. To obtain histological confirmation, transbronchial lung biopsy was performed, which revealed unspecific fibrotic changes. Since the patient rejected open lung biopsy, we could not specify the histopathologic patterns. MTX (15 mg/week) and prednisolone treatment (30 mg per day) were initiated. We choose MTX because at that time that patient mainly suffered from joint symptoms but presented only marginally impaired lung function. However, the patient subsequently developed pulmonary infection with rapid improvement with antibiotic therapy despite lacking device of an infectious agent. Since we could not exclude MTX-mediated worsening of the lung disease, MTX was terminated after only three

TABLE 1: Development of laboratory and clinical parameters in response to different immunosupressive agents.

Parameter	Treatment		
	MTX + prednisolone (baseline)	Cyclophophamide + prednisolone (week 18)	Rituximab + MTX + prednisolone (week 59)
6MWT (% of debit)	380 m (63.60%)	436 m (79.39%)	536 m (90.44%)
FVC (% of debit)	2.49 L (56.8%)	3.36 L (76%)	3.49 L (87%)
BGA			
pO_2	53 mmHg	62 mmHg	63 mmHg
pCO_2	35 mmHg	38 mmHg	36 mmHg
DAS 28	7.47	7.7	2.8
CRP	131 mg/L	72 mg/L	1.7 mg/L
Ultrasound synovitis Score (PIP II–V)	10	7	4

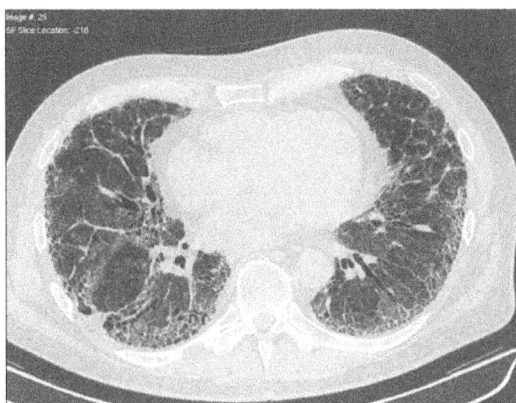

FIGURE 1: HR-CT-scan of the thorax revealed pronounced signs of pulmonary fibrosis including consolidations and honeycombing especially in basal areas.

applications. With steroids as the remaining therapy, disease deteriorated rapidly with polysynovitis and high levels of systemic inflammation (CRP 120 mg/L), and therefore multiple intra-articular steroid injections were performed. At that time, pulmonary involvement had progressed to a partial respiratory insufficiency with the requirement of home oxygen supplementation. Arterial blood gas analysis (BGA) revealed a pO_2 of 53 mmHg, a pCO_2 of 35 mmHg, and O_2-saturation of 88%. Distance in the 6-minute walk test (6MWT) as a specific measurement for the functional pulmonary capacity was significantly reduced to 380 m (normal values for untrained man: 600–700 m). In addition, the forced vital capacity (FVC) of the lung was reduced to 2.49 L. Despite the lack of evidence in RA-ILD, we decided to install cyclophosphamide (CYC) in combination with high dose prednisolone, which has been suggested as a treatment option in patients suffering from idiopathic pulmonary fibrosis as well as patients with scleroderma-associated lung disease.

However, after three courses of CYC the patient presented with persistently high disease activity (DAS28: 7.7; CRP 72 mg/L), and the respiratory situation had only been slightly improved (Table 1). At this point, we combined CYC with

rituximab (RTX). Within the next 12 weeks, profound improvement of joint manifestations in combination with stable pulmonary function could be observed (DAS28: 4.5; CRP 39 mg/L), so that we were able to reduce the prednisolone dose to 7.5 mg daily. Due to this improvement, the patient stopped CYC therapy after a total of 6 infusions by himself and also rejected other DMARD therapy. Eight weeks following reduction of prednisolone to 5 mg per day, RA exacerbated again, and the patient was again admitted to our outpatient clinic with polysynovitis (DAS28: 6.3; CRP 65 mg/L). Immunophenotyping revealed complete peripheral B cell reconstitution, and therefore prednisolone was increased up to 20 mg per day, and a combination therapy of MTX (10 mg/week) and RTX (2 × 1000 mg within 2 weeks) was started. Again, successful depletion of peripheral B-cells could be confirmed by FACS-analysis, and RA disease activity declined within the next 16 weeks (DAS28: 2.8; CRP 1.7 mg/L). Most surprisingly, the pulmonary situation improved dramatically as demonstrated at a follow-up visit 12 weeks after the second RTX course by normal values for the BGA with a pO_2 of 63 mmHg and a pCO_2 of 36 mmHg. This striking recovery could be confirmed by an almost normal value for the 6MWT of 563 m. In addition, lung function testing showed a stabilization of the FVC at 3.49 L. Furthermore, the patient's quality of life had significantly improved since home oxygen supplementation could be discontinued (Table 1).

Pulmonary involvement in RA is directly responsible for 10–20% of all mortality [1–4]. Despite this adverse impact solid treatment recommendations for RA-ILD are still lacking. In contrast, drug-induced worsening of pulmonary function in RA patients is well known [5, 6]. Combined CYC and steroid therapy does not substantially improve survival in IPF patients [7]. RA-ILD has similar features with regard to histopathology as well as gene expression profile, but the clinical course seems to be milder. However, in our case we could not definitively exclude a response to treatment with CYC alone but the lack of significant improvement of 6MWT under CYC makes this unlikely.

RTX is known to be an effective therapeutic instrument in joint diseases. Here, we present a remarkable response of RA-ILD to RTX. With regard to the histopathologic finding of peribronchial infiltration with B-lymphocytes in RA-ILD, we propose that B cells are critically involved in the pathogenesis of RA-ILD. We therefore regard RTX as an alternative treatment for RA-ILD in patients with primary failure of conventional DMARD therapy. Nevertheless, further studies are warranted to substantiate our observation, and to enlarge our therapeutic armamentarium for this severe disorder.

References

[1] M. Hakala, "Poor prognosis in patients with rheumatoid arthritis hospitalized for interstitial lung fibrosis," *Chest*, vol. 93, no. 1, pp. 114–118, 1988.

[2] N. J. Minaur, R. K. Jacoby, J. A. Cosh, G. Taylor, and J. J. Rasker, "Outcome after 40 years with rheumatoid arthritis: a prospective study of function, disease activity, and mortality," *Journal of Rheumatology*, vol. 31, no. 69, pp. 3–8, 2004.

[3] S. Sihvonen, M. Korpela, P. Laippala, J. Mustonen, and A. Pasternack, "Death rates and causes of death in patients with rheumatoid arthritis: a population-based study," *Scandinavian Journal of Rheumatology*, vol. 33, no. 4, pp. 221–227, 2004.

[4] A. Suzuki, Y. Ohosone, M. Obana et al., "Cause of death in 81 autopsied patients with rheumatoid arthritis," *Journal of Rheumatology*, vol. 21, no. 1, pp. 33–36, 1994.

[5] O. Lateef, N. Shakoor, and R. A. Balk, "Methotrexate pulmonary toxicity," *Expert Opinion on Drug Safety*, vol. 4, no. 4, pp. 723–730, 2005.

[6] J. K. Dawson, D. R. Graham, J. Desmond, H. E. Fewins, and M. P. Lynch, "Investigation of the chronic pulmonary effects of low-dose oral methotrexate in patients with rheumatoid arthritis: a prospective study incorporating HRCT scanning and pulmonary function tests," *Rheumatology*, vol. 41, no. 3, pp. 262–267, 2002.

[7] H. R. Collard, J. H. Ryu, W. W. Douglas et al., "Combined corticosteroid and cyclophosphamide therapy does not alter survival in idiopathic pulmonary fibrosis," *Chest*, vol. 125, no. 6, pp. 2169–2174, 2004.

11

CVID Associated with Systemic Amyloidosis

Saliha Esenboga,[1] **Deniz Çagdas Ayvaz,**[1] **Arzu Saglam Ayhan,**[2] **Banu Peynircioglu,**[3]
Ozden Sanal,[1] **and Ilhan Tezcan**[1]

[1]*Division of Immunology, Department of Pediatrics, Hacettepe University Faculty of Medicine, 06100 Ankara, Turkey*
[2]*Department of Pathology, Hacettepe University Faculty of Medicine, 06100 Ankara, Turkey*
[3]*Department of Medical Biology and Genetics, Hacettepe University Faculty of Medicine, 06100 Ankara, Turkey*

Correspondence should be addressed to Saliha Esenboga; salihaeren@yahoo.com

Academic Editor: Vassilios Lougaris

Common variable immunodeficiency (CVID) is a frequent primary immune deficiency (PID), which consists of a heterogeneous group of disorders and can present with recurrent infections, chronic diarrhea, autoimmunity, chronic pulmonary and gastrointestinal diseases, and malignancy. Secondary amyloidosis is an uncommon complication of CVID. We report an unusual case of a 27-year-old male patient who presented with recurrent sinopulmonary infections, chronic diarrhea, and hypogammaglobulinemia and was diagnosed with CVID. The patient was treated with intravenous immunoglobulin (IVIg) therapy once every 21 days and daily trimethoprim-sulfamethoxazole for prophylaxis. Two years after initial diagnosis, the patient was found to have progressive decline in IgG levels (as low as 200–300 mg/dL) despite regular Ig infusions. The laboratory tests revealed massive proteinuria and his kidney biopsy showed accumulation of AA type amyloid. We believe that the delay in the diagnosis of CVID and initiation of Ig replacement therapy caused chronic inflammation due to recurrent infections in our patient and this led to an uncommon and life-threatening complication, amyloidosis. Patients with CVID require regular follow-up for the control of infections and assessment of adequacy of Ig replacement therapy. Amyloidosis should be kept in the differential diagnosis when managing patients with CVID.

1. Introduction

Common variable immunodeficiency (CVID) is a frequent primary immune deficiency (PID) which consists of a heterogeneous group of disorders. It is more frequently seen in adults and characterized by impaired B cell differentiation resulting in hypogammaglobulinemia, normal or low numbers of B cells, and poor antibody response [1]. As the "variable" term implies, its clinical manifestation is heterogenous and includes recurrent infections, chronic pulmonary and gastrointestinal diseases, and chronic diarrhea as well as autoimmunity and increased susceptibility to malignancy [2].

Secondary amyloidosis, mostly reported in middle-aged men, is an uncommon complication of CVID [2]. Chronic and recurrent infections in patients with CVID may lead to extracellular deposition of serum amyloid A (SAA) protein fibrils [3]. Infectious diseases, bronchiectasis, cor pulmonale, respiratory distress, or tuberculosis, are the predisposing conditions for the development of amyloidosis in patients with CVID [4, 5]. Delay in the diagnosis of CVID or initiation of immunoglobulin replacement therapy or administration of insufficient doses of IVIg may contribute to the development of amyloidosis secondary to poor infection control [5].

In this paper, we describe an unusual case of a man with CVID who developed renal amyloidosis during his follow-up under IVIg replacement therapy.

2. Case Report

A 27-year-old male patient was referred to the division of Pediatric Immunology at Hacettepe University for further evaluation of recurrent sinopulmonary infections, chronic diarrhea, and hypogammaglobulinemia. He had been followed up with the diagnosis of bronchiectasis (Figure 1) since the age of 7 years and undergone two separate pulmonary lobectomy surgeries at the ages of 15 and 18 years. On presentation, his chief complaints were diarrhea for

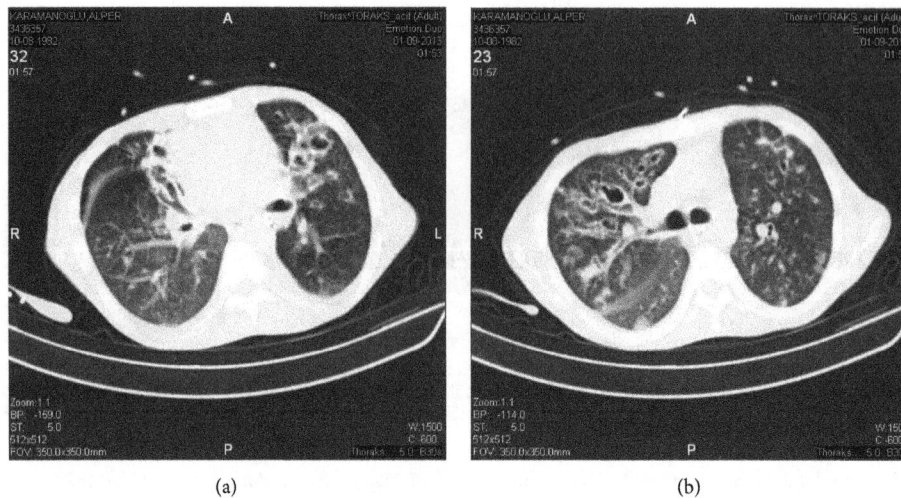

(a)

(b)

FIGURE 1: Thoracal CT of the patient shows bilateral bronchiectatic segments.

9 months and loss of weight (~10 Kg) within the past 6 months. The microbiological evaluation of stool was negative for a bacteria, parasite, or *Cryptosporidium*. He had been evaluated by a colonoscopy at outside hospital and this was reportedly normal. His physical examination revealed normal vital signs, body mass index of 14 (weight: 43 Kg, height: 175 cm), clubbing in both hands and feet, right sided rales on lung auscultation, perforated nasal septum and left tympanic membrane, and diffuse erythematous, squamous plaques on the trunk, hands, and behind the ears, compatible with psoriasis. The family history revealed consanguinity.

Laboratory tests on admission showed hypogammaglobulinemia (IgG, 290 mg/dL [n: 913–1884]; IgA, 75 mg/dL [n: 139–378]; IgM, 314 mg/dL [n: 88–322]; total IgE, 1.93 mg/dL), anemia, and elevated erythrocyte sedimentation rate (65 mm/hr [n: 0–20]), and CRP level (16.25 mg/dL [n: 0–0.8]). There was no lymphopenia (ALC: 2600) or neutropenia (ANC: 8500) in the complete blood count. Total protein and serum albumin were normal (6.5 and 4.3 g/dL, resp.). Urine analysis was negative for proteinuria. Flow cytometry of peripheral blood revealed CD3 of 90%, CD4 of 19%, CD8 of 60%, CD16 + 56 of 7%, CD19 of 0%, and CD20 of 0%. In order to rule out X-linked agammaglobulinemia, Bruton tyrosine kinase (BTK) mutation was tested and found to be negative. Pneumococcal antibody response was absent. The clinical findings and laboratory workup did not let us to classify as CVID or combined immunodeficiency (the molecular analysis did not result yet). He was evaluated under the CVID umbrella and was treated with intravenous immunoglobulin therapy (IVIg) with the dose of 400 mg/kg once every 21 days for hypogammaglobulinemia and daily trimethoprim-sulfamethoxazole prophylactically for CD4 + T cell lymphopenia (absolute count: 392/mm³). The patient initially responded to the treatment well with cessation of pneumonia episodes and requirement for hospitalizations. He gained 10 Kg during the first year of follow-up (from 43 to 53 Kg). Two years later, at the age of 29 years, his IgG levels started declining progressively to levels around 200–300 mg/dL despite regular IVIg infusions. His serum albumin

level decreased to 3.2 g/dL (n: 3.4–4.8) and he was found to have massive proteinuria with 1726.4 mg/day protein loss on a 24-hour urine collection. Urinary ultrasonography demonstrated increased echogenicity of renal parenchyma (grade 1). Rectal and gingival biopsies were performed with the suspicion of amyloidosis; however, this was negative. A renal biopsy was performed and pathology analysis revealed focal segmental accumulation of AA type amyloidosis in glomeruli and focal accumulation in the interstitium and vessel walls accompanied by tubular atrophy and increased mononuclear cells in the interstitium (Figure 2). Serum amyloid A (SAA) protein level was 330 mg/L (n: 0–10). Familial mediterranean fever was excluded with the absence of MEFV mutation. The patient was started on angiotensin receptor blocker and colchicine, since some previous reports showed decrease in proteinuria with colchicine treatment in patients with isolated renal amyloidosis [6, 7]. Three months/years later, the patient presented to our hospital with pneumonia leading to acute hypoxemic respiratory failure. He was treated with broad spectrum IV antibiotics, intubated and mechanically ventilated. Because of severe protein loss secondary to amyloidosis, his IVIg replacement dose was increased to 200 mg/kg twice monthly. His serum albumin levels progressively decreased to 1.3 g/dL despite all the aggressive measures and albumin infusions. The patient expired from sepsis and ARDS at the age of 33 years.

3. Discussion

SAA are acute phase proteins in the form of apolipoproteins associated with specific high-density lipoprotein (HDL), and they are expressed extrahepatically in the absence of HDL. Several cytokines (mainly IL-1, IL-6, and TNF), lipopolysaccharides, and transcription factors can induce SAA deposition [8]. During acute phase response, SAA increases the affinity of HDL for macrophages and adipocytes, binds to the extracellular matrix, shows chemoattractant activity for monocytes and lymphocytes, and stimulates the release of proinflammatory cytokines [9].

(a)

(b)

(c)

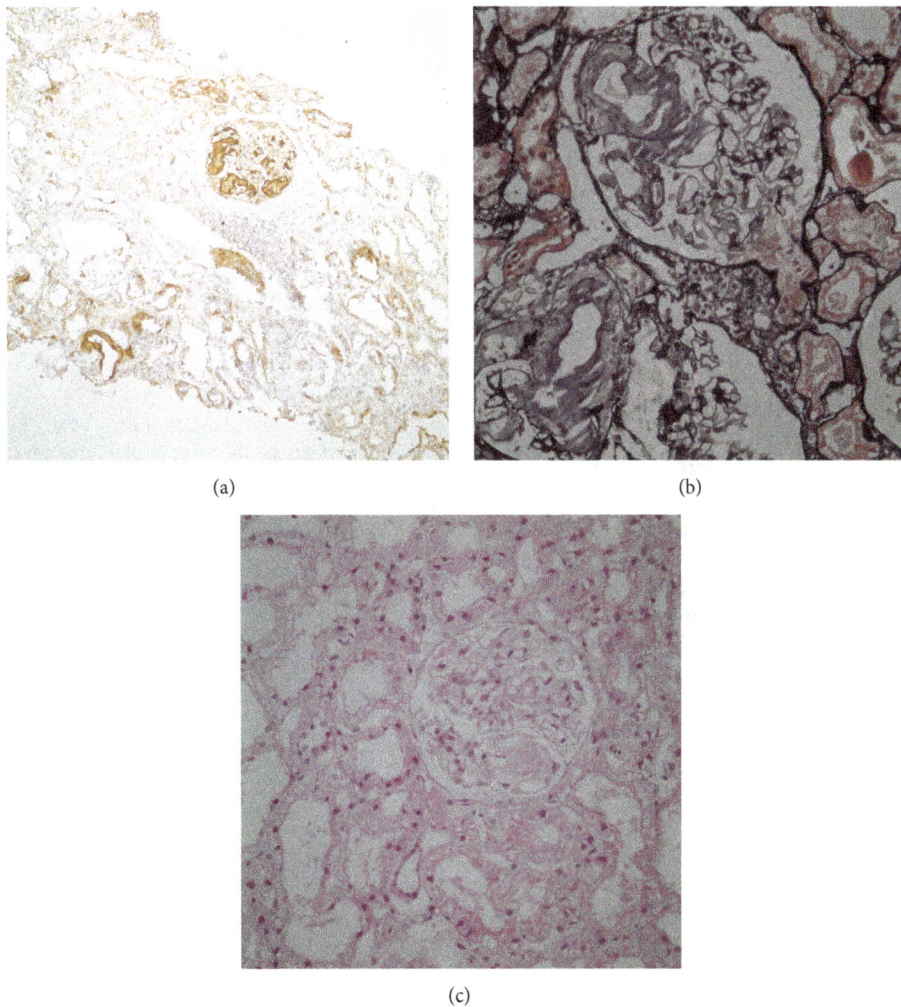

FIGURE 2: Immunohistochemical reactivity of deposited material with anti-amyloid A protein, note staining of glomeruli and vascular walls (a). Negative staining of deposited material (consistent with amyloid) silver stain (b). Focal mesangial widening due to deposition of amorphous acellular eosinophilic material consistent with amyloid. Note deposition of amyloid along the hilar arterioles (c).

AA amyloidosis is well known to be a complication of chronic or recurrent inflammatory states seen with rheumatoid arthritis, inflammatory bowel disease, chronic infections, or periodic fever syndromes [9, 10]. The clinical important major sites for amyloid deposition are the kidneys, heart, gut, and liver. Renal involvement of amyloidosis may present with a range from symptomatic proteinuria to clinically apparent nephrotic syndrome [9]. If a patient's history and clinical manifestations raise suspicion for amyloidosis, a tissue biopsy should be performed in order to confirm the diagnosis. In case of a single organ involvement, tissue biopsy should be taken from the involved site. A fat pad aspiration biopsy is suggested as the initial biopsy technique for patients with more extensive involvement [11]. In our patient, renal biopsy was positive despite rectal and gingival biopsies negative for SAA deposition because the kidneys were the primarily affected organs. Increased SAA production and deposition in patients with CVID are most likely triggered by a defect in the control of inflammation in patients with CVID. Renal and/or intestinal loss of immunoglobulins due to involvement of

these organs with amyloidosis leads to further worsening of hypogammaglobulinemia and subsequently increased frequency of infections despite IVIg replacement [12]. At the late course of the disease, our patient suffered from recurrent pulmonary infections and died from ARDS which can raise the suspicion for pulmonary amyloidosis which was reported in the literature before [13]. However, no tissue biopsy was performed to rule in or exclude this diagnosis in our patient.

Our patient had had several clinical features consistent with CVID since the age of 7 years. However, he was officially diagnosed with this disease at the age of 27 years. We believe that the years-long chronic and recurrent infections due to prolonged delay (~20 years) in the diagnosis and appropriate treatment of CVID led to renal amyloidosis and unfortunately subsequent mortality in our patient. Although the time course is still not well known, it is estimated that development of clinical amyloidosis may last for 8 to 14 years which is shorter than the untreated course in our patient [14]. Early diagnosis of primary immunodeficiency has prime importance in patients with recurrent symptoms.

Ig replacement therapy is the mainstay of the management of PIDs and it should be started at appropriate doses and intervals as soon as possible after the diagnosis in order to prevent chronic inflammation and its complications. Patients should be kept under regular control by monitoring serum IgG levels and replacement with adequate Ig doses and prophylactic antibiotherapy to prevent infections. The possibility of amyloidosis should be suspected when the IgG levels cannot be maintained above 500 mg/dL.

Although Ig replacement therapy is generally started with the doses of 400 to 600 mg/kg every 21 or 30 days, for patients with bronchiectasis or chronic sinusitis, the dose can be as high as 600 to 800 mg/kg every 21 days as recommended in the literature [13]. Intravenous (iv) and subcutaneous (sc) routes of Ig replacement therapies have different pharmacokinetic profiles, and sc route may be preferred in patients with CVID, since IgG is first locally distributed, followed by slow diffusion into extravascular space from vascular space [14].

Delay in the diagnosis of CVID and initiation of IVIg replacement therapy in patients with recurrent infections can increase the risk of chronic inflammation resulting in an uncommon but life-threatening complication, amyloidosis. We believe that regular clinical follow-ups, control of infections, and adequate replacement of Ig may seem to prevent development of amyloidosis in patients with CVID. However, further research is needed to shed more light on the epidemiology, pathogenesis, screening, and management of amyloidosis in patients with CVID.

Conflict of Interests

The authors declare that they have no conflict of interests.

References

[1] B. Gathmann, N. Mahlaoui, L. Gérard et al., "Clinical picture and treatment of 2212 patients with common variable immunodeficiency," *Journal of Allergy and Clinical Immunology*, vol. 134, no. 1, pp. 116–126, 2014.

[2] P. Kotilainen, K. Vuori, L. Kainulainen et al., "Systemic amyloidosis in a patient with hypogammaglobulinaemia," *Journal of Internal Medicine*, vol. 240, no. 2, pp. 103–106, 1996.

[3] G. Merlini and V. Bellotti, "Molecular mechanisms of amyloidosis," *The New England Journal of Medicine*, vol. 349, no. 6, pp. 583–596, 2003.

[4] A. F. Çelik, M. R. Altiparmak, G. E. Pamuk, Ö. N. Pamuk, and F. Tabak, "Association of secondary amyloidosis with common variable immune deficiency and tuberculosis," *Yonsei Medical Journal*, vol. 46, no. 6, pp. 847–850, 2005.

[5] D. Soysal, E. Türkkan, V. Karakuş, E. Tatar, Ö. Y. Kabayeğit, and A. Avci, "A case of common variable immunodeficiency disease and thyroid amyloidosis," *Turkish Journal of Medical Sciences*, vol. 39, no. 3, pp. 467–473, 2009.

[6] S. Unverdi, S. Inal, M. Ceri et al., "Is colchicine therapy effective in all patients with secondary amyloidosis?" *Renal Failure*, vol. 35, no. 8, pp. 1071–1074, 2013.

[7] C. F. Meneses, C. A. Egües, M. Uriarte, J. Belzunegui, and M. Rezola, "Colchicine use in isolated renal AA amyloidosis," *Reumatología Clínica*, vol. 11, no. 4, pp. 242–243, 2015.

[8] V. Bellotti, M. Nuvolone, S. Giorgetti et al., "The workings of the amyloid diseases," *Annals of Medicine*, vol. 39, no. 3, pp. 200–207, 2007.

[9] H. J. Lachmann, H. J. B. Goodman, J. A. Gilbertson et al., "Natural history and outcome in systemic AA amyloidosis," *The New England Journal of Medicine*, vol. 356, no. 23, pp. 2361–2371, 2007.

[10] I. Tezcan, F. Ersoy, O. Sanal, E. N. Gönc, M. Arici, and I. Berkel, "A case of X linked agammaglobulinaemia complicated with systemic amyloidosis," *Archives of Disease in Childhood*, vol. 79, no. 1, article 94, 1998.

[11] N. Kurita, N. Kotera, Y. Ishimoto et al., "AA amyloid nephropathy with predominant vascular deposition in Crohn's disease," *Clinical Nephrology*, vol. 79, no. 3, pp. 229–232, 2013.

[12] D. Firinu, L. Serusi, M. M. Lorrai et al., "Systemic reactive (AA) amyloidosis in the course of common variable immunodeficiency," *Amyloid*, vol. 18, supplement 1, pp. 214–216, 2011.

[13] S. Arslan, R. Ucar, D. M. Yavsan et al., "Common variable immunodeficiency and pulmonary amyloidosis: a case report," *Journal of Clinical Immunology*, vol. 35, no. 4, pp. 344–347, 2015.

[14] S. Nishi, B. Alchi, N. Imai, and F. Gejyo, "New advances in renal amyloidosis," *Clinical and Experimental Nephrology*, vol. 12, no. 2, pp. 93–101, 2008.

12

Allergen Immunotherapy in an HIV+ Patient with Allergic Fungal Rhinosinusitis

Ian A. Myles[1] and Satyen Gada[2]

[1]*Bacterial Pathogenesis Unit, Laboratory of Clinical Infectious Diseases, National Institute of Allergy and Infectious Diseases, National Institutes of Health, 9000 Rockville Pike, Building 33, Room 2W10A, Bethesda, MD 20892, USA*
[2]*Allergy/Immunology/Immunization Service, Department of Medicine, Walter Reed National Military Medical Center, 8901 Wisconsin Avenue, Bethesda, MD 20889, USA*

Correspondence should be addressed to Ian A. Myles; mylesi@niaid.nih.gov

Academic Editor: Jiri Litzman

Patients with HIV/AIDS can present with multiple types of fungal rhinosinusitis, fungal balls, granulomatous invasive fungal rhinosinusitis, acute or chronic invasive fungal rhinosinusitis, or allergic fungal rhinosinusitis (AFRS). Given the variable spectrum of immune status and susceptibility to severe infection from opportunistic pathogens it is extremely important that clinicians distinguish aggressive fungal invasive fungal disease from the much milder forms such as AFRS. Here we describe a patient with HIV and AFRS to both remind providers of the importance of ruling out invasive fungal disease and outline the other unique features of fungal sinusitis treatment in the HIV-positive population. Additionally we discuss the evidence for and against use of allergen immunotherapy (AIT) for fungal disease in general, as well as the evidence for AIT in the HIV population.

1. Introduction

A recent review by Callejas and Douglas outlined five major types of fungal rhinosinusitis [1]. Fungal balls are dense growths mainly of *Aspergillus* species that afflict mostly middle-aged to elderly women; the disorder can occur in both immunocompromised and immunocompetent hosts and has excellent surgical cure rates. Another potential fungal sinus disease found in immunocompetent hosts is the far less common granulomatous invasive fungal rhinosinusitis. This disorder is geographically limited mostly to Sudan, India, Pakistan, and Saudi Arabia, most often caused by *Aspergillus flavus*, and is treated with a combination of surgery and itraconazole. Immunosuppressed patients may present with acute or chronic invasive fungal rhinosinusitis, with the distinguishing feature being the severity of the immunologic defect. In chronic invasive disease, the defect tends to be subtle such as the immune dysfunction seen in poorly controlled diabetics and patients on low-dose corticosteroids. In contrast, the acute form tends to manifest in patients with severe reduction in neutrophil numbers

or function, such as patients undergoing chemotherapy or afflicted with blood-based cancers. Chronic invasive fungal rhinosinusitis is considered a medical emergency due to the potential for rapid invasion into the central nervous system imparting a high mortality rate. *Aspergillus* and *Mucorales* are the most common causative agents identified in both acute and chronic invasive diseases, and both forms are treated with immune reconstitution (if possible), surgical debridement, and systemic antifungals. Allergic fungal rhinosinusitis (AFRS) is also most often caused by *Aspergillus* species but may be due to *Alternaria*, *Bipolaris*, or *Curvularia* species. Atopic yet immunocompetent patients often present with this disorder and treatment includes surgery, nasal steroids, and perhaps the addition of allergen immunotherapy (AIT). Given the variable spectrum of immune status and susceptibility to severe infection from opportunistic pathogens, patients with HIV/AIDS can present with any of the five types of fungal rhinosinusitis. It is thus extremely important when seeing a patient with HIV and fungal sinus disease to distinguish aggressive fungal disease such as acute invasive fungal rhinosinusitis from the much milder forms such

TABLE 1: Review of sinus disease categories and features.

Sinus diseases of immunocompetent hosts				
Type	Pathogen	Host features	Treatment	Pearls
Fungal ball	*Aspergillus* species	Females over ~50 years of age	Outpatient surgery	High cure rate
Granulomatous invasive fungal rhinosinusitis	*Aspergillus flavus*	All demographics, in Sudan, India, Pakistan, and Saudi Arabia	Outpatient surgery and systemic antifungals	Postoperative itraconazole may reduce relapse rate
Allergic fungal rhinosinusitis	*Aspergillus* sp., *Alternaria* sp., *Bipolaris* sp., and *Curvularia* sp.	Atopic patient	Outpatient surgery, allergic treatments (nasal steroids), and considering allergen immunotherapy	Best evidence is for allergen immunotherapy initiation 4–6 weeks after surgery
Sinus diseases limited to immunocompromised hosts				
Type	Pathogen	Host features	Treatment	Pearls
Acute invasive fungal rhinosinusitis	*Aspergillus* species, *Rhizopus* sp., and *Mucor* sp.	Reduced neutrophil number of functions, HIV	Inpatient surgery, systemic antifungals, and immune reconstitution	Must be distinguished from noninvasive disease in immunocompromised host, high mortality
Chronic invasive fungal rhinosinusitis	*Aspergillus* species, *Rhizopus* sp., and *Mucor* sp.	Less severe impairment such as diabetes, systemic corticosteroids, and HIV	Outpatient surgery, systemic antifungals, and immune reconstitution	Must be distinguished from noninvasive disease in immunocompromised host; recurrence is possible

Modified from Callejas and Douglas, 2013 [1].

as AFRS (Table 1). Here we describe a patient with HIV and AFRS to remind providers of the importance of ruling out invasive fungal disease and other unique features of fungal sinusitis treatment in the HIV-positive population. Additionally we discuss the evidence for and against use of AIT for fungal disease in general, as well as the evidence for AIT in the HIV population.

2. Case Presentation

A 40-year-old male presented for evaluation with 15–20 years of congestion, headache, and anosmia. He reported a variable response to nasal steroids and oral antihistamines. In 1994, he underwent sinus surgery for sinus polyposis, after which his symptoms improved. Despite continued treatment with daily loratadine and then later fexofenadine, he required repeat sinus surgery in 2000. He was then placed on cetirizine with improved and stable symptoms for several months. However, around this time he was found to be HIV-positive and cetirizine was discontinued due to concern for drug interaction with his antiretroviral medications. Given continued symptoms and limited oral treatment options due to lack of efficacy or potential medication interactions, he was treated with allergen immunotherapy (AIT) from 2000 to 2003 to molds and dust mite per self-report. While he described symptomatic improvement on AIT, his treatment was interrupted after moving and was not restarted. After reporting worsening of symptoms including chronic nasal congestion with acute episodes of worsening when exposed to "moldy rooms" and cats, a repeat CT demonstrated evidence of recurrent pansinusitis. Subsequent MRI confirmed CT findings of pansinusitis with no evidence of invasive disease, prompting a third sinus surgery in late 2009. Thick,

inspissated "allergic" mucin and nasal polyposis were noted intraoperatively, consistent with the diagnosis of AFS. Tissue examination revealed fungal elements by GMS/PAS stain and numerous eosinophils with growth of *Curvularia* on culture. His symptoms included stable, daily nasal congestion with exacerbations. The recurrent nature of his allergic fungal sinusitis raised the question of whether he would be best treated with reinitiation AIT, and thus he was referred to our allergy clinic for evaluation.

His past medical history was positive for adult attention deficit hyperactivity disorder and HIV with a CD4 count of 397 and an undetectable viral load. He denied any respiratory complaints and had no history of asthma. Vital signs were within normal limits. Physical exam was significant for surgical removal of much of the middle turbinates and dry nasal mucosa without erythema, edema, or nasal polyposis. There was no sinus tenderness. His medications included daily lamivudine, abacavir, raltegravir, efavirenz, methylphenidate, calcium supplements, budesonide suspension used in conjunction with nasal sinus saline rinse, azelastine, and mometasone nasal sprays. He had no history of ever receiving antifungal medications.

Our evaluation revealed negative skin prick testing to all relevant trees and grasses, as well as cat, dog, cockroach, and dust mite. He had positive skin prick testing to *Curvularia spicifera*, *Alternaria tenuis*, *Helminthosporium mix*, *Penicillium notatum*, and ragweed mix. Intradermal skin tests were positive to *Aspergillus fumigatus*, *Cladosporium mix*, and *Epicoccum nigrum*. Total serum immunoglobulin E (IgE) was 298.2 mg/dL. Serum sensitization was confirmed for *Cladosporium herbarum*, *Alternaria*, and *Aspergillus*. He had mild specific IgE elevations to ragweed and elder marsh. Specific IgE to grasses (Bermuda, Johnson, Kentucky

TABLE 2: Maintenance allergy immune-therapy dose composition for our presented case report.

Species	Concentration (weight/volume)	Volume
Alternaria	1 : 20	0.5 mL
Aspergillus fumigatus	1 : 20	0.5 mL
Helminthosporium	1 : 10	0.5 mL
Hormodendrum/Cladosporium	1 : 20	0.5 mL
Curvularia	1 : 20	0.5 mL
Epicoccum	1 : 40	0.5 mL
Penicillium	1 : 20	0.5 mL
Diluent	—	6.5 mL
Total	1 : 200	10 mL

Blue), elm, juniper, oak, olive tree, dust mite, cat, dog, and cockroach were all negative. Having established clinically relevant fungal sensitization and after discussing risks and potential benefits, AIT against the sensitized fungal allergens was initiated. He tolerated AIT without serious reactions, achieving maintenance after a one-year period of buildup (Table 2). At that time, repeat CT of sinuses revealed stable postoperative changes with no finding of recurrent fungal disease. He continued on maintenance AIT for two years and then discontinued due to his work schedule preventing compliance with monthly maintenance injections. He has remained on daily mometasone nasal spray as well as budesonide suspension with saline sinus lavage. Despite only two years of maintenance AIT, he has remained stable, with minimal symptoms and a recent endoscopy demonstrated only small, asymptomatic polyps.

3. Discussion

This case highlights the unique issues related to fungal sinus disease. Although this patient's clinical course ended up to be one of the successful treatments, as soon as fungal sinus disease is suspected in an immunocompromised patient, invasive disease should be excluded immediately, especially if neutropenia is also present [2, 3]. Bone erosion and extrasinus extension do not manifest until late in the course of invasive disease, and thus lack of such findings should not dissuade further work-up [4]. In one study the most suggestive (albeit nonspecific) finding in HIV patients with invasive disease was severe unilateral mucosal thickening [5].

Overall, up to 68% of HIV patients report some form of sinus disease [4, 6]. Part of the pathogenesis may be reduced ciliary clearance seen in HIV-positive individuals [7] perhaps leading to mucus stasis [4]. While the evaluation of sinus disease in the HIV-positive population is often similar to seronegative patients, in addition to ruling out invasive disease clinicians should ensure that any sinus cultures are sent for all possible cultures including fungal, viral, aerobic, anaerobic, and mycobacterial ones [4]. The most common pathogens causing acute sinusitis in the HIV-positive population are *S. pneumoniae*, *H. influenza*, *M. catarrhalis*,

and *S. viridans*, whereas chronic sinus disease in HIV-positive individuals is most often *S. aureus*, *S. epidermidis*, or anaerobic bacteria [1, 4]. When invasive fungal disease is encountered, clinicians must understand that mortality is high and thus aggressive, and open surgical debridement with adjunct liposomal amphotericin B is indicated [3].

In contrast with invasive disease, allergic fungal sinusitis in patients with HIV is addressed identically to seronegative patients. Diagnosis may involve the Bent III and Kuhn criteria [8]: (1) nasal polyps, (2) sinus content positive for fungi on staining and/or cultures, (3) eosinophil rich mucin, (4) no evidence of invasive disease but positive CT findings of sinus expansion or opacification, and (5) evidence of allergic sensitivity in either skin testing or serum IgE specific to fungi (with skin testing showing greater sensitivity than serum IgE testing [1]). Unlike our patient, total IgE is typically elevated over 1000 IU/mL; however, unlike in a similar disease ABPA (allergic bronchopulmonary aspergillosis) following IgE levels does not appear to provide clinical benefit [1]. Treatment involves nasal saline irrigation, nasal corticosteroids, and consideration for short-courses of systemic corticosteroids [1, 9–12]. Of note, our patient's systemic antihistamines were discontinued at the time of his HIV diagnosis yet while antiretroviral medications carry a general interaction cytochrome p450 warning with antihistamines (presumably the reason for the discontinuation), the specific interactions are described for H-1 antagonists such as astemizole and there are no contraindications to H-2 receptor blocker use in the presence of antiretroviral therapy [13]. There are conflicting recommendations for use of systemic antifungals in AFRS [9, 14]; however one recent study reported significant reduction in recurrence of AFRS with postoperative use of intranasal fluconazole [9]. Surgical treatment involving functional endoscopic sinus surgery (FESS) may also be indicated; however patients should be informed that recurrence is high even with surgical intervention [15, 16] and many patients require several surgeries before clinical resolution is obtained [17, 18].

This case also highlights another potential therapeutic intervention, one with far less clarity on utility, allergen immunotherapy. The use of AIT in allergic fungal sinusitis started on shaky ground when a study of 7 patients reported that only 2 patients improved while 5 had worsening of symptoms [19, 20]. Furthermore, the researchers uncovered induction of fungal-specific IgG, raising the possibility of inducing a type III immune-complex reaction [20]. However, further investigation revealed that the two patients that showed improvement started AIT after surgery, whereas the five that worsened started prior to their operation [20, 21] and further investigation has failed to show any signs of the theorized immune-complex induction [21]. A recent review recommends waiting 4–6 weeks after surgery to begin AIT, surmising that AIT may worsen symptoms in those with active disease but may aide those in a disease-free postsurgical window [20]. Other early reports of treatment failure were subsequently shown to have been using end-point concentrations of antigens far below what would be recommended in modern AIT and thus may be explained simply by dose limitations [21]. The largest evaluation, a retrospective evaluation of 36 post-FESS patients treated with AIT compared to 24 controls, found that AIT imparted a threefold reduction in the need for repeat surgery (11% versus 33%) at a mean follow-up of about four years [17]. In a clinical trial including 22 patients' status after FESS, the 11 subjects that received AIT had significantly better outcomes on quality of life surveys, endoscopic mucosal staging, and reduced use of systemic and nasal steroids at their mean follow-up of 33 months [22]; however, this study did not include a placebo control. Overall, these studies and others examining AIT for allergic fungal sinus disease show promise when correctly timed and targeted; however much work is still needed to elucidate the optimal timing, dose, and duration.

Given that our patient had a personal history of benefit from AIT we elected to resume treatment and will need to monitor despite little literature guidance on duration. However, the literature does not offer any better data for pollen and venom AIT in HIV-positive patients than what it offers for fungal sinus disease. In addition, although the recommendation for AIT is 3–5 years when treating allergic rhinitis and allergic asthma, there are no specific recommendations for length of treatment in AFS. A potential, yet theoretical, complication of AIT in HIV-positive patients would be the expansion of memory CD4+ T cells and a subsequent increase in viral proliferation [23, 24]. Yet one case report [25] and another care series [26] have described a total of four patients treated for periods ranging from 24 to 102 weeks, and none showed any evidence of either increased viral load or instability in their CD4+ counts. Despite this evidence of benefit, a survey of providers revealed that when treating HIV-positive patients, 26% would not perform skin testing and 60% were less likely to treat with AIT due to seropositivity [27, 28]. While we lack comparative controls, treatment in our patient for allergic sinus disease with 24 months of maintenance AIT was well tolerated and demonstrated benefit, adding to the case reports of safe AIT treatment in patients with HIV.

Consent

The patient gave consent for publication of these findings.

Conflict of Interests

The authors declare that there is no conflict of interests regarding the publication of this paper.

Acknowledgments

This research was supported by the Intramural Research Program of National Institutes of Health and National Institute of Allergy and Infectious Disease. The authors would like to thank Dr. Susan Laubach for her preliminary work with the case description.

References

[1] C. A. Callejas and R. G. Douglas, "Fungal rhinosinusitis: what every allergist should know," *Clinical and Experimental Allergy*, vol. 43, no. 8, pp. 835–849, 2013.

[2] G. Y. Minamoto, T. F. Barlam, and N. J. Vander Els, "Invasive aspergillosis in patients with AIDS," *Clinical Infectious Diseases*, vol. 14, no. 1, pp. 66–74, 1992.

[3] S. M. Hunt, R. C. Miyamoto, R. S. Cornelius, and T. A. Tami, "Invasive fungal sinusitis in the acquired immunodeficiency syndrome," *Otolaryngologic Clinics of North America*, vol. 33, no. 2, pp. 335–347, 2000.

[4] A. R. Shah, J. A. Hairston, and T. A. Tami, "Sinusitis in HIV: microbiology and therapy," *Current Allergy and Asthma Reports*, vol. 5, no. 6, pp. 495–499, 2005.

[5] J. M. DelGaudio, R. E. Swain Jr., T. T. Kingdom, S. Muller, and P. A. Hudgins, "Computed tomographic findings in patients with invasive fungal sinusitis," *Archives of Otolaryngology—Head and Neck Surgery*, vol. 129, no. 2, pp. 236–240, 2003.

[6] T. A. Gurney and A. H. Murr, "Otolaryngologic manifestations of human immunodeficiency virus infection," *Otolaryngologic Clinics of North America*, vol. 36, no. 4, pp. 607–624, 2003.

[7] L. M. Milgrim, J. S. Rubin, and C. B. Small, "Mucociliary clearance abnormalities in the HIV-infected patient: a precursor to acute sinusitis," *Laryngoscope*, vol. 105, no. 11, pp. 1202–1208, 1995.

[8] J. P. Bent III and F. A. Kuhn, "Diagnosis of allergic fungal sinusitis," *Otolaryngology—Head and Neck Surgery*, vol. 111, no. 5, pp. 580–588, 1994.

[9] Y. Khalil, A. Tharwat, A. G. Abdou et al., "The role of antifungal therapy in the prevention of recurrent allergic fungal rhinosinusitis after functional endoscopic sinus surgery: a randomized, controlled study," *Ear, Nose and Throat Journal*, vol. 90, no. 8, pp. E1–E7, 2011.

[10] D. A. Stevens, H. J. Schwartz, J. Y. Lee et al., "A randomized trial of itraconazole in allergic bronchopulmonary aspergillosis," *The New England Journal of Medicine*, vol. 342, no. 11, pp. 756–762, 2000.

[11] P. A. B. Wark, M. J. Hensley, N. Saltos et al., "Anti-inflammatory effect of itraconazole in stable allergic bronchopulmonary aspergillosis: a randomized controlled trial," *Journal of Allergy and Clinical Immunology*, vol. 111, no. 5, pp. 952–957, 2003.

[12] P. A. Wark, P. G. Gibson, and A. J. Wilson, "Azoles for allergic bronchopulmonary aspergillosis associated with asthma," *Cochrane Database of Systematic Reviews*, no. 3, Article ID CD001108, 2004.

[13] S. C. Armstrong and K. L. Cozza, "Antihistamines," *Psychosomatics*, vol. 44, pp. 430–434, 2003.

[14] E. C. Gan, A. Thamboo, L. Rudmik, P. H. Hwang, B. J. Ferguson, and A. R. Javer, "Medical management of allergic fungal rhinosinusitis following endoscopic sinus surgery: an evidence-based review and recommendations," *International Forum of Allergy & Rhinology*, vol. 4, no. 9, pp. 702–715, 2014.

[15] V. Rupa, M. Jacob, M. S. Mathews, and M. S. Seshadri, "A prospective, randomised, placebo-controlled trial of postoperative oral steroid in allergic fungal sinusitis," *European Archives of Oto-Rhino-Laryngology*, vol. 267, no. 2, pp. 233–238, 2010.

[16] S. B. Kupferberg, J. P. Bent III, and F. A. Kuhn, "Prognosis for allergic fungal sinusitis," *Otolaryngology—Head and Neck Surgery*, vol. 117, no. 1, pp. 35–41, 1997.

[17] B. A. Bassichis, B. F. Marple, R. L. Mabry, M. T. Newcomer, and N. D. Schwade, "Use of immunotherapy in previously treated

patients with allergic fungal sinusitis," *Otolaryngology—Head and Neck Surgery*, vol. 125, no. 5, pp. 487–490, 2001.

[18] B. Marple, M. Newcomer, N. Schwade, and R. Mabry, "Natural history of allergic fungal rhinosinusitis: a 4- to 10-year follow-up," *Otolaryngology—Head and Neck Surgery*, vol. 127, no. 5, pp. 361–366, 2002.

[19] B. J. Ferguson, "What role do systemic corticosteroids, immunotherapy, and antifungal drugs play in the therapy of allergic fungal rhinosinusitis?" *Archives of Otolaryngology—Head and Neck Surgery*, vol. 124, no. 10, pp. 1174–1178, 1998.

[20] A. G. Hall and R. D. DeShazo, "Immunotherapy for allergic fungal sinusitis," *Current Opinion in Allergy and Clinical Immunology*, vol. 12, no. 6, pp. 629–634, 2012.

[21] M. S. Doellman, G. R. Dion, E. K. Weitzel, and E. G. Reyes, "Immunotherapy in allergic fungal sinusitis: the controversy continues. A recent review of literature," *Allergy & Rhinology*, vol. 4, no. 1, pp. e32–e35, 2013.

[22] R. J. Folker, B. F. Marple, R. L. Mabry, and C. S. Mabry, "Treatment of allergic fungal sinusitis: a comparison trial of postoperative immunotherapy with specific fungal antigens," *Laryngoscope*, vol. 108, no. 11, pp. 1623–1627, 1998.

[23] M. A. Ostrowski, S. K. Stanley, J. S. Justement, K. Gantt, D. Goletti, and A. S. Fauci, "Increased in vitro tetanus-induced production of HIV type 1 following in vivo immunization of HIV type 1-infected individuals with tetanus toxoid," *AIDS Research and Human Retroviruses*, vol. 13, no. 6, pp. 473–480, 1997.

[24] K. R. Fowke, R. D'Amico, D. N. Chernoff et al., "Immunologic and virologic evaluation after influenza vaccination of HIV-1-infected patients," *AIDS*, vol. 11, no. 8, pp. 1013–1021, 1997.

[25] I. S. Randhawa, I. Junaid, and W. B. Klaustermeyer, "Allergen immunotherapy in a patient with human immunodeficiency virus: effect on T-cell activation and viral replication," *Annals of Allergy, Asthma and Immunology*, vol. 98, no. 5, pp. 495–497, 2007.

[26] J. Fodeman, S. Jariwala, G. Hudes, E. Jerschow, and D. Rosenstreich, "Subcutaneous allergen immunotherapy in 3 patients with HIV," *Annals of Allergy, Asthma and Immunology*, vol. 105, no. 4, pp. 320–321, 2010.

[27] C. Saltoun and P. C. Avila, "Advances in upper airway diseases and allergen immunotherapy in 2007," *Journal of Allergy and Clinical Immunology*, vol. 122, no. 3, pp. 481–487, 2008.

[28] R. E. Coifman and L. S. Cox, "2006 American Academy of Allergy, Asthma & Immunology member immunotherapy practice patterns and concerns," *Journal of Allergy and Clinical Immunology*, vol. 119, no. 4, pp. 1012–1013, 2007.

13

Combined Treatment with Antiviral Therapy and Rituximab in Patients with Mixed Cryoglobulinemia: Review of the Literature and Report of a Case Using Direct Antiviral Agents-Based Antihepatitis C Virus Therapy

Teresa Urraro, Laura Gragnani, Alessia Piluso, Alessio Fabbrizzi, Monica Monti, Elisa Fognani, Barbara Boldrini, Jessica Ranieri, and Anna Linda Zignego

Center for Systemic Manifestations of Hepatitis Viruses (MASVE), Department of Experimental and Clinical Medicine, University of Florence, Lagro Brambilla 3, 50134 Florence, Italy

Correspondence should be addressed to Anna Linda Zignego; a.zignego@dmi.unifi.it

Academic Editor: Lenin Pavón

Mixed cryoglobulinemia (MC) is an autoimmune/B-cell lymphoproliferative disorder associated with Hepatitis C Virus (HCV) infection, manifesting as a systemic vasculitis. In the last decade, antiviral treatment (AT) with pegylated interferon (Peg-IFN) plus ribavirin (RBV) was considered the first therapeutic option for HCV-MC. In MC patients ineligible or not responsive to antivirals, the anti-CD20 monoclonal antibody rituximab (RTX) is effective. A combined AT plus RTX was also suggested. Since the introduction of direct acting antivirals (DAAs), few data were published about MC and no data about a combined schedule. Here, we report a complete remission of MC after a sustained virological response following a combined RTX/Peg-IFN+RBV+DAA (boceprevir) treatment and review the literature about the combined RTX/AT.

1. Introduction

Mixed cryoglobulinemia (MC) is both an autoimmune and B-cell lymphoproliferative disorder (LPD) characterized by immune complexes (cryoglobulins, CGs) that reversibly precipitate at low temperature [1].

In the large majority of cases, MC is triggered by Hepatitis C Virus (HCV) infection.

HCV is both a hepatotropic and lymphotropic virus and may lead not only to liver diseases, but also to some lymphoproliferative disorders ranging from the benign MC to malignant B-cell non-Hodgkin's lymphoma [2].

Small-to-medium sized vessel vasculitis is the pathological substrate of the MC-related clinical syndrome (MCS) [1].

Antiviral therapy (AT) has been indicated as first-line therapy in patients with mild-to-moderate HCV-related MCS. The use of IFN-α to treat MC was successfully proposed, even before HCV discovery, because of its antiproliferative and immunomodulatory effects [3]. However,

the benefit was transient and relapses were very frequent after treatment discontinuation when viral eradication was not achieved [4–6].

Starting with the IFN monotherapy, the efficacy of AT progressively increased during two decades thanks to the use of Peg-IFN and RBV. The increased antiviral activity was associated with an increased clinical effectiveness in patients with MCS [2, 7, 8].

In severe cases and/or in patients intolerant or ineligible to AT, the usefulness and safety of anti-CD20 monoclonal antibody rituximab (RTX) have been clearly shown in several studies. RTX was shown to be highly effective in modifying the dynamics of B cells by deleting expanded clones and markedly improving MCS in most cases [9–11].

Peg-IFN plus RBV has been considered the standard AT for about a decade [12]. Recently, the direct acting antiviral drugs (DAAs), inhibitor of the nonstructural 3/4A HCV protease, boceprevir (BOC), and telaprevir, in combination with Peg-IFN and RBV, have consistently increased the likelihood

Table 1: Main clinical and laboratory data before rituximab (RTX-baseline), 2 months after rituximab cycle (BOC-baseline), and at the end of follow-up after boceprevir-based antiviral therapy (post-BOC).

	RTX-baseline (June 2011)	BOC-baseline (September 2011)	Post-BOC (November 2013)
Gender	Female		
Age (years)	63		
IL28b rs12979860	T/T		
Stiffness (kPa)	14.5	12	11.7
HCV titer (IU $\times 10^6$/mL)	0.98	1.39	NEG
ALT (IU/L)[†]	44	37	19
MC manifestations			
Clinical			
Purpura	++	−	−
Arthralgia	++	+	−
Weakness	++	−	−
Peripheral neuropathy	−	−	−
Raynaud syndrome	−	−	−
Nephritis	−	−	−
Sicca syndrome	++	+	+
Laboratory			
Cryocrit (%)	5	0	0
RF (IU/mL)[§]	24	<10	<10
C4 (mg/dL)[‡]	9	16	25

RTX: rituximab; BOC: boceprevir; MC: mixed cryoglobulinemia; IL28B: polymorphism of interleukin-28B; stiffness: liver stiffness as evaluated by transient elastography; kPa: kilopascal; IU: international units; ALT: alanine aminotransferase; RF: rheumatoid factor. [†]Normal values: <40 IU/L; [§]normal values: <10 IU/mL; [‡]normal values: from 10 to 40 mg/dL.

of response in patients infected with HCV genotype 1 (Gt 1a or 1b) [13, 14]. Few data are still available for patients with HCV-related MCS treated with DAAs [15–18] and no clear information exists about the combination with RTX.

Here we describe, for the first time, a case of HCV-related MCS treated with the combination of RTX and BOC-based triple AT and review the available literature about the combination of RTX and anti-HCV therapy.

2. Case Report

In May, 2010, a 63-year-old woman with a 30-year history of HCV (Gt 1b) chronic infection and harboring compensated liver cirrhosis with normal liver function tests and no signs of portal hypertension was evaluated at the MASVE Center of the University of Florence. The main clinical and laboratory data are detailed in Table 1. The analysis of cryocrit was performed in the MASVE laboratory at every medical appointment. Briefly, the patient blood was kept at 37°–40°C to avoid CGs precipitation; immediately after centrifugation, a special graduated glass tube (Wintrobe tube) has been filled

with 1.0 mL of serum, placed at 4°C, and examined after at least 7 days to assess the percentage of packed cryoglobulins.

The reduction of C4 complement component and the RF levels was performed as routine tests by the Centralized Diagnostic Laboratory of the Careggi Hospital, Florence, Italy, by immunoturbidimetric method and immunoenzymatic assay, respectively.

Since 2008, the patient showed a typical MCS [19] characterized by recurrent lower limb purpura, arthralgia/arthritis of hands and shoulders, and burning paresthesia with "bootie" distribution. She repeatedly scored positive for mixed type II (polyclonal IgG/monoclonal IgMk) cryoglobulins as well as rheumatoid factor (RF), increased inflammatory markers, and low C4. The patient previously failed two Peg-IFNα-2b+RBV treatments. Her interleukin-28b (IL28b) genotype (rs12979860) was T/T, a negative predictor of response to IFN-based therapy [20]. In June 2010, the patient underwent treatment with RTX (1 g twice monthly) which led to a complete MCS clinical response, with improvement in all baseline clinical manifestations [21]. After recurrence of symptoms in July 2011, the treatment was repeated. Clinical conditions consistently improved and in September 2011 the patient underwent AT. The BOC-based treatment was chosen on the basis of negative predictors of response [12] and higher efficacy of triple therapy compared to dual one.

After a 4-week lead-in phase with Peg-IFNα-2b (1.5 μg/Kg/week, subcutaneously) plus RBV (800 mg/daily, orally), BOC was added (800 mg three times daily, orally) and triple therapy was continued for 44 weeks.

Viremia disappeared 1 week after BOC administration and remained negative throughout therapy and follow-up (sustained virological response).

The cryocrit scored negative during therapy and follow-up and C4 and RF remained persistently normal (Table 1 and Figure 1).

During treatment, the patient did not experience purpura or arthritis. She developed anemia and neutropenia requiring administration of erythropoietin and granulokines and reduction of RBV (600 mg/daily).

After therapy, the patient was regularly checked up every three months. During every scheduled check-up C4, RF, cryocrit levels as well as liver functional parameters, and viremia were evaluated (data not shown).

We observed long-term clinical and virological response: after a 15-month follow-up, the patient no longer had purpura, arthritis, or other baseline symptoms. Persistence of mild xerostomia and xerophthalmia was occasionally treated with symptomatic drugs (Table 1).

3. Review of the Literature

We performed a literature search on PubMed about combined/sequential treatment of MC (Table 2).

In the first pilot study, Saadoun et al. treated 16 consecutive, unselected refractory HCV-MC patients with RTX followed by AT with Peg-IFN and RBV. 15/16 patients showed clinical improvement, with a good profile of safety [22].

(a)

(b)

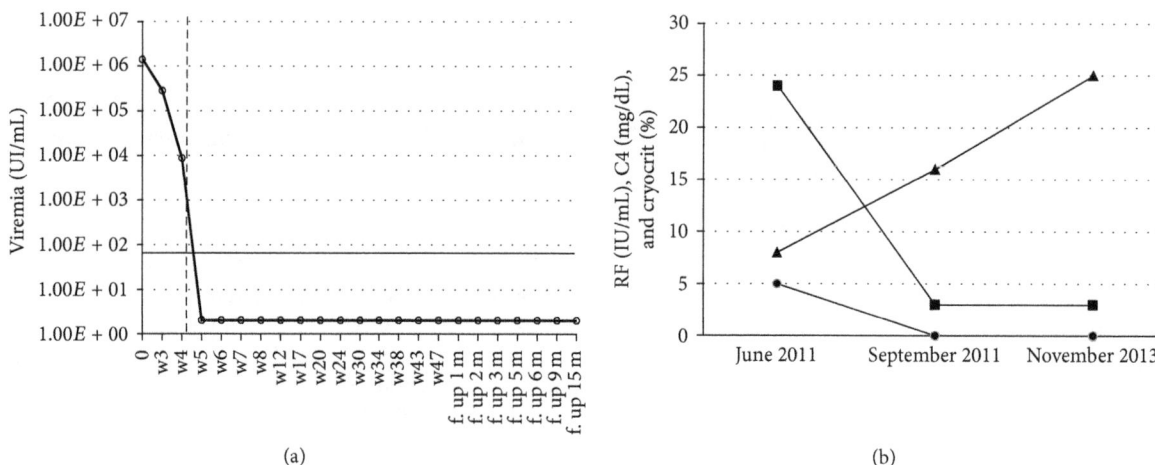

FIGURE 1: (a) Viral kinetics: a slight decrease in serum HCV RNA values was observed during the lead-in phase. Soon after the introduction of boceprevir (week 4), a drastic reduction in viremia was observed, with complete negativization at week 5. The vertical dashed line represents the introduction of boceprevir; the horizontal continuous line indicates the detection limit of the HCV RNA test (15 IU/mL). IU: international units; mL: milliliter; w: week; f. up: follow up; m: month. (B) Cryocrit C4 and RF kinetics during the combined therapy (RTX+Peg-IFN+RBV+BOC). The time points considered are (1) before rituximab (June 2011), (2) two months after rituximab cycle (September 2011; triple therapy baseline), and (3) end of the follow-up after boceprevir-based antiviral therapy (November 2013). After RTX therapy cryocrit, C4 and RF normalized and remained persistently normal. (●) Cryocrit; (■) rheumatoid factor; (▲) C4. RF: rheumatoid factor; normal values: <10 IU/mL; normal values of C4: from 10 to 40 mg/dL.

TABLE 2: Combined treatment with antiviral therapy and rituximab in MC patients: review of the literature.

Author	Patients	Main indication	Regimen	Therapy outcome (CR/PR/NR)	AEs
Saadoun et al., 2008 [22]	16	Refractory MC	ST (RTX 375 mg/sqm × 4 Peg IFNα2b[+] + RBV[++] after a month)	(10/6/1)	2°
Terrier et al., 2009 [23]	20	Severe MC	ST (RTX 375 mg/sqm × 4 or 1 gr × 2 Peg IFNα2b[+] + RBV[++] after a month)	(16/3/1)	4°°
Dammacco et al., 2010 [24]	22	MC (naïve patients)	CT (RTX 375 mg/sqm × 4 weekly + two 5 monthly inf. + Peg IFNα2b[+] or α2a[+++] + RBV[++])	(12/5/5)	3°°°
Saadoun et al., 2010 [25]	38	MC (unselected)	ST (RTX 375 mg/sqm × 4 or 1 gr × 2 Peg IFNα2b[+] or α2a[+++] + RBV[++] after a month)	(28/9/1)	5°°+
Ignatova et al., 2014 [26]	6	Severe MC	ST (RTX n.d. dose Peg IFNα + RBV[++] after a month)	(n.d./n.d./n.d.)	n.d.

MC: mixed cryoglobulinemia; ST: sequential treatment; CT: combined treatment; CR: complete response, PR: partial response, NR: no response; AEs: adverse events (requiring antiviral treatment interruption); n.d.: not determined.
[+]1.5 mcg/kg weekly; [++]weight-based; [+++]180 mcg weekly.
°One worsening of peripheral neuropathy case and 1 flare of psoriasis case.
°°Two hematologic toxicity cases; 1 flare of psoriasis case; 1 hepatocarcinoma case.
°°°One severe anemia case; 2 grade 4 neutropenia cases.
°°+Two hematologic toxicity cases; 1 depression case; 1 flare of psoriasis cases; 1 neuropathy case.

A subsequent study of Terrier et al. comprised 32 severe HCV-MCS patients, treated either with RTX monotherapy (12 patients) or with RTX followed by AT (20 patients, 11 already included in the previous pilot study). The authors reported the efficacy of RTX, with a better response in RTX/Peg-IFN+RBV group [23].

In 2010 Dammacco et al. and Saadoun et al. published two studies on the use of RTX and AT with Peg-IFN+RBV according to a combined [24] or sequential [25] scheme.

In the first study, 37 HCV-MCS patients, naïve for IFNs or previous administration of immunosuppressive drugs, were randomized to get a RTX/Peg-IFN+RBV treatment (22 patients) or Peg-IFN+RBV (15 patients, controls) [24]. Patients in the first group obtained a significantly higher rate of complete and sustained response, without increase of adverse events.

In the second study, a prospective, nonrandomised cohort study of 93 patients, Saadoun et al. found that combined therapy reduced the clinical remission time, improved renal response rate, and led to higher rates of cryoglobulin clearance and clonal VH1-69+B cell suppression than Peg-IFN+RBV alone [25].

In a recent letter, Ignatova and coworkers described 18 patients who underwent AT with Peg-IFN+RBV. In six subjects, RTX was administered 1 month before AT in order to treat severe MC. Data of this report confirm that AT increases the relapse-free survival compared with standard immunosuppression or RTX alone and that combined RTX/AT schedule can be useful in moderate/severe MC [26, 27].

4. Discussion

Patients' response to AT has been shown to be lower in HCV patients with MC than without, after both double (Peg-IFN+RBV) and BOC-based triple therapy [15, 28]. The reasons for a lower propensity to eradicate HCV are unknown but are possibly related to a stronger involvement of lymphatic cells (especially B-cell) by the infection in MC [1] leading to more consistent viral reservoirs and, when using DAAs, a higher risk of viral mutations.

The usefulness and safety of RTX in MC have been clearly shown in numerous studies, including also patients with advanced liver disease [11, 21, 29–31], even if most patients treated with RTX-monotherapy experienced vasculitis relapse following B-cell recovery [23].

Combined therapy with RTX plus Peg-IFN+RBV, according to a sequential or contemporary scheme, has previously provided an improvement of clinical response and higher cryoglobulin clearance than Peg-IFN+RBV, in the absence of increasing adverse events [23–25, 32]. The pathogenetic bases could be linked to the association of cooperating mechanisms, like the viral eradication and the depletion of the pathological B-cell clones. Furthermore, the B-cell depletion could favor the elimination of a viral reservoir. On the other hand, the clinical improvement obtained with RTX treatment could make eligible to AT patients previously not eligible.

Interestingly, in our previous study on 35 HCV chronically infected subjects, the only MCS patient who persistently responded to treatment was the one excluded from the comparative analysis owing to a recent treatment with RTX [15].

In the same study we showed a sudden decrease in cryocrit together with the rapid decrease of viremia due to the introduction of BOC, stressing the role exerted by viral replication in MC pathogenesis [15].

In conclusion, we are reporting here the first description of a safe and highly efficacious combination of RTX and BOC-based AT in a patient with cryoglobulinemic vasculitis. The persistent response was both virological and clinical. Our previous observation of a low rate of virological response in MCS patients may increase the interest of this report which seems to agree with the hypothesis of a key role played by B cells as HCV reservoirs. Such an observation appears to confirm the positive effect of a combined therapeutic approach also when using DAA-dependent AT.

These results were, however, obtained in a single case and further studies based on significant numbers of patients are needed in order to confirm our observations in the specific setting of patients with HCV-related MC.

Conflict of Interests

All the authors declare no conflict of interests.

Acknowledgments

This work was supported by grants from the "Istituto Toscano Tumori" (ITT) and "Ente Cassa di Risparmio di Firenze"; Laura Gragnani is supported by a 2015 fellowship "Fondazione Umberto Veronesi"; Elisa Fognani is supported by an AIRC fellowship.

References

[1] A. L. Zignego, L. Gragnani, C. Giannini, and G. Laffi, "The hepatitis C virus infection as a systemic disease," *Internal and Emergency Medicine*, vol. 7, supplement 3, pp. S201–S208, 2012.

[2] A. L. Zignego, C. Giannini, and L. Gragnani, "HCV and lymphoproliferation," *Clinical and Developmental Immunology*, vol. 2012, Article ID 980942, 8 pages, 2012.

[3] L. Bonomo, M. Casato, A. Afeltra, and D. Caccavo, "Treatment of idiopathic mixed cryoglobulinemia with alpha interferon," *The American Journal of Medicine*, vol. 83, no. 4, pp. 726–730, 1987.

[4] C. Ferri, E. Marzo, G. Longombardo et al., "Interferon-α in mixed cryoglobulinemia patients: a randomized, crossover-controlled trial," *Blood*, vol. 81, no. 5, pp. 1132–1136, 1993.

[5] R. Misiani, P. Bellavita, D. Fenili et al., "Interferon alfa-2a therapy in cryoglobulinemia associated with hepatitis C virus," *The New England Journal of Medicine*, vol. 330, no. 11, pp. 751–756, 1994.

[6] V. M. Lauta and A. de Sangro, "Long-term results regarding the use of recombinant interferon alpha-2b in the treatment of II type mixed essential cryoglobulinemia," *Medical Oncology*, vol. 12, no. 4, pp. 223–230, 1995.

[7] P. Cacoub, L. Gragnani, C. Comarmond, and A. L. Zignego, "Extrahepatic manifestations of chronic hepatitis C virus infection," *Digestive and Liver Disease*, vol. 46, pp. S165–S173, 2014.

[8] A. L. Zignego, L. Gragnani, A. Piluso et al., "Virus-driven autoimmunity and lymphoproliferation: the example of HCV infection," *Expert Review of Clinical Immunology*, vol. 11, no. 1, pp. 15–31, 2015.

[9] F. Zaja, S. de Vita, C. Mazzaro et al., "Efficacy and safety of rituximab in type II mixed cryoglobulinemia," *Blood*, vol. 101, no. 10, pp. 3827–3834, 2003.

[10] M. Pietrogrande, S. de Vita, A. L. Zignego et al., "Recommendations for the management of mixed cryoglobulinemia syndrome in hepatitis C virus-infected patients," *Autoimmunity Reviews*, vol. 10, no. 8, pp. 444–454, 2011.

[11] S. De Vita, L. Quartuccio, M. Isola et al., "A randomized controlled trial of rituximab for the treatment of severe cryoglobulinemic vasculitis," *Arthritis and Rheumatism*, vol. 64, no. 3, pp. 843–853, 2012.

[12] European Association for the Study of the Liver, "EASL clinical practice guidelines: management of hepatitis C virus infection," *Journal of Hepatology*, vol. 55, no. 2, pp. 245–264, 2011.

[13] F. Poordad, J. McCone Jr., B. R. Bacon et al., "Boceprevir for untreated chronic HCV genotype 1 infection," *The New England Journal of Medicine*, vol. 364, no. 13, pp. 1195–1206, 2011.

[14] I. M. Jacobson, J. G. McHutchison, G. Dusheiko et al., "Telaprevir for previously untreated chronic hepatitis C virus infection," *The New England Journal of Medicine*, vol. 364, no. 25, pp. 2405–2416, 2011.

[15] L. Gragnani, A. Fabbrizzi, E. Triboli et al., "Triple antiviral therapy in hepatitis C virus infection with or without mixed cryoglobulinaemia: a prospective, controlled pilot study," *Digestive and Liver Disease*, vol. 46, no. 9, pp. 833–837, 2014.

[16] D. Saadoun, M. R. Rigon, V. Thibault et al., "Peg-IFNα/ribavirin/protease inhibitor combination in hepatitis C virus associated mixed cryoglobulinemia vasculitis: results at week 24," *Annals of the Rheumatic Diseases*, vol. 73, no. 5, pp. 831–837, 2014.

[17] S. De Nicola, A. Aghemo, M. R. Campise et al., "Telaprevir in a patient with chronic hepatitis C and cryoglobulinemic glomerulonephritis," *Antiviral Therapy*, vol. 19, no. 5, pp. 527–531, 2014.

[18] D. Saadoun, M. Resche Rigon, S. Pol et al., "PegIFNα/ribavirin/protease inhibitor combination in severe hepatitis C virus-associated mixed cryoglobulinemia vasculitis," *Journal of Hepatology*, vol. 62, no. 1, pp. 24–30, 2015.

[19] S. De Vita, F. Soldano, M. Isola et al., "Preliminary classification criteria for the cryoglobulinaemic vasculitis," *Annals of the Rheumatic Diseases*, vol. 70, no. 7, pp. 1183–1190, 2011.

[20] A. Piluso, C. Giannini, E. Fognani et al., "Value of IL28B genotyping in patients with HCV-related mixed cryoglobulinemia: results of a large, prospective study," *Journal of Viral Hepatitis*, vol. 20, no. 4, pp. e107–e114, 2013.

[21] A. Petrarca, L. Rigacci, P. Caini et al., "Safety and efficacy of rituximab in patients with hepatitis C virus-related mixed cryoglobulinemia and severe liver disease," *Blood*, vol. 116, no. 3, pp. 335–342, 2010.

[22] D. Saadoun, M. Resche-Rigon, D. Sene, L. Perard, A. Karras, and P. Cacoub, "Rituximab combined with Peg-interferon-ribavirin in refractory hepatitis C virus-associated cryoglobulinaemia vasculitis," *Annals of the Rheumatic Diseases*, vol. 67, no. 10, pp. 1431–1436, 2008.

[23] B. Terrier, D. Saadoun, D. Sène et al., "Efficacy and tolerability of rituximab with or without PEGylated interferon alfa-2b plus ribavirin in severe hepatitis C virus-related vasculitis: a long-term followup study of thirty-two patients," *Arthritis & Rheumatism*, vol. 60, no. 8, pp. 2531–2540, 2009.

[24] F. Dammacco, F. A. Tucci, G. Lauletta et al., "Pegylated interferon-α, ribavirin, and rituximab combined therapy of hepatitis C virus-related mixed cryoglobulinemia: a long-term study," *Blood*, vol. 116, no. 3, pp. 343–353, 2010.

[25] D. Saadoun, M. R. Rigon, D. Sene et al., "Rituximab plus Peg-interferon-alpha/ribavirin compared with Peg-interferon-alpha/ribavirin in hepatitis C-related mixed cryoglobulinemia," *Blood*, vol. 116, no. 3, pp. 326–334, 504–505, 2010.

[26] T. Ignatova, O. Chernova, P. Novikov, and S. Moiseev, "HCV-associated cryoglobulinaemic vasculitis: triple/dual antiviral treatment and/or rituximab?" *Annals of the Rheumatic Diseases*, vol. 73, no. 9, article e58, 2014.

[27] D. Saadoun and P. Cacoub, "HCV-associated cryoglobulinemic vasculitis: triple/dual antiviral treatment and/or rituximab? Reply to the comment by Ignatova et al," *Annals of the Rheumatic Diseases*, vol. 73, no. 9, article e59, 2014.

[28] L. Gragnani, E. Fognani, A. Piluso et al., "Long-term effect of HCV eradication in patients with mixed cryoglobulinemia: A prospective, controlled, open-label, cohort study," *Hepatology*, 2015.

[29] F. Zaja, D. Russo, G. Fuga, F. Patriarca, A. Ermacora, and M. Baccarani, "Rituximab for the treatment of type II mixed cryoglobulinemia," *Haematologica*, vol. 84, no. 12, pp. 1157–1158, 1999.

[30] D. Sansonno, V. de Re, G. Lauletta, F. A. Tucci, M. Boiocchi, and F. Dammacco, "Monoclonal antibody treatment of mixed cryoglobulinemia resistant to interferon α with an anti-CD20," *Blood*, vol. 101, no. 10, pp. 3818–3826, 2003.

[31] C. Ferri, P. Cacoub, C. Mazzaro et al., "Treatment with rituximab in patients with mixed cryoglobulinemia syndrome: results of multicenter cohort study and review of the literature," *Autoimmunity Reviews*, vol. 11, no. 1, pp. 48–55, 2011.

[32] E. Mauro, M. Pedata, A. Ermacora, and C. Mazzaro, "An additional line of therapy with pegylated interferon and ribavirin after rituximab in a patient with hepatitis C virus-related mixed cryoglobulinaemia and indolent non-Hodgkin's lymphoma previously treated with interferon," *Blood Transfusion*, vol. 10, no. 1, pp. 101–103, 2012.

14

Infectious and Noninfectious Granulomatosis in Patient with Multiple Sclerosis: Diagnostic Dilemmas and Followup

Jelena Paovic,[1] **Predrag Paovic,**[1] **and Vojislav Sredovic**[2]

[1] *University Eye Clinic, Clinical Center of Serbia, Pasterova 2, 11000 Belgrade, Serbia*
[2] *Primary Health Care Center, Jove Negusevica 5, 22140 Pecinci, Serbia*

Correspondence should be addressed to Jelena Paovic; maliceda@eunet.rs

Academic Editors: A. M. Mansour and A. Vojdani

Patient was followed up over the course of 30 years. In 1978, after severe systemic infection followed by fever, pulmonary edema, and numerous neurological manifestations, patient was differentially diagnosed with apoplectic form of multiple sclerosis (MS), which was confirmed a year later via neurological and MRI findings. Approximately 20 years following the initial attack, sarcoidosis was diagnosed during the regular preoperative procedures required for cataract surgery. As consequence of lower immune system, infectious granulomatosis in form of pulmonary tuberculosis developed. Ophthalmological findings revealed bilateral retrobulbar neuritis (RBN) approximately six years after initial attack. This developed into total uveitis with retinal periphlebitis and anterior granulomatous uveitis—all of which are clinically similar in both MS and sarcoidosis.

1. Introduction

Sarcoidosis and multiple sclerosis (MS) belong to a group of systemic vasculitides.

Besides trauma, MS as chronic inflammation with demyelination and scarring is the most frequent cause of neurologic disability. It occurs more commonly in young middle aged females. MS, disease disseminated in time and space, is characterized by frequent recidivism. If full recovery has not been achieved, definitive neurological deficits persist. During the course of the disease, magnetic resonance imaging (MRI) reveals presence of demyelinating plaques, while liquor analysis shows oligoclonal response [1–4]. Lesions that occur in MS are characterized by perivenous cuffing and tissue infiltration by mononuclear cells (predominantly T lymphocytes and macrophages). Demyelination appears as disease progresses and as macrophages and microglial cells form the myelin debris. Due to proliferation of astrocytes, scarring occurs. Damage of myelin sheet can in most cases be connected to previous viral infection. It is believed that stress is also one of the important triggering factors [5–8].

Initial symptoms of the disease are muscle weakness in one or more limbs, blurred vision (secondary to optic neuritis), sensory disturbances, ataxia, diplopia, and so forth.

However, no clinical signs or findings from diagnostic procedures are unique to MS [9, 10].

Ocular manifestations such as retrobulbar neuritis (RBN), retinal vasculitis (RV), and anterior granulomatous uveitis occur as part of MS. According to some authors, RV (periphlebitis) is a primary inflammation subsequent to vitreal inflammation and snow bank formation [3, 11].

Sarcoidosis is a multisystemic, granulomatous disease of unknown etiology. As of yet, no incriminating antigens have been proven. However, there exists an autoimmune disorder which can be manifested as noncaseating granuloma in all organs and tissue types. Due to its similarity to tuberculosis (TBC), a granulomatous infective disease characterized by caseating granulomas, many authors suggest that *Mycobacterium tuberculosis* or *Propionibacterium acnes* can influence appearance of sarcoidosis [12–14].

There are three forms of sarcoidosis: acute, subacute, and chronic. Most common systemic manifestation is pulmonary sarcoidosis, which can be manifested in four stages, that is, hilar adenopathy, pulmonary parenchyma involvement, interstitial lung changes, and chronic pulmonary fibrosis. Other forms of sarcoidosis, according to frequency of occurrence, are skin, bones and joint, mucosa, and salivary gland. Neurosarcoidosis (presence of granulomas in central nervous system (CNS)) can be manifested similarly to demyelinating diseases [15–18].

Ocular sarcoidosis occurs in 20–25% of cases who have systemic sarcoidosis. All structures of the eye can be involved, that is, cornea (dry-eye, marginal corneal infiltrates), anterior uvea (anterior granulomatous uveitis similar in characteristics to MS, viral or tuberculous anterior uveitis), and posterior segment (intermediate uveitis with both peripheral basal exudates and RV/periphlebitis) [3, 19].

There are no major differences in clinical manifestations on the eye fundus between MS and sarcoidosis in their developed states, and one can say that there is a certain degree of mimicry between the two. Intermediate uveitis and RV are ocular manifestations which occur as part of both MS and sarcoidosis but have different pathophysiological mechanisms and thus present a differential, diagnostic problem when ocular manifestations are concerned. Another differential diagnostic problem occurs due to similar appearance of inflammation on the anterior segment in a form of anterior granulomatous uveitis with mutton-fat precipitates and fibrinous exudates. There is, however, a major distinction between MS and sarcoidosis in that multifocal granulomatous posterior uveitis appears in sarcoidosis, whereas initially bilateral RBN occurs as part of MS. In both cases, late stages of disease are manifested with RV.

Ocular complications on the anterior segment in both MS and sarcoidosis are secondary glaucoma and complicated cataract. Band keratopathy is one of the complications which are characteristic for sarcoidosis alone. Possible complications on the posterior eye segment are macular edema (ME), disc atrophy, and peripheral retinal ischemia with retinal breaks and retinoschisis as a consequence. We are of the opinion that ME always occurs as complication of retinal periphlebitis, while certain authors suggest that ME occurs due to RBN [20]. In case of MS, disc atrophy can be consequence of RBN as primary ocular manifestation.

Importance of this case report lies in the fact that there are three disorders involved in case of one patient. Two of them are systemic infectious and noninfectious granulomatous diseases and one is demyelinating in nature. All three have been proven via vast clinical examinations, numerous laboratory tests, various imaging techniques (X-ray, MSCT, and MRI), histological analysis (lung biopsy), and ophthalmological examinations in one patient followedup for over 30 years (in the period from 1978 until today).

2. Case Report

2.1. 1978. Twenty-one-year old female patient was admitted to an emergency room with clinical signs of lung edema and circulatory collapse. She also had strong headache and was vomiting. Fifteen days previous to this, this female patient had suffered from strong headache, fatigue, nausea, and instability while walking. Upon admission there was no verbal communication established between her and the medical staff, and contact was highly febrile. She had problems breathing (wheezing), and was coughing up foamy, bloody, yellowish/greenish mucus. All symptoms were highly suggestive of acute pulmonary edema.

She also had tachycardia and neurological signs: right central facial palsy, left facial hyperesthesia; nystagmus; heterotopia; anisocoric pupils; asymmetric pallet and tongue deviating to the left; nasal speech; problems whilst swallowing suggestive of microlesions of the brain stem. MRI of brain and lumbar puncture revealed no pathological findings.

Laboratory analysis showed high white blood cell count, glucose level, and transaminase. Results of immunological tests for collagen and viral diseases were performed and at normal levels.

Audiometric examination pointed toward central vestibular neuritis. Ophthalmological findings were normal.

Differential diagnosis was apoplectic form of multiple sclerosis (MS).

Patient underwent treatment for pulmonary edema and tachycardia (diuretics, bronchospasmolytics, cardiotonics, corticosteroids, and antibiotics). Following treatment commencement suggestive of full recovery, there were however certain clinical signs as a repercussion of primary attack which had occurred in 1978. These repercussions were neurological in nature such as mild left facial hyperesthesia: left pallet and lip paresis; bladder incoordination; speech problems which were indicative of damage of the myelin sheath.

2.2. 1979. Patient returned to the emergency room with neurological symptoms similar to those she had one year earlier, but in lower intensity. She was examined by neurologist who ordered MRI and laboratory tests to exclude or confirm systemic collagen diseases or MS. MRI findings showed demyelinating changes for the first time. According to all examinations, demyelinating changes are confirmed (MS was diagnosed), while collagen diseases are excluded. She underwent systemic corticosteroid therapy which resulted in partial recovery of neurological signs.

2.3. 1979–1984. In this period there was no reactivation of primary disease and patient went on with normal every day activities. Two years following pregnancy, clinical signs started to appear again and subsequent ocular manifestations were evident.

2.4. 1984. Ocular manifestations such as painful eye movements, acute decrease of visual acuity (VA) started to appear. Complete ophthalmological examination was performed.

In April, patient's VA had slightly decreased: right eye VA from 1.0 to 0.7 and left eye VA from 1.0 to 0.9. Bilateral RBN was diagnosed. Uveitis was not found. Patient received pulse doses of corticosteroid agent (repeated doses of metilprednisolone, 1000 mg, intravenous).

In October second lumbar puncture was performed due to confirming diagnosis of MS. Intrathecal synthesis antibodies were not confirmed.

Six months after diagnosis of RBN, first bilateral inflammatory changes of uveal tissue in form of total uveitis were diagnosed—proteins and cellular Tyndall in anterior chamber and vitreous, inflamed retinal blood vessels (mostly veins), papillitis, and macular (ME) and retinal edema (RE). According to all these ocular manifestations, disease was diagnosed as neurouveitis. Treatment consisted of systemic and local application of corticosteroid agents.

2.5. 1989.

After 5 years of remission, patient was admitted to the neurology ward because of transitory speech problems, weakness of right hand, and urine incontinency. MRI was performed once again and showed diffused, high intensity, bilateral, periventricular, subcortical, and deep changes in white matter of CNS. NMR finding in conjunction with neurological signs indicated that there was MS present (approximately 11 years following an initial diagnosis when it was assumed that the patient had apoplectic form of MS).

Ophthalmological manifestations were persistent, recurrent, bilateral uveitis, ME (as consequence of RV), and disc atrophy (as consequence of RBN) which lead to decrease of visual acuity. Once again, patient received repeated pulse doses of corticosteroids.

2.6. 1989–2003.

During this period, patient did not consult neurologist. She had had, however, regular consultations with an ophthalmologist regarding uveitis.

2.7. 2003.

It was noted that besides other symptoms patient still had some speech impairment; paresthesias; impaired muscle coordination; from time to time loss of sensation; impaired vision; urinary incontinence and additional tests were performed in order to once again check the etiology of the disease. Immunological tests for collagen and viral diseases were repeated and only antinuclear antibody-HEp-2 test was positive.

Progressions of uveitis lead to development of bilateral complicated cataract.

2.8. 2004.

While undergoing tests required for cataract surgery it was suspected that the patient might be suffering from sarcoidosis. Among other tests, chest X-ray revealed fibrinous, bilateral, lung changes and subsequently granulomatosis and chronic lung sarcoidosis of 3rd degree. Angiotensin converting enzyme (ACE) was noted to be 68 U/L (normal range 8–52 U/L).

Biopsy finding of bronchial mucosa showed pathophysiological changes in lamina propria (basement membrane) in form of small granulomas consisting of few changed histiocytes, lymphocyte, individual Langerhans type giant cells, plasma cells eosinophils, and granulocytes. Necrosis has not been noted. Mild interstitial fibrosis was present in the pulmonary/lung parenchyma typical for noncaseating granulomatosis (sarcoidosis). Tuberculosis (TB) was excluded.

Due to presence and confirmation of pulmonary sarcoidosis, CNS MRI was repeated in order to investigate neurosarcoidosis. MRI revealed diffused, multifocal lesions which affected both cerebral hemispheres and cerebellum (its' white matter was depicted). These changes were assumed to be demyelinating in nature as there was presence of consecutive, second degree, global, white matter atrophy. Active lesions or manifestations of neurosarcoidosis were not found. Seeing that liquor test was negative and that there

was a benign clinical picture but that there was evidence of demyelination, secondary, CNS, demyelinating vasculitis was suspected.

As part of preoperative management, patient received local and systemic corticosteroid drugs after which bilateral phacoemulsification cataract surgery was performed.

2.9. 2004–2009.

During this period patient consulted pulmonologist regarding lung sarcoidosis, and ophthalmologist regarding ocular manifestations and received systemic as well as local treatments as per protocol (corticosteroid and/cytostatic drugs). No neurological consultations were performed during this period.

Over the course of this period, patient experienced recurrent bilateral uveitis and thus as a consequence had secondary cataract and posterior capsulotomy was performed (Figures 1 and 2). There were repeated cycles of RV as well (Figures 3 and 4). Periphlebitis occurred more frequently than periarteritis. ME and epiretinal membranes appeared as complications of RV (Figures 5 and 6). Repeated sub-Tenon's injections of triamcinolone acetonide (40 mg every 3-4 weeks) were used in treatment of these complications (Figure 7).

2.10. 2009.

In order to confirm sarcoidosis extensive testing was performed among which were chest X-ray and MSCT scan. MSCT imaging showed intense condensation of pulmonary tissue of the right top lobule in form of mixed reticular/nodular type with pronounced fibrosis of rarer, nodular fields predominantly peripherally located. Peribronchial fibrosis, with hilo lateral as well as hilo apical, multidirectional, distribution was noted. Partially wet necrotic lymphoid nodules were present in both the subcarinal right side of mediastinum and along the spine. Two laboratory readings showed increased levels of ACE in serum (86 U/L, 65 U/L, resp.).

2.11. 2010.

During the course of the year, patient exhibited neurological problems, while towards the end of the year she noted blood in sputum which led to further testing for sarcoidosis. ACE serum level was 68 U/L. As there were signs indicative of neurosarcoidosis, MRI was repeated and revealed presence of consequential, supratentorial lesions of open etiology, which could differentially point towards periventricular leukoencephalopathy. Due to this, neurosarcoidosis was not confirmed, but it rather stayed as differential diagnosis.

2.12. 2011.

Due to additional clinical signs indicative of pulmonary tuberculosis (TBC), additional tests were performed. Microscopic sputum examination confirmed presence of acid-fast bacilli. Laboratory tests showed high blood sedimentation rate, CRP, and leukocyte count. Based on previous results and current examinations, patient was diagnosed with pulmonary TBC and underwent anti-TBC treatment (as per protocol). Initial treatment during the period of 2 months consisted of isoniazid, rifampicin, pyrazinamide, and ethambutol. For the next four months isoniazid and rifampicin were applied. Patients liver and kidney functions

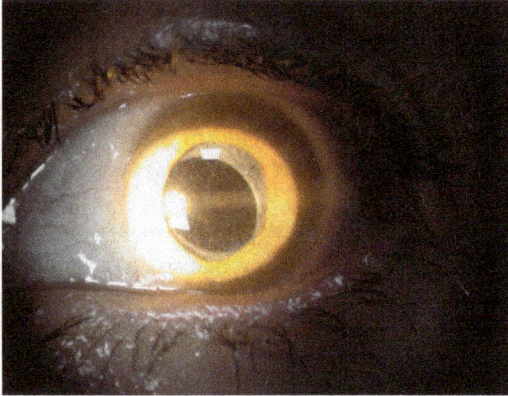

FIGURE 1: Pseudophakia, secondary cataract, and anterior granulomatous uveitis in MS (right eye).

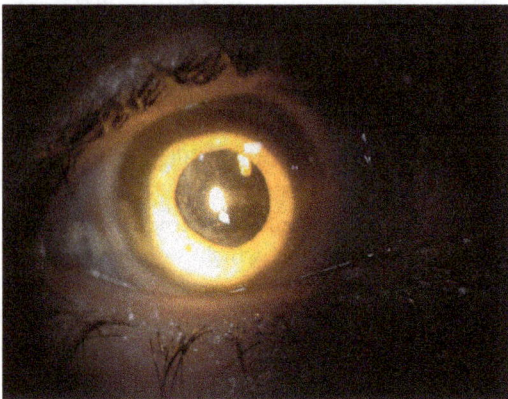

FIGURE 2: Pseudophakia, secondary cataract, and anterior granulomatous uveitis in MS (left eye).

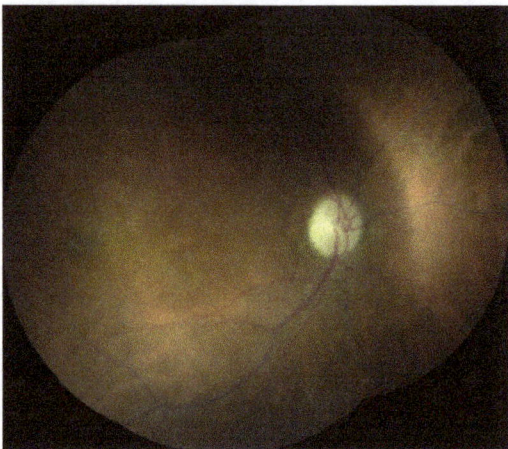

FIGURE 3: Retinal vasculitis, disc atrophy, and macular edema in patient with MS (right eye).

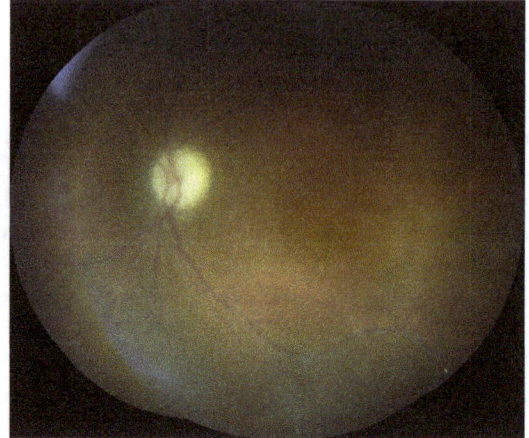

FIGURE 4: Retinal vasculitis, disc atrophy, and macular edema in patient with MS (left eye).

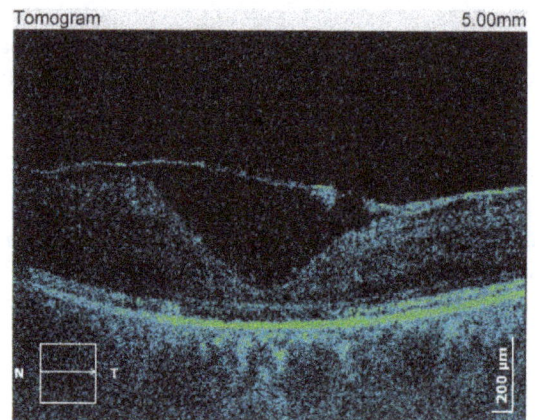

FIGURE 5: Macular edema and epiretinal membrane as complication of periphlebitis in patient with MS (right eye).

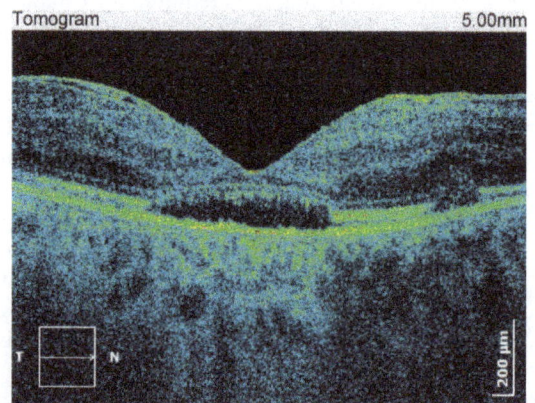

FIGURE 6: Macular edema and epiretinal membrane as complication of periphlebitis in patient with MS (left eye).

were monitored regularly during this period. Within three months, remission of the disease was noted.

From onset of the disease until today, ophthalmological examinations revealed no TBC ocular manifestations present.

2.13. 2013. In August of this year, due to exacerbation of old and appearance of new neurological symptoms (such as uncoordinated movements), patient was admitted to neurology ward and subjected to further examinations. Latest MRI images showed no new changes as compared to previous findings from 2010. Patient was released from hospital with intent to return in 3-4 months in order to undergo further diagnostic testing. During this period she was advised to

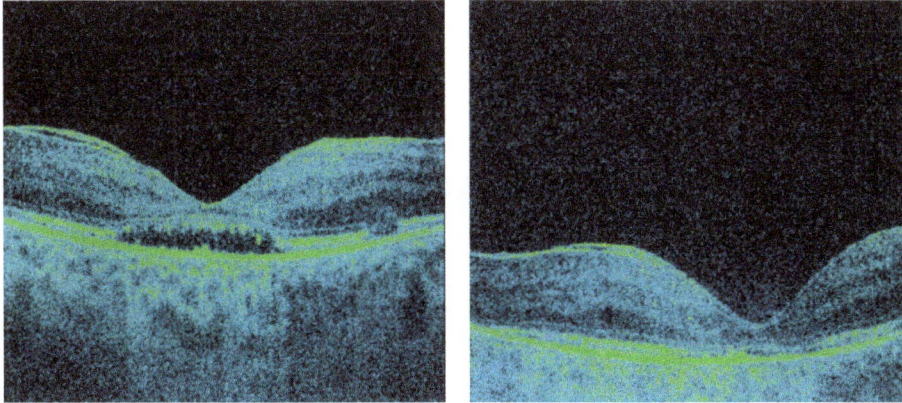

FIGURE 7: Macular edema, subretinal fluid, and epiretinal membrane treated with sub-Tenon's triamcinolone acetonide injections in patient with retinal vasculitis in MS (followup).

monitor her physical condition and take therapy required for circulatory disease (Ginkgo biloba extract, 40 mg every 8 hours) and spasmolytic drugs (tolterodine tartrate, 2 mg every 12 hours).

3. Discussion

This case report is indicative of a complex diagnostic problem which can present itself in the field of medicine. Here we have a case where the onset of the disease was acute in nature and in a manner that is typical for a systemic infection that led to substantial damage of various CNS structures and a suspicion of apoplectic form of MS.

Even though the first (initial) diagnostic procedures such as MRI did not fully prove demyelinating changes, neurologically persistent changes and later confirmation of demyelinating plaque all point towards the fact that the patient had MS from the very beginning. Demyelinating optic neuritis is often a herald of MS but is only one of many possible neuroophthalmologic abnormalities which may occur. Demyelinating white matter lesions that can be present in the brain MRI at the time of presentation of optic neuritis are the strongest predictor for development of clinically definite MS. In most cases with optic neuritis there are white matter lesions that are present and are consistent with this diagnosis. In favor of a MS is also the fact that there was RBN present at the time and this is one of the most common and amongst the first ocular manifestation of MS. It is possible that one of the pathogens, most probably of viral etiology, caused damage to the myelin sheath and led to development of the demyelination.

Few years later pulmonary sarcoidosis which has been proven via X-ray, MSCT and has histological proof to back it up cannot be connected to MS, but it can, however, be connected to previous systemic infection. So, this poses a differentially diagnostic problem. Namely, bearing in mind that sarcoidosis and MS have similar MRI and neurological manifestations, and that there have been certain CNS symptoms noted, was there actually neurosarcoidosis present as part of systemic sarcoidosis at the time?

During the course of the disease, pulmonary TB developed and was proven via numerous laboratory tests and microscopic analysis, only to be resolved six months following its initial appearance and prescribed treatment. Such outcome could be attributed to the fact that there was a decline in patients' immune response due to a lengthy immunosuppressive therapy consisting of various corticosteroids and cytostatic drugs. Besides diagnostic and differentially diagnostic issues which have arisen in this case, a particular problem lies in application of treatment between the two diseases. In particular we have noninfectious granulomatosis, where primary therapy consists of corticosteroids, and infectious granulomatosis, where primary therapy consists of agents belonging to a completely opposite group of medicaments (noncorticosteroid therapy). Problem lies in the fact that corticosteroids are contraindicative in treatment of TBC. Thus it is particularly interesting that there is incidence of both infective and noninfective granulomatosis present at the same time in the same individual.

Ophthalmic assessment was very interesting in itself and suggested that the disease began as bilateral RBN followed by optic disc atrophy and a later development of neurouveitis, all typical for infectious diseases and of demyelinating processes. Later on, the main ocular, clinical manifestation was in form of bilateral RV (predominantly periphlebitis) as well as anterior granulomatous uveitis (which can develop as part of both MS and sarcoidosis).

Clinical signs are suggestive of the fact that there was an inflammation caused by systemic infection or autoimmune process in the eye where the pathogenic reagent was a trigger factor, whereas inflammation of the optic disc and retinal blood vessels points towards a demyelinating process (a fact which was proven correct via an MRI imaging performed in 1989, which was nearly 11 years following the initial attack).

Recurrent and progressive course of disease has resulted in severe complications some of which are in form of a complicated cataract (which was operated on) and ME, all of which seem to respond well to local (sub-Tenon's injections of triamcinolone acetonide) and systemic (mainly corticosteroid) therapy. Patient's history as well as clinical signs of the disease represents a major diagnostic and therapeutic challenge requiring multidisciplinary approach and frequent monitoring.

Until today, in this particular case one cannot say with 100% certainty that ocular and other manifestations are typical signs of MS and sarcoidosis but are rather a possible consequence of a systemic infection which had started in 1978 and developed into these, previously mentioned diseases.

Conflict of Interests

The authors declare that there is no conflict of interests regarding the publication of this paper.

Acknowledgment

The authors of this paper would like to give special acknowledgment to Professor Dr. Anka Stanojević-Paović, the chief medical officer at Uvea Center, for the scientific and professional help and support that she has provided.

References

[1] C. H. Polman, S. C. Reingold, B. Banwell et al., "Diagnostic criteria for multiple sclerosis: 2010 revisions to the McDonald criteria," *Annals of Neurology*, vol. 69, no. 2, pp. 292–302, 2011.

[2] J. Graves and L. J. Balcer, "Eye disorders in patients with multiple sclerosis: natural history and management," *Clinical Ophthalmology*, vol. 4, no. 1, pp. 1409–1422, 2010.

[3] L. Chen and L. K. Gordon, "Ocular manifestations of multiple sclerosis," *Current Opinion in Ophthalmology*, vol. 16, no. 5, pp. 315–320, 2005.

[4] A. Stanojevic-Paovic, "Chapter II," in *Uveitis*, A. Stanojevic-Paovic, Ed., pp. 105–144, School of Medicine, University of Belgrade, Belgrade, Serbia, 2008.

[5] A. Langer-Gould, K. B. Albers, S. K. van den Eeden, and L. M. Nelson, "Autoimmune diseases prior to the diagnosis of multiple sclerosis: a population-based case-control study," *Multiple Sclerosis*, vol. 16, no. 7, pp. 855–861, 2010.

[6] J. P. Campbell, H. A. Leder, Y. J. Sepah et al., "Wide-field retinal imaging in the management of noninfectious posterior Uveitis," *American Journal of Ophthalmology*, vol. 154, no. 5, pp. 908–911, 2012.

[7] K. Turaka and J. S. Bryan, "Does fingolimod in multiple sclerosis patients cause macular edema?" *Journal of Neurology*, vol. 259, no. 2, pp. 386–388, 2012.

[8] N. Jain and M. T. Bhatti, "Fingolimod-associated macular edema: incidence, detection, and management," *Neurology*, vol. 78, no. 9, pp. 672–680, 2012.

[9] K. M. Galetta, J. Graves, L. S. Talman et al., "Visual pathway axonal loss in benign multiple sclerosis: a longitudinal study," *Journal of Neuro-Ophthalmology*, vol. 32, no. 2, pp. 116–123, 2012.

[10] L. S. Talman, E. R. Bisker, D. J. Sackel et al., "Longitudinal study of vision and retinal nerve fiber layer thickness in multiple sclerosis," *Annals of Neurology*, vol. 67, no. 6, pp. 749–760, 2010.

[11] J. M. Gelfand, R. Nolan, D. M. Schwartz, J. Graves, and A. J. Green, "Microcystic macular oedema in multiple sclerosis is associated with disease severity," *Brain*, vol. 135, part 6, pp. 1786–1793, 2012.

[12] A. D. Birnbaum, F. S. Oh, A. Chakrabarti, H. H. Tessler, and D. A. Goldstein, "Clinical features and diagnostic evaluation of biopsy-proven ocular sarcoidosis," *Archives of Ophthalmology*, vol. 129, no. 4, pp. 409–413, 2011.

[13] C. P. Herbort, N. A. Rao, M. Mochizuki et al., "International criteria for the diagnosis of ocular sarcoidosis: results of the first international workshop on ocular sarcoidosis (IWOS)," *Ocular Immunology and Inflammation*, vol. 17, no. 3, pp. 160–169, 2009.

[14] G. W. Hunninghake, U. Costabel, M. Ando et al., "ATS/ERS/WASOG statement on sarcoidosis. American Thoracic Society/European Respiratory Society World Association of Sarcoidosis and other Granulomatous Disorders," *Sarcoidosis, Vasculitis and Diffuse Lung Diseases*, vol. 16, no. 2, pp. 149–173, 1999.

[15] R. P. Baughman, A. S. Teirstein, M. A. Judson et al., "Clinical characteristics of patients in a case control study of sarcoidosis," *American Journal of Respiratory and Critical Care Medicine*, vol. 164, no. 10 I, pp. 1885–1889, 2001.

[16] K. Babu, R. Kini, R. Mehta, M. P. Abraham, D. Subbakrishna, and K. R. Murthy, "Clinical profile of ocular sarcoidosis in a South Indian patient population," *Ocular Immunology and Inflammation*, vol. 18, no. 5, pp. 362–369, 2010.

[17] M. Evans, O. Sharma, L. LaBree, R. E. Smith, and N. A. Rao, "Differences in clinical findings between Caucasians and African Americans with biopsy-proven sarcoidosis," *Ophthalmology*, vol. 114, no. 2, pp. 325–333, 2007.

[18] S. R. Boyd, S. Young, and S. Lightman, "Immunopathology of the noninfectious posterior and intermediate Uveitides," *Survey of Ophthalmology*, vol. 46, no. 3, pp. 209–233, 2001.

[19] E. E. Lower, J. P. Broderick, T. G. Brott, and R. P. Baughman, "Diagnosis and management of neurological sarcoidosis," *Archives of Internal Medicine*, vol. 157, no. 16, pp. 1864–1868, 1997.

[20] B. M. Burkholder and J. P. Dunn, "Multiple Sclerosis-associated Uveitis," *Expert Review of Ophthalmology*, vol. 7, no. 6, pp. 587–594, 2012.

15

Immunodeficiency in a Child with Rapadilino Syndrome: A Case Report and Review of the Literature

M. M. G. Vollebregt,[1] A. Malfroot,[1] M. De Raedemaecker,[2] M. van der Burg,[3] and J. E. van der Werff ten Bosch[4]

[1]Department of Pediatrics, University Hospital Brussels, 1090 Brussels, Belgium
[2]Department of Genetics, University Hospital Brussels, 1090 Brussels, Belgium
[3]Department of Immunology, Erasmus MC, 3015 CN Rotterdam, Netherlands
[4]Department of Pediatric Hematology, Oncology and Immunology, University Hospital Brussels, 1090 Brussels, Belgium

Correspondence should be addressed to J. E. van der Werff ten Bosch; jvdwerff@uzbrussel.be

Academic Editor: Jiri Litzman

Rapadilino syndrome is a genetic disease characterized by a characteristic clinical tableau. It is caused by mutations in RECQL4 gene. Immunodeficiency is not described as a classical feature of the disease. We present a 2-year-old girl with Rapadilino syndrome with important lymphadenopathies and pneumonia due to disseminated *Mycobacterium lentiflavum* infection. An immunological work-up showed several unexpected abnormalities. Repeated blood samples showed severe lymphopenia. Immunophenotyping showed low T, B, and NK cells. No Treg cells were seen. T cell responses to stimulations were insufficient. The IL12/IL23 interferon gamma pathway was normal. Gamma globulin levels and vaccination responses were low. With this report, we aim to stress the importance of screening immunodeficiency in patients with RECQL4 mutations for immunodeficiency and the need to further research into its physiopathology.

1. Introduction

Rapadilino syndrome (RS) is a genetic disease with a characteristic clinical tableau. The name is an acronym standing for radial (hypo)aplasia, patellae (hypo)aplasia and cleft or highly arched palate, diarrhoea and dislocated joints, little size and limb malformation, and nose slender and normal intelligence [1]. Like Rothmund-Thomson syndrome (RTS) and Baller-Gerold syndrome (BGS), the syndrome is caused by mutations in *RECQL4* gene. This gene encodes a protein that plays a role in the initiation of DNA replication as well as in DNA repair. Immunodeficiency has not been described as a prominent clinical feature in any of the 3 syndromes. RTS is a rare autosomal recessively inherited genodermatosis with a heterogeneous clinical presentation. It is characterized by a characteristic facial rash appearing in infancy (poikiloderma), short stature, radial ray defects, variable degree of osteopenia, sparse scalp hair, eyelashes, and eyebrows, dental abnormalities, and cataract. Moreover, RTS

patients are at increased risk of cancer, especially osteosarcoma and nonmelanoma skin cancer, but also leukemia and a range of others tumors [2]. RTS is a very rare disease and reliable data on its prevalence are not available. To date, approximately 300 patients have been recorded in the medical literature [3]. BGS is characterized by a combination of coronal craniosynostosis, manifesting as abnormal shape of the skull (brachycephaly) with ocular proptosis and bulging forehead, and radial ray defect, manifesting as oligodactyly (reduction in number of digits), aplasia or hypoplasia of the thumb, and/or aplasia or hypoplasia of the radius. The prevalence of BGS is unknown; it is probably less than 1 : 1.000.000 [4].

We present a now 4-year-old girl diagnosed with RS presenting with significant lymphadenopathies and pneumonia due to disseminated *Mycobacterium lentiflavum* infection. An immunological work-up showed several unexpected abnormalities. The child was treated and the clinical condition

TABLE 1: Immunological work-up.

			Normal values
White blood cells	$4,7 \times 10^3/mm^3$		$4,0–10,0 \times 10^3/mm^3$
Neutrophils	$2,8 \times 10^3/mm^3$		$1,5–8,5 \times 10^3/mm^3$
Lymphocytes	$1,0 \times 10^3/mm^3$		$2,3–5,6 \times 10^3/mm^3$
Immunoglobulin G	2,5 g/L		4,0–11,0 g/L
Immunoglobulin A	1,01 g/L		0,1–1,6 g/L
Immunoglobulin M	0,75 g/L		0,5–1,8 g/L
CD3+	$411/mm^3$		$900–4500/mm^3$
CD4+	$279/mm^3$		$500–2400/mm^3$
CD4RA	$140/mm^3$		
CD4RO	$139/mm^3$		
CD8	$124/mm^3$		$300–1600/mm^3$
CD8RA	$52/mm^3$		
CD8RO	$72/mm^3$		
CD25+CD127−FoxP3+	0		
CD19	$84/mm^3$		$200–1300/mm^3$
CD3−CD16+CD56+	$5/mm^3$		$100–1000/mm^3$
Response of T cells to PHA	low		
	Before vaccination	After vaccination	Normal values
Anti-pneumococcal AB	<3 IE/mL	<3 IE/mL	>19/mL
Anti-tetanos AB	<0.01 IE/mL	0.1 IE/mL	>0.1 IE/mL
Anti-poliovirus AB	Absent	Present	
Anti-rubella AB	300 IE	—	Positive
Anti-mumps AB	Negative	—	Positive

gradually improved. We suggest screening children with RECQL4 mutations for immunodeficiency and stress the need for further research into its physiopathology.

2. Case Report

A 2-year-old girl was admitted because of severe lymphadenopathies. She had been diagnosed with RS at birth. No important infections occurred in the first years of life until these unexplained lymphadenopathies. Because an increased risk of lymphoma at a young age has been documented in patients with RS [6], a biopsy was taken, excluding a malignancy. For the 8 months that followed, the girl was lost to follow-up in our center, but she represented later that year with cough, fever, and dyspnea requiring oxygen. Lymphadenopathies persisted in all regions. There were no signs of hepatosplenomegaly. Chest X-ray showed mediastinal enlargement and bilateral infiltrates (Figure 1).

Cultures from bronchoalveolar lavage remained negative for bacteria, including mycobacteria. PCR for viruses (CMV, EBV) and mycoplasma were negative. Because a slight lymphopenia was observed in the routine blood sample, an immunological work-up was performed (Table 1). Hypogammaglobulinemia was observed. Antibodies against the received childhood vaccinations (pneumococcus, tetanus, rubella, polio, and hepatitis B) were all negative. Revaccination with Pneumo 23 and tetanus did not lead to an increase in the antibody titers. T cell numbers were

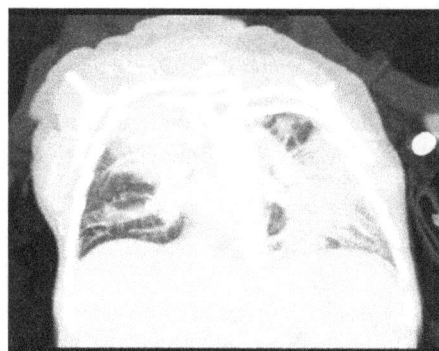

FIGURE 1: CT scan showing mediastinal enlargement and bilateral infiltrates.

low, with a slightly diminished function. The number of CD4+CD25+FoxP3+ regulatory T cells was remarkably low (Table 1). Switched memory B cells were slightly low according to the Euroclass criteria [7]. The number of double negative T cells, vitamin B12, and Fas mediated apoptosis were normal. The interferon gamma/interleukin 23 pathway was intact. Expression of IL-12 receptor beta 1 and IFN-gamma receptor expression were analysed by flow cytometry. The production of IFN-gamma was measured after stimulation of white blood cells with phytohaemagglutinin and staphylococcal enterotoxin B.

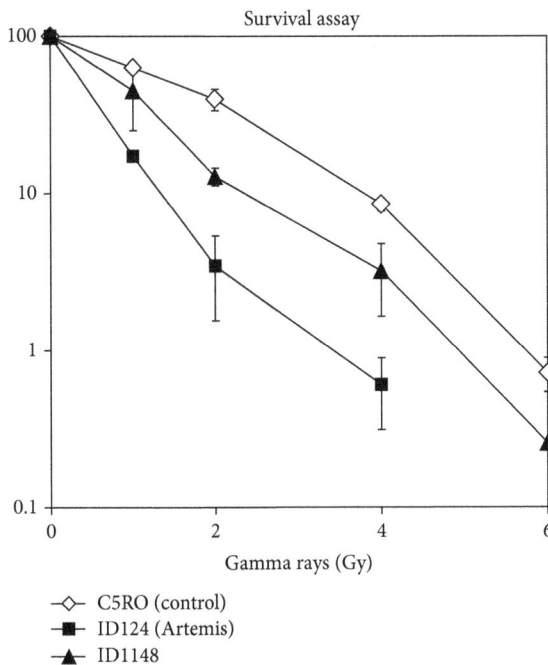

FIGURE 2: Radiosensitivity assay. Clonogenic survival assays with primary skin were performed as described in Noordzij et al., Blood 2003 [5]. In short, primary skin fibroblasts in exponential growth were trypsinized, and 1000–2,000 cells (10,000–20,000 cells for the highest doses) were seeded into 10 cm plastic dishes (2 dishes per dose) and irradiated at room temperature with 0, 1,2,4 or 6 Gy. After 12–14 days, the cells were rinsed with 0.9% NaCl and stained with 0.25% methylene blue for survival assessment. Two independent survival experiments were performed.

HIV screening was negative. Radiosensitivity was mildly increased (Figure 2).

A lymph node biopsy showed signs of follicular and interfollicular hyperplasia as well as granulomas. Ziehl-Nielssen staining and IGRA (Interferon Gamma Release Assay) test were negative. PCR for CMV and EBV were negative as were cultures for bacteria. Finally, a culture from the bone marrow became positive for *Mycobacterium lentiflavum*. The child was treated accordingly and gradually improved, although the lymphadenopathies persisted.

Because of the poor responses to vaccination, the child is receiving intravenous immunoglobulin substitution therapy. Until now, the patient is still dependent on immunoglobulin substitution therapy. Moreover, she now receives *Pneumocystis jiroveci* prophylaxis. Ionizing radiation is used as little as possible. Under these circumstances, the child is doing well. No more invasive infections were observed so far.

3. Discussion

RS, RTS, and BGS are caused by mutations in *RECQL4* gene. The RecQ family of helicases is a group of proteins that play a role in genomic stability. The family contains 5 members, 3 of which are involved in disorders characterized by genomic instability. RecQL4 seems to be involved in more

than one cellular pathway involved in DNA repair, but the exact function is not well understood [8]. There is evidence that RECQL4 plays multiple key roles in DNA metabolism, as it is involved in single-stranded DNA annealing activity, DNA replication, double strand break repair, and repair of UV or ionizing radiation induced DNA damage [2]. How defects in these proteins can lead to such a broad spectrum of clinical manifestations needs further to be investigated. How defects in this protein lead to immunodeficiency is even less clear [9].

Immunodeficiency is a well described feature of other chromosomal breakage syndromes such as ataxia telangiectasia (AT) and Bloom syndrome. In Bloom syndrome, the clinical phenotype is variable, with prolonged panhypogammaglobulinaemia, severe respiratory infection causing chronic lung disease, and sinopulmonary infection being the most common manifestations. In AT, the immunodeficiency is characterized by both cellular and humoral impairment, but clinical manifestations are extremely variable, ranging from normal to profoundly reduced responses to bacterial antigens. Recurrent sinopulmonary infection is common and is associated with hypogammaglobulinaemia due to B cell maturation defects. Cellular immunodeficiency is characterized by defective thymic development, with macroscopic absence of the thymus at postmortem examination. Another hypothesis can be postulated in a defective class switch mechanism. Class switch recombination is known to be defective in other DNA repair syndromes and could be deficient in lymphocytes from patients with RS [10]. The fact that the patient had low switched memory B cells could be compatible with this hypothesis but further research will have to show whether or not this hypothesis is correct.

There are only few data on the quality of the immune system in children with RECQL4 mutations. There is an increasing number of reports on increased susceptibility to infections and immunodeficiency in RTS [10–14]. Our patient presented with an intriguing immunological phenotype, which was very similar to the phenotype described by de Somer et al. [2]. Our patient had low T and B as well as a low percentage of switched memory B cells and NK cells. The patient with RTS described by de Somer et al. [2] also revealed by immunophenotyping low T and NK cells and a low number of class switched B cells and diminished specific antibody response. The low T cells might be partially due to diminished thymic output. RECQL4 is highly expressed in the thymus and KO mice have smaller thymi, suggesting a role for RECQL4 in T cell development [15]. The finding that regulatory T cells were absent in our patient is intriguing, although it is unclear if this phenomenon is typical for patients with Recq4 mutations or a result of the severe infection. The finding that in Mycobacterium tuberculosis infection regulatory T cells are high instead of low makes the second hypothesis less probable [16]. Further research would help to clarify this issue.

The diminished thymic output cannot explain the defects in the other lymphocytes nor the low percentage of switched memory B cells. This finding is observed in AT patients as well. Specific antibodies against poliovirus, measles, and hepatitis B virus were lacking in our patient, as in the patient described by de Somer et al. [2], despite adequate immunization. Anti-pneumococcal antibody response to vaccination with the polysaccharide pneumococcal vaccine was also low.

Granulomas in a variety of organs are not uncommon in patients with a wide range of immunodeficiencies of different origins, [17, 18] as well as in some infections, such as mycobacteria. In the group of patients with DNA repair problems, this phenomenon has been described as well [2, 19]. This finding could thus be interpreted as a sign of the underlying infection and further support the diagnosis of an immunodeficient state.

Although our patient had no antibodies against the pneumococcal vaccinations she had received, she did not suffer from recurrent ear infections or other pneumococcal infections. In contrast, her presenting infection, disseminated *Mycobacterium lentiflavum*, has been the only important infection in this patient. Disseminated mycobacterial infections usually point to a defect in the Interferon gamma/IL12/23 pathway, which was normal in our patient. This further stresses the need for further investigation in these patients to try to determine the exact mechanism leading to this immunodeficiency.

This case report suggests that immunodeficiency can occur in children with REQL4 mutations and that immunological screening should be performed as a standard of care. RTS, RS, and BGS are genetically related disorders with mutations in the same gene but each a partly overlapping but distinct clinical phenotype. In literature, a number of reports on increased susceptibility to infections or abnormalities in the immune system of patients with RTS have appeared recently [10–14]; also one case of a patient with BGS is reported [20]. But so far, this has not been reported in patients with RS. Larger studies will be necessary to conclude if the immunological abnormalities found in this patient are indeed common in children with RS as well.

Conflict of Interests

The authors declare that there is no conflict of interests regarding the publication of this paper.

References

[1] H. A. Siitonen, O. Kopra, H. Kääriäinen et al., "Molecular defect of RAPADILINO syndrome expands the phenotype spectrum of RECQL diseases," *Human Molecular Genetics*, vol. 12, no. 21, pp. 2837–2844, 2003.

[2] L. de Somer, C. Wouters, M.-A. Morren et al., "Granulomatous skin lesions complicating Varicella infection in a patient with Rothmund-Thomson syndrome and immune deficiency: case report," *Orphanet Journal of Rare Diseases*, vol. 5, no. 1, article 37, 2010.

[3] L. Larizza, G. Roversi, and L. Volpi, "Rothmund-thomson syndrome," *Orphanet Journal of Rare Diseases*, vol. 5, no. 1, article 2, 2010.

[4] L. van Maldergem, "Baller-Gerold syndrome," in *GeneReviews*, R. A. Pagon, M. P. Adam, T. D. Bird, C. R. Dolan, C. T. Fong, and K. Stephens, Eds., University of Washington, Seattle, Wash, USA, 2007.

[5] J. G. Noordzij, N. S. Verkaik, M. van der Burg et al., "Radiosensitive SCID patients with Artemis gene mutations show a complete B-cell differentiation arrest at the pre-B-cell receptor checkpoint in bone marrow," *Blood*, vol. 101, no. 4, pp. 1446–1452, 2003.

[6] A. H. Siitonen, J. Sotkasiira, M. Biervliet et al., "The mutation spectrum in RECQL4 diseases," *European Journal of Human Genetics*, vol. 17, no. 2, pp. 151–158, 2009.

[7] C. Wehr, T. Kivioja, C. Schmitt et al., "The Euroclass trial: defining subgroups in common variable immunodeficiency," *Blood*, vol. 111, no. 1, pp. 77–85, 2008.

[8] T. Dietschy, I. Shevelev, and I. Stagljar, "The molecular role of the Rothmund-Thomson-, RAPADILINO- and Baller-Gerold-gene product, RECQL4: recent progress," *Cellular and Molecular Life Sciences*, vol. 64, no. 7-8, pp. 796–802, 2007.

[9] D. L. Croteau, M. L. Rossi, J. Ross et al., "RAPADILINO RECQL4 mutant protein lacks helicase and ATPase activity," *Biochimica et Biophysica Acta—Molecular Basis of Disease*, vol. 1822, no. 11, pp. 1727–1734, 2012.

[10] A. R. Gennery, A. J. Cant, and P. A. Jeggo, "Immunodeficiency associated with DNA repair defects," *Clinical and Experimental Immunology*, vol. 121, no. 1, pp. 1–7, 2000.

[11] M. Kubota, M. Yasunaga, H. Hashimoto et al., "IgG4 deficiency with Rothmund-Thomson syndrome: a case report," *European Journal of Pediatrics*, vol. 152, no. 5, pp. 406–408, 1993.

[12] T. Ito, Y. Tokura, S. I. Moriwaki et al., "Rothmund-Thomson syndrome with herpes encephalitis," *European Journal of Dermatology*, vol. 9, no. 5, pp. 354–356, 1999.

[13] M. A. Broom, L. L. Wang, S. K. Otta et al., "Successful umbilical cord blood stem cell transplantation in a patient with Rothmund-Thomson syndrome and combined immunodeficiency," *Clinical Genetics*, vol. 69, no. 4, pp. 337–343, 2006.

[14] P. Reix, J. Derelle, H. Levrey-Hadden, H. Plauchu, and G. Bellon, "Bronchiectasis in two pediatric patients with Rothmund-Thomson syndrome," *Pediatrics International*, vol. 49, no. 1, pp. 118–120, 2007.

[15] N. M. Lindor, Y. Furuichi, S. Kitao, A. Shimamoto, C. Arndt, and S. Jalal, "Rothmund-Thomson syndrome due to *RECQ4* helicase mutations: report and clinical and molecular comparisons with Bloom syndrome and Werner syndrome," *American Journal of Medical Genetics*, vol. 90, no. 3, pp. 223–228, 2000.

[16] R. P. Larson, S. Shafiani, and K. B. Urdahl, "Foxp3(+) regulatory T cells in tuberculosis," *Advances in Experimental Medicine and Biology*, vol. 783, pp. 165–180, 2013.

[17] Y. Morimoto and J. M. Routes, "Granulomatous disease in common variable immunodeficiency," *Current Allergy and Asthma Reports*, vol. 5, no. 5, pp. 370–375, 2005.

[18] L. J. Mechanic, S. Dikman, and C. Cunningham-Rundles, "Granulomatous disease in common variable immunodeficiency," *Annals of Internal Medicine*, vol. 127, no. 8, pp. 613–617, 1997.

[19] L. Y. T. Chiam, M. M. M. Verhagen, A. Haraldsson et al., "Cutaneous granulomas in ataxia telangiectasia and other primary immunodeficiencies: reflection of inappropriate immune regulation?" *Dermatology*, vol. 223, no. 1, pp. 13–19, 2011.

[20] S. G. Golombek, S. Brook, L. T. Clement, M. Begleiter, and W. E. Truog, "Immunodeficiency in a patient with Baller-Gerold syndrome: a reason for early demise?" *Southern Medical Journal*, vol. 91, no. 10, pp. 966–969, 1998.

16

Intravenous Immunoglobulin and Mycophenolate Mofetil for Long-Standing Sensory Neuronopathy in Sjögren's Syndrome

Maria Giovanna Danieli,[1] Lucia Pettinari,[2] Ramona Morariu,[1] Fernando Monteforte,[3] and Francesco Logullo[4]

[1] Clinica Medica, Dipartimento di Scienze Cliniche e Molecolari,
  Università Politecnica delle Marche & Ospedali Riuniti, Via Tronto 10, 60126 Ancona, Italy
[2] U.O. di Medicina-LPA, Presidio di Loreto, 66025 Loreto, Italy
[3] U.O. di Radiodiagnostica, Ospedale di Casarano, 73042 Lecce, Italy
[4] Clinica Neurologica, Dipartimento di Medicina Sperimentale e Clinica, Polo Didattico Scientifico,
  Università Politecnica delle Marche & Azienda Ospedali Riuniti, Via Tronto 10, 60126 Ancona, Italy

Correspondence should be addressed to Maria Giovanna Danieli, mgdanieli@mail.com

Academic Editors: N. Kutukculer, Y. Nozaki, B. Sarov, and A. Vojdani

Sensory neuronopathy is described in association with the Sjögren's syndrome (SS). We studied a 55-year-old woman with a 4-year history of progressive asymmetric numbness, distal tingling, and burning sensation in upper and lower limbs. In a few months, she developed ataxia with increased hypoanaesthesia. Electrodiagnostic tests revealed undetectable distal and proximal sensory nerve action potential in upper and lower limbs. Cervical spine magnetic resonance showed a signal hyperintensity of posterior columns. Previous treatment with high-dose glucocorticoids and azathioprine was ineffective. A combined treatment with intravenous immunoglobulin and mycophenolate mofetil was followed by a progressive and persistent improvement. This case documented the efficacy and the safety of the coadministration of intravenous immunoglobulin and mycophenolate mofetil in sensory neuronopathy associated with SS refractory to conventional immunosuppressive therapy.

1. Introduction

Central nervous system involvement in Sjögren's syndrome (SS) is rarely reported and may be severe and varied [1]. Sensory neuronopathy (or sensory ganglionopathy, SN) is a distinctive neuropathy of SS, accounting for 15–20% of all neuropathies seen in this condition [2]. A sensory neuropathy is often the presenting feature of SS, and, therefore, a high index of suspicion is required, particularly in female patients with non-length-dependent, painful, or ataxic sensory neuropathy or those with trigeminal sensory and autonomic involvement [3]. At the onset of SN, numbness, tingling, burning, and pain sensations are reported in all limbs, usually with asymmetric distribution. With the disease progression, the sensory disturbances can involve the trunk, the face or they develop into a symmetric way. On examination, degeneration of large sensory neurons leads to gait ataxia, proprioceptive sensory loss, and widespread deep tendon areflexia [3]. When smaller sensory neurons are affected, deficits are those of hypoesthesia to pain and thermal stimuli with hyperacute pain. Autonomic nervous system involvement may cause fixed tachycardia, orthostatic hypotension, and gastrointestinal pseudo-obstruction. The response to treatment is usually poor, even with glucocorticoids, immunosuppressants, and plasmapheresis [3].

Here we report the case of a woman with primary SS who presented with SN that was successfully managed with intravenous immunoglobulin and mycophenolate mofetil coadministration.

2. Case Report

In 2001, a 55-year-old woman presented with progressive asymmetric numbness distal tingling and burning sensation in upper limbs associated with xerostomia and xerophtalmia. Antibodies to SS-A/Ro and anti-SS-B/La were positive. A minor salivary gland biopsy showed mononuclear cells with prominent lymphocyte infiltration with glandular cell atrophy. Nerve conduction studies showed a "sensory axonal neuropathy." The diagnosis of SS was made according to the criteria of American-European Community [4], and she was treated with anti-inflammatory drugs. In 2003, distal sensory deficits aggravated and extended to the lower limbs with increased hypo-anaesthesia and unsteady gait. In spite of treatment with oral prednisone (1 mg/kg/day) and azathioprine (2 mg/kg/day), distal sensory deficits progressed. Thus, she was admitted to our hospital in June, 2005.

On admission she was bedridden and she could not ambulate independently. A global impairment of sensation was detected as a profound loss in all lower limbs and, as moderate reduction, in the upper limbs. Deep tendon reflexes were absent. No autonomic symptoms were detected. Neurological examination of the cranial nerves was normal. Muscle strength was normal in all of the four limbs. Severe sensory ataxia was present in assisted gait. Romberg's sign was positive.

We documented a mild normocytic anaemia with lymphopenia with high erythrocyte sedimentation rate. The antinuclear antibody titre was elevated with positive anti-SS-A/Ro and anti-SS-B/La by fluorescence enzyme immunoassay. Levels of immunoglobulins (IgG, IgM, and IgA) and serum concentrations of complement levels (C3 and C4) measured by nephelometry were normal. As for serological autoimmune markers, immunofixation did not detect monoclonal immunoglobulins; cryoglobulins were negative, as ANA and rheumatoid factors (IgM-RF) and anti-CCP antibodies. HBV and HCV markers were negative. Electrodiagnostic studies revealed undetectable distal and proximal sensory nerve action potential (SNPAs) in upper and lower limbs. Nerve conduction studies were normal. Concentric needle examination of distal and proximal muscles was normal. Somatosensory-evoked potentials were absent with distal stimulation, both in upper and lower limbs. Spinal cord magnetic resonance disclosed high signal intensity without gadolinium enhancement in posterior columns of the cervical spinal cord (Figure 1), findings consisting with the diagnosis of neuronopathy.

We started a combined treatment with intravenous immunoglobulin and oral mycophenolate mofetil. Intravenous immunoglobulin was infused at 1 g/kg/day (5 g/hour) on two consecutive days each month for six months, followed by further cycles every other month for six months. Oral mycophenolate mofetil was started at 500 mg/day and then titrated to the definite dosage of 30 mg/kg/day. Oral prednisone was slowly tapered from the initial dose of 1 mg/kg/day to an average of 0.25 mg/kg every other day.

Within three months, the patient presented a marked improvement in sensory symptoms, in gait and in the functional status. No modification of *sicca syndrome* was reported. She continued with MMF for one year more and with IVIg with decreased doses and longer intervals between courses for two years. At last followup she was ataxic but she can ambulate without support, and the sensory loss in upper

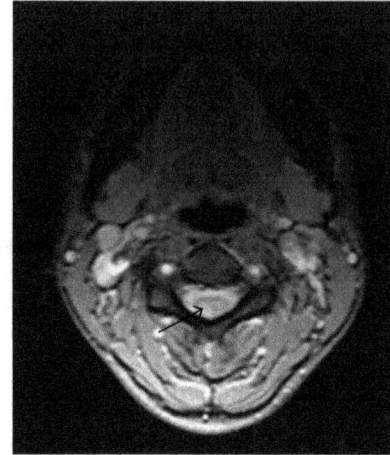

FIGURE 1: MRI 1.5T Axial section obtained with sequence GRE-T2 at C4 level showing a signal hyperintensity of posterior columns.

and lower limbs was notably reduced. Magnetic resonance features were unchanged.

3. Discussion

We report a case of a long-standing severe ganglionopathy in the context of SS for which the combined treatment with intravenous immunoglobulin and mycophenolate mofetil was remarkably and persistently successful. The pathogenic mechanism responsible for the neuronopathy is still debated. Some authors have postulated that the dorsal root ganglion damage is associated with loss of neurons and mononuclear inflammatory infiltrates without vasculitis [5]. In the literature, few studies, mainly case reports or small series, investigated the therapeutic options for neuronopathy. More studies are available for nonvasculitic neuropathies associated with SS. For both forms, the response to traditional glucocorticoids and immunosuppressants is generally poor [5]. Cyclophosphamide, used preferentially in vasculitic neuropathies, is linked to a certain degree of toxicity. In sensory neuropathy associated with SS, positive results have been reported following the use of IVIg, with long-term sustained improvement and a reduction in the rate and severity of glucocorticoids-related adverse effects [6, 7]. In a retrospective national multicentric study, Rist et al. [8] documented the benefit of IVIg in 19 patients with SS-related neuropathy without any necrotizing vasculitis. The clinical response was observed after two courses of IVIg administration, thus underlying the necessity to evaluate the treatment response only after two courses.

As for MMF in SS, we found in the literature only a small pilot trial in patients refractory to other immunosuppressants. The authors documented an improvement in xerophthalmia as well in some laboratory parameters (reduction of gamma globulins and IgM-RF titre, increase of C3 and C4 complement levels and white blood cell count) [9].

No data are available on the use of coadministration of intravenous immunoglobulin and mycophenolate mofetil in SS. In neuronopathy, the rationale of using intravenous immunoglobulin and mycophenolate mofetil involves the cell-mediated [5] and humoral [10] immunological mechanisms underlying the ganglionopathy. Immunoglobulin is widely used in autoimmune diseases, intravenously and subcutaneously [11, 12]. Among other mechanisms, intravenous immunoglobulin can affect T regulatory cells by increasing their suppressive function [13] and accelerate the rate of the pathogenic IgG catabolism [11, 14]. Mycophenolate mofetil affects the *de novo* synthesis of guanosine nucleotides thus inhibiting a crucial pathway for DNA synthesis in lymphocytes. The synergism between the action of intravenous immunoglobulin and mycophenolate mofetil in suppressing the activation and the proliferation of lymphocytes could explain the favourable response and the long-term remission we observed.

We choose to continue the IVIg administration at monthly intervals, since in previous reports only repeated doses of IVIg permitted the maintenance of the clinical response [6]. Moreover, the use of IVIg enables a reduction of the infective risk in subjects treated with immunosuppressant. This point is of particular interest since immunodeficiency states are increasingly recognised in patients with immune-mediated diseases and they are due to intrinsic defect linked to the disease itself and/or to the immunosuppressant employed throughout the disease management.

In conclusion, we documented a distinct improvement of the disability linked to ganglionopathy within the first three months of intravenous immunoglobulin coadministered with mycophenolate mofetil treatment. The better neurological condition was maintained over a period of more than 4 years. The coadministration of intravenous immunoglobulin and mycophenolate mofetil was demonstrated to be beneficial and safe in a case of sensory neuronopathy associated with SS refractory to conventional immunosuppressive therapy.

Take Home Messages

(i) Intravenous immunoglobulin has been widely used in the treatment of immune-mediated diseases.

(ii) Not many reports described the intravenous immunoglobulin application in Sjögren's syndrome, and even fewer are related to mycophenolate mofetil.

(iii) The use of intravenous immunoglobulin co-administered with mycophenolate mofetil permitted to attain a complete remission with a relevant functional recovery in a subject with long-standing refractory neuronopathy.

(iv) No side effects were linked to this combined treatment.

References

[1] G. J. Tobón, J. O. Pers, V. Devauchelle-Pensec et al., "Neurological disorders in primary Sjögren's syndrome," *Autoimmune Diseases*, vol. 2012, Article ID 645967, 11 pages, 2012.

[2] S. I. Mellgren, L. G. Göransson, and R. Omdal, "Primary Sjögren's syndrome associated neuropathy," *Canadian Journal of Neurological Sciences*, vol. 34, no. 3, pp. 280–287, 2007.

[3] A. Sghirlanzoni, D. Pareyson, and G. Lauria, "Sensory neuron diseases," *Lancet Neurology*, vol. 4, no. 6, pp. 349–361, 2005.

[4] C. Vitali, S. Bombardieri, R. Jonsson et al., "Classification criteria for Sjögren's syndrome: a revised version of the European criteria proposed by the American-European Consensus Group," *Annals of the Rheumatic Diseases*, vol. 61, no. 6, pp. 554–558, 2002.

[5] J. W. Griffin, D. R. Cornblath, E. Alexander et al., "Ataxic sensory neuropathy and dorsal root ganglionitis associated with Sjögren's syndrome," *Annals of Neurology*, vol. 27, no. 3, pp. 304–315, 1990.

[6] J. A. Molina, J. Benito-Leon, F. Bermejo, F. J. Jimenez-Jimenez, and J. Olivan, "Intravenous immunoglobulin therapy in sensory neuropathy associated with Sjögren's syndrome," *Journal of Neurology Neurosurgery and Psychiatry*, vol. 60, no. 6, p. 699, 1996.

[7] Y. Takahashi, T. Takata, M. Hoshino, M. Sakurai, and I. Kanazawa, "Benefit of IVIG for long-standing ataxic sensory neuronopathy with Sjögren's syndrome," *Neurology*, vol. 60, no. 3, pp. 503–505, 2003.

[8] S. Rist, J. Sellam, E. Hachulla et al., "Experience of intravenous immunoglobulin therapy in neuropathy associated with primary Sjögren's syndrome: a national multicentric retrospective study," *Arthritis Care & Research*, vol. 63, pp. 1339–1344, 2011.

[9] P. Willeke, B. Schlüter, H. Becker, H. Schotte, W. Domschke, and M. Gaubitz, "Mycophenolate sodium treatment in patients with primary Sjögren's syndrome: a pilot trial," *Arthritis Research and Therapy*, vol. 9, no. 6, pp. 115–121, 2007.

[10] Y. Murata, K. Maeda, H. Kawai et al., "Antiganglion neuron antibodies correlate with neuropathy in Sjögren's syndrome," *NeuroReport*, vol. 16, no. 7, pp. 677–681, 2005.

[11] J. F. Seite, Y. Shoenfeld, P. Youinou, and S. Hillion, "What is the contents of the magic draft IVIg?" *Autoimmunity Reviews*, vol. 7, no. 6, pp. 435–439, 2008.

[12] M. G. Danieli, L. Pettinari, R. Moretti, F. Logullo, and A. Gabrielli, "Subcutaneous immunoglobulin in polymyositis and dermatomyositis: a novel application," *Autoimmunity Reviews*, vol. 10, no. 3, pp. 144–149, 2011.

[13] A. Kessel, H. Ammuri, R. Peri et al., "Intravenous immunoglobulin therapy affects t regulatory cells by increasing their suppressive function," *Journal of Immunology*, vol. 179, no. 8, pp. 5571–5575, 2007.

[14] J. Vani, S. Elluru, V. S. Negi et al., "Role of natural antibodies in immune homeostasis: IVIg perspective," *Autoimmunity Reviews*, vol. 7, no. 6, pp. 440–444, 2008.

17

Variant of X-Linked Chronic Granulomatous Disease Revealed by a Severe *Burkholderia cepacia* Invasive Infection in an Infant

Saul Oswaldo Lugo Reyes,[1,2] **Nizar Mahlaoui,**[3,4] **Carolina Prando,**[5,6]
Lizbeth Blancas Galicia,[1,2] **Marjorie Hubeau,**[2] **Stéphane Blanche,**[4] **Capucine Picard,**[2,3,4]
Jean-Laurent Casanova,[2,4,5] **and Jacinta Bustamante**[2,3]

[1] *Immunodeficiencies Research Unit, National Institute of Pediatrics, Coyoacan, 04530 Mexico City, DF, Mexico*
[2] *Laboratory of Human Genetics of Infectious Diseases, INSERM U980, University Paris Descartes, Paris Sorbonne Cité,*
75014 Paris, France
[3] *French Reference Center for Primary Immune Deficiencies (CEREDIH), Necker-Enfants Malades University Hospital,*
AP-HP, 75015 Paris, France
[4] *Pediatric Immunology-Hematology Unit, Necker-Enfants Malades University Hospital, AP-HP, 75015 Paris, France*
[5] *St. Giles Laboratory of Human Genetics of Infectious Diseases, Rockefeller University, New York, NY 10065, USA*
[6] *Bioinformatics Laboratory, Pelé Pequeno Principe Research Institute, 80250-060 Curitiba, PR, Brazil*

Correspondence should be addressed to Jacinta Bustamante; jacinta.bustamante@inserm.fr

Academic Editors: V. Lougaris, N. Martinez-Quiles, Y. Nozaki, and A. Vojdani

Chronic granulomatous disease (CGD) is a primary immunodeficiency characterized by increased susceptibility to bacteria and fungi since early in life, caused by mutations in any of the five genes coding for protein subunits in NADPH oxidase. X-linked variant CGD can be missed during routine evaluation or present later in life due to hypomorphic mutations and a residual superoxide production. The case of a 10-month-old boy who died of pneumonia is reported. The isolation of *Burkholderia cepacia* from his lung, together with a marginally low nitroblue tetrazolium reduction assay (NBT), made us suspect and pursue the molecular diagnosis of CGD. A postmortem genetic analysis finally demonstrated CGD caused by a hypomorphic missense mutation with normal gp91^{phox} expression. In a patient being investigated for unusually severe or recurrent infection, a high index of suspicion of immunodeficiency must be maintained.

1. Introduction

Chronic granulomatous disease (CGD) is a rare primary immunodeficiency that affects microbial killing by phagocytes, resulting in bacterial, fungal, and/or mycobacterial infections since early life [1, 2]. The superoxide production by NADPH oxidase is markedly reduced or absent due to mutations in any of the five genes coding for protein subunits of the enzymatic complex [3]. Mutations in *CYBB*, coding for gp91^{phox}, result in the most common X-linked CGD (65%–70% of all cases) [4]. Hypomorphic mutations (Xgp91^{+} and Xgp91^{-}) may result in X-linked variant CGD [5, 6]. Patients with variant CGD express the gp91^{phox} protein and produce decreased but detectable superoxide, which allow the defect to manifest later in life with a milder history of infections. By far, the most common micro-organisms causing infections in CGD are *Staphylococcus aureus* and *Aspergillus* species; other agents include *Pseudomonas*, *Serratia*, *Salmonella*, and *Candida* species. *Burkholderia cepacia* infection is frequently associated to CGD diagnosis (6–8). Here, we present the case of a patient who died of *Burkholderia cepacia* lung infection, in whom the diagnosis of X-CGD could only be attained postmortem due to residual superoxide production and normal protein expression.

2. Case Report

A 10-month-old boy, the first child of nonconsanguineous parents living in the Tahiti archipelago (French Polynesia), was referred for severe pneumonia. The father is from Europe and the mother is from Oceania; there was no relevant family history. During the first months of life, the patient had experienced some infections, mostly of the upper airways, as well as bronchitis and diarrhea. He received all the immunizations according to his age (including BCG) with no adverse events. He developed a failure to thrive at the age of 3 months. One month before admission he had a severe lung infection with fever, cough, dyspnea, and diarrhea, unresponsive to an empiric oral macrolide (josamycin). Upon admission to his local hospital, he had fever (39.5°C), mild respiratory distress, and crackles on auscultation. Oxygen saturation was 95% in room air. Complete blood count (CBC) reported marked leukocytosis (36,600/mL) with neutrophilia (29,000 polymorphonuclear cells (PMN)/mL) and anemia (Hb = 7.6 g/dL); serum immunoglobulin levels were as follows: IgG = 1,900 mg/dL (reference value for 7–12 months: 661 ± 219 mg/dL), IgA = 166 mg/dL (37 ± 18), IgM = 220 mg/dL (54 ± 23), and IgE 43 IU/mL (normal < 20 IU/mL). Chloride sweat test and tuberculin skin test were negative. Chest X-ray and computed tomography scan (CT) revealed bilateral pneumonia with multiple excavations in both lungs. Intravenous (IV) cefotaxime and fosfomycin were started for suspected staphylococcal pneumonia. Bronchoscopy showed diffuse edema of the trachea and bronchi. Bronchoalveolar lavage (BAL) and Gram stain reported 1,100 cells (97% PMN) and abundant Gram negative bacteria that grew Burkholderia cepacia (10^7 CFU, >25 white cells). Antibiotherapy was then switched to IV rifamycin and trimethoprim/sulfamethoxazole.

After a transient improvement, the patient's condition deteriorated, and he was referred to our hospital, where he was found to be small for his age and cachectic, with severe respiratory distress and hepatosplenomegaly. Lung CT scan revealed extensive destruction of the lungs with multiple bullous lesions and opacification of the left lung; the right lung had multiple nodular lesions and opacified upper lobe. Immunological workup confirmed marked leukocytosis with neutrophilia and anemia, elevated serum C-reactive protein (CRP = 165 mg/L), and fibrinogen (6 g/L). BAL retrieved Burkholderia cepacia (10^6 CFU/mL, >25 white cells/field). Lymphocyte subset counts, T lymphocytes proliferation, and specific antibody production assays were all normal. Nitroblue tetrazolium reduction (NBT) test and luminol chemiluminescence to assess reactive oxygen species (ROS) production in PMNs repeatedly showed a baseline activity level at around 45% (low but detectable), and response to stimulation was poor. Chemotaxis chamber assay was normal, as well as CD18 and CD11a,b,c expression on PMNs. When a peripheral blood smear reported vacuolized enlarged PMNs, dense granule disease was suspected and ruled out: normal secretory vesicles, secondary granules, azurophile granules, and myeloperoxidase production; normal specific staining of secondary granule proteases (neutrophil elastase, myeloperoxidase, Cathepsin G, and Lactoferrin). Despite intensive supportive care, including broad-spectrum antibiotics and daily granulocyte transfusions, his lung infection worsened, and he finally died of acute respiratory distress and multiorgan dysfunction in the intensive care unit. Permission to perform an autopsy was refused by his parents.

The clinical presentation and the impaired NBT reduction assays of this boy were consistent with a primary phagocyte defect. We assessed superoxide (O_2^-) production in PMNs from the patient as measured by the cytochrome-c reduction assay, compared to another patient with known X-linked CGD (−) and a healthy control (+), following stimulation with phorbol myristate acetate (PMA). Residual NADPH oxidase activity was detected in the PMNs of the patient (Figure 1(a)). In addition, 123-dihydrorhodamine (DHR) oxidation assay by flow cytometry revealed a partial deficiency of ROS production in the patient's PMN, while his mother had two granulocyte populations: one strongly rhodamine-positive (reactive) and the other rhodamine-low fluorescence intensity (Figure 1(b)). These results again suggested that our patient had a partial defect in the respiratory burst. We next investigated the H_2O_2 production upon milder activation, involving priming with TNF-α, IL-1β, or cytochalasin b, followed by fMLF (formyl-methionyl-leucyl-phenylalanine) stimulation. PMNs from the patient produced detectable but low H_2O_2 (Figure 1(c)).

Genomic sequencing of CYBB revealed a hemizygous A > G substitution in exon 9, generating the replacement of a histidine by an arginine residue (H338R) in the FAD binding domain (FADBR), a probably damaging substitution according to the PolyPhen-2 prediction website (http://genetics.bwh.harvard.edu/pph2/). The patient's mother was heterozygous, and his brother (born after the patient's death) was hemizygous for the mutation. The mutation was confirmed also in cDNA from the patient (c.1013A > G). We investigated the molecular basis of the germline H338R mutation through detection of flavocytochrome b$_{558}$ expression by flow cytometry, using the monoclonal antibody 7D5 (MBL, Nagasaki, Japan), which recognizes residues [160]IKNP[163] and [226]RIVRG[230] on gp91^{phox} in the presence of p22^{phox}. Protein expression in Epstein-Barr virus transformed B cells (EBV-B cells) from the patient was similar to the healthy control (Figure 2).

3. Discussion

The isolation of Burkholderia cepacia from lung secretion or blood of a previously healthy patient is strongly suggestive of CGD. Aside from it, lung infections caused by Burkholderia species can be seen in patients with existing bronchiectasis (lung epithelial damage is a prerequisite for Burkholderia invasiveness), including notably patients with cystic fibrosis [7] and in some immunocompromised and hospitalised patients [8, 9]. In a child being investigated for recurrent infections, isolation of Burkholderia should always raise the suspicion of CGD [10–12]. For some patients with normal gp91^{phox} expression and residual superoxide production as measured by conventional assays, a milder activation assay with fMLF might be needed to demonstrate low ROS production.

(a)

(b)

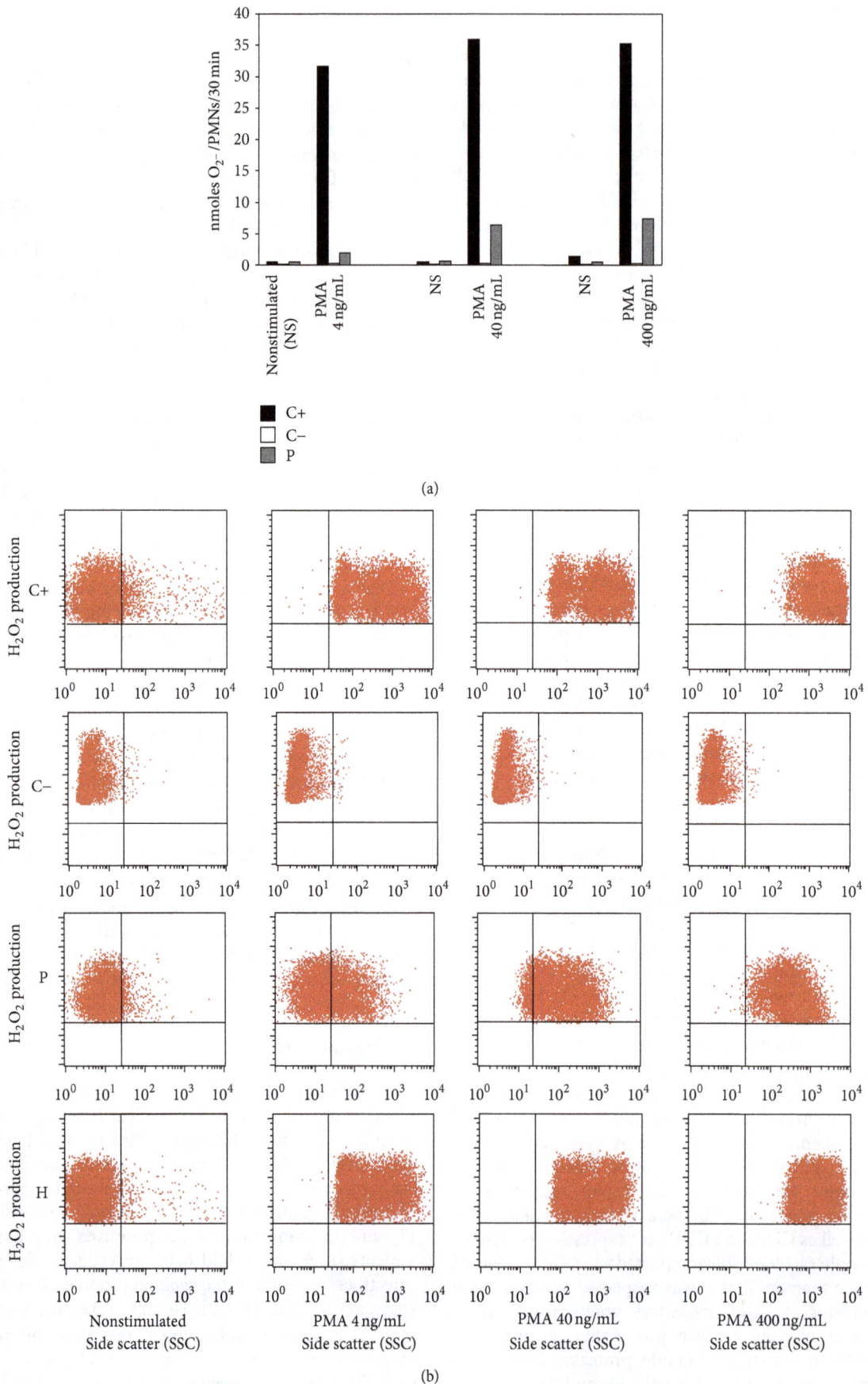

FIGURE 1: Continued.

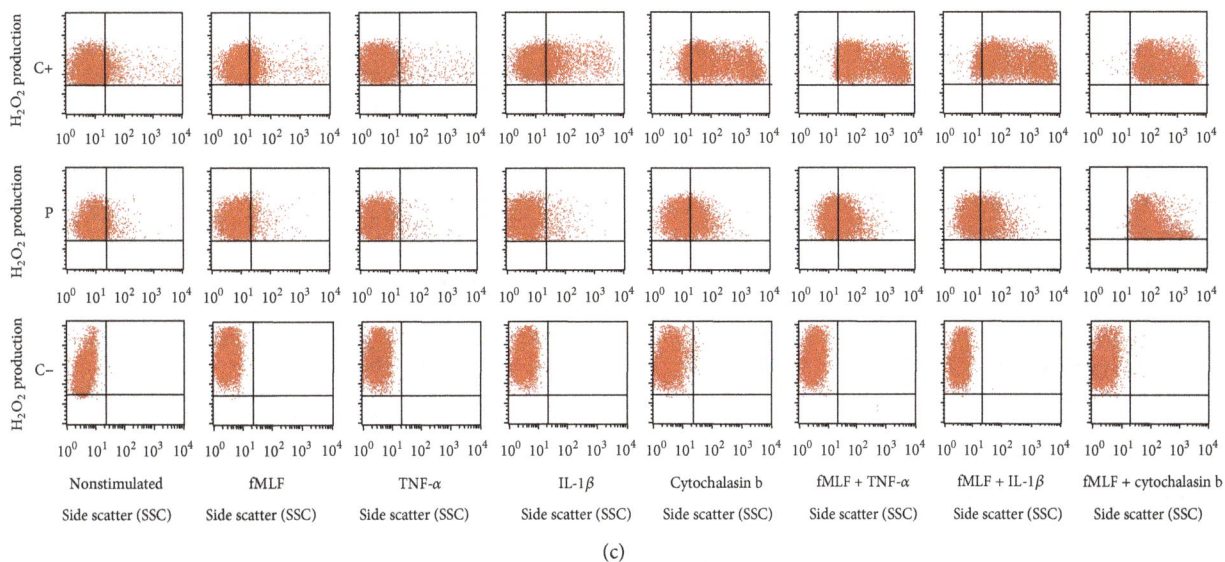

(c)

FIGURE 1: NADPH oxidase activity evaluation in PMNs. (a) Superoxide generation was measured by assaying superoxide dismutase-inhibitable cytochrome-*c* reduction in PNMs after adding three doses of PMA (4, 40, and 400 ng/mL), for healthy controls (C+), CGD patient (C−), and our patient (P). (b) Histograms for the flow cytometric analysis of intracellular H_2O_2 production, using the fluorescent 123DHR probe in PMNs from a healthy control (C+), an X-linked CGD patient (C−), the proband (P), and the mother (H), before (NS) and after stimulation with PMA (4, 40, and 400 ng/mL). (c) PMNs from C+, C−, and P were left untreated or treated with TNF-α, IL-1β, and cytochalasin b and then stimulated with fMLF. The results shown are representative of two independent experiments.

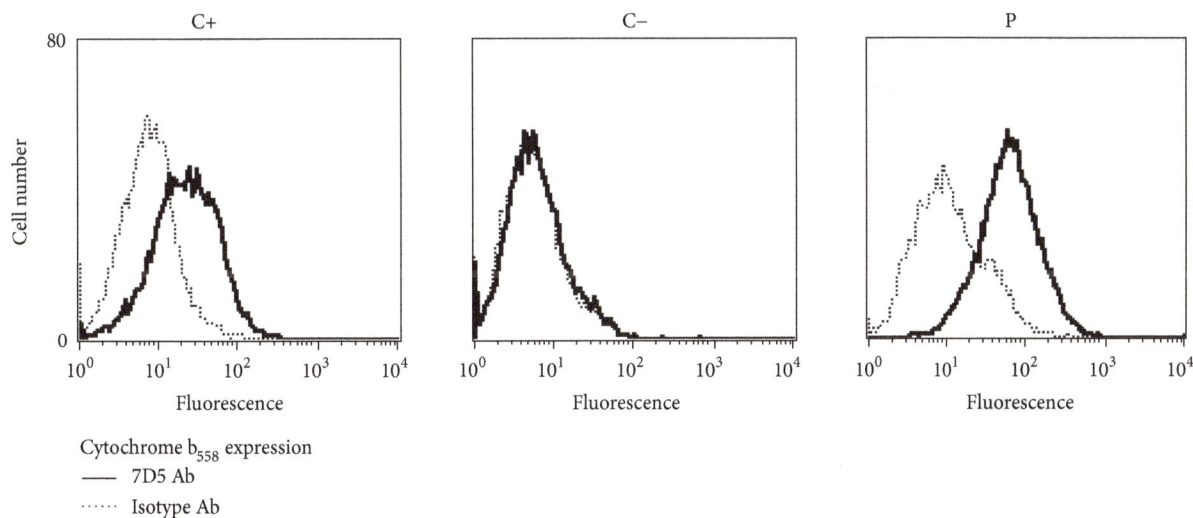

Cytochrome b$_{558}$ expression
—— 7D5 Ab
······ Isotype Ab

FIGURE 2: Expression of gp91^{phox} in a patient with the H338R *CYBB* mutation. Immunostaining of cytochrome b$_{558}$ in EBV-B cells from a healthy control (C+), an X-linked CGD patient (C−), and the patient (P). Cell surface staining with mAb7D5 (an antibody specific for the extracellular epitope of gp91^{phox}; solid lines); an isotype IgG1 (dotted lines) followed by staining with an Alexa Fluor 488 goat anti-mouse Ig secondary antibody. The results shown are representative of two independent experiments.

Missense mutations beyond aminoacid 309 of gp91^{phox} usually allow normal protein expression but result in null superoxide production. The patient's residual ROS generation is thus different from the thorough survival analysis by Kuhns et al. [3]. Also, given this infant's residual superoxide production, a severe course with early demise is surprising.

In conclusion, we identified *postmortem* a point mutation in a CGD causing gene from a 10-month-old boy who presented with a *Burkholderia* spp. overwhelming lung infection. X-CGD diagnosis was delayed because of initial normal results. A high index of suspicion for CGD must be maintained in patients with *Burkholderia* isolates and close to normal values of usual CGD diagnostic tests such as NBT.

An early and accurate diagnosis can lead to genetic counselling, to family screening, and to a timely intervention.

Abbreviations

CGD: Chronic granulomatous disease
PID: Primary immune deficiency
NADPH: Nicotinamide adenine dinucleotide phosphate hydrogen
BCG: Bacillus Calmette-Guérin.

Conflict of Interests

The authors declare no conflict of interests.

Authors' Contributions

Saul Oswaldo Lugo Reyes and Nizar Mahlaoui equally contributed to this work.

Acknowledgments

The authors thank the patient's family members for their willingness to participate in this study. The authors thank Michelle N'Guyen, Martine Courat, and Tony Leclerc for secretarial and technical assistance. The Laboratory of Human Genetics of Infectious Diseases is supported in part by grants from BNP-Paribas and Schlumberger Foundations, the March of Dimes, the Dana Foundation, the St. Giles Foundation, and the Agence Nationale de la Recherche Médicale. The Immunodeficiencies Research Unit is supported in part by Fundacion Mexicana para Niñas y niños con Inmunodeficiencias Primarias (FUMENI). Marjorie Hubeau is supported by a fellowship grant from the Société Française d'Hématologie.

References

[1] J. Bustamante, G. Aksu, G. Vogt et al., "BCG-osis and tuberculosis in a child with chronic granulomatous disease," *Journal of Allergy and Clinical Immunology*, vol. 120, no. 1, pp. 32–38, 2007.

[2] J. Bustamante, A. A. Arias, G. Vogt et al., "Germline CYBB mutations that selectively affect macrophages in kindreds with X-linked predisposition to tuberculous mycobacterial disease," *Nature Immunology*, vol. 12, no. 3, pp. 213–221, 2011.

[3] D. B. Kuhns, W. G. Alvord, T. Heller et al., "Residual NADPH oxidase and survival in chronic granulomatous disease douglas," *The New England Journal of Medicine*, vol. 363, no. 27, pp. 2600–2610, 2010.

[4] D. Roos, D. B. Kuhns, A. Maddalena et al., "Hematologically important mutations: X-linked chronic granulomatous disease (third update)," *Blood Cells, Molecules, and Diseases*, vol. 45, no. 3, pp. 246–265, 2010.

[5] B. Boog, A. Quach, M. Costabile et al., "Identification and functional characterization of two novel mutations in the α-helical loop (residues 484–503) of CYBB/gp91^{phox} resulting in the rare X91+ variant of chronic granulomatous disease," *Human Mutation*, vol. 33, no. 3, pp. 471–475, 2012.

[6] M. J. Stasia, B. Lardy, A. Maturana et al., "Molecular and functional characterization of a new X-linked chronic granulomatous disease variant (X91+) case with a double missense mutation in the cytosolic gp91^{phox} C-terminal tail," *Biochimica et Biophysica Acta*, vol. 1586, no. 3, pp. 316–330, 2002.

[7] D. E. Greenberg, J. B. Goldberg, F. Stock, P. R. Murray, S. M. Holland, and J. J. Lipuma, "Recurrent Burkholderia infection in patients with chronic granulomatous disease: 11-Year experience at a large referral center," *Clinical Infectious Diseases*, vol. 48, no. 11, pp. 1577–1579, 2009.

[8] S. G. Avgeri, D. K. Matthaiou, G. Dimopoulos, A. P. Grammatikos, and M. E. Falagas, "Therapeutic options for Burkholderia cepacia infections beyond co-trimoxazole: a systematic review of the clinical evidence," *International Journal of Antimicrobial Agents*, vol. 33, no. 5, pp. 394–404, 2009.

[9] V. Gautam, L. Singhal, and P. Ray, "Burkholderia cepacia complex: Beyond pseudomonas and acinetobacter," *Indian Journal of Medical Microbiology*, vol. 29, no. 1, pp. 4–12, 2011.

[10] R. Lakshman, S. Bruce, D. A. Spencer et al., "Postmortem diagnosis of chronic granulomatous disease: how worthwhile is it?" *Journal of Clinical Pathology*, vol. 58, no. 12, pp. 1339–1341, 2005.

[11] J. L. Madden, M. E. Schober, R. L. Meyers et al., "Successful use of extracorporeal membrane oxygenation for acute respiratory failure in a patient with chronic granulomatous disease," *Journal of Pediatric Surgery*, vol. 47, pp. e21–e23, 2012.

[12] R. Renella, J. Perez, S. Chollet-Martin et al., "Burkholderia pseudomallei infection in chronic granulomatous disease," *European Journal of Pediatrics*, vol. 165, no. 3, pp. 175–177, 2006.

Refractory Immunological Thrombocytopenia Purpura and Splenectomy in Pregnancy

Santiago Bernal-Macías,[1] **Laura-Marcela Fino-Velásquez,**[1] **Felipe E. Vargas-Barato,**[2,3] **Lucio Guerra-Galue,**[4] **Benjamín Reyes-Beltrán,**[1] **and Adriana Rojas-Villarraga**[1]

[1]*Center for Autoimmune Diseases Research (CREA), School of Medicine and Health Sciences, Universidad del Rosario, Bogotá, Colombia*
[2]*Surgery Department, School of Medicine and Health Sciences, Universidad del Rosario, Bogotá, Colombia*
[3]*Surgery Department, Hospital Universitario Mayor-Mederi (HUM), Bogotá, Colombia*
[4]*Gynaecology Department, Hospital Universitario Mayor-Mederi (HUM), Bogotá, Colombia*

Correspondence should be addressed to Santiago Bernal-Macías; bernal.santiago@urosario.edu.co

Academic Editor: Christian Drouet

Thrombocytopenia is defined as a platelet count of less than 100,000 platelets per microlitre (mcL). Thrombocytopenia develops in approximately 6-7% of women during pregnancy and at least 3% of these cases are caused by immunological platelet destruction. Herein, we present a pregnant woman who develops at the first trimester autoimmune thrombocytopenia purpura associated with positive antiphospholipid antibodies. The disease was refractory to pharmacological treatments but had a favourable response to splenectomy. The patient carried the pregnancy to term without complication and gave birth to a healthy baby girl.

1. Introduction

The immunological thrombocytopenic purpura (ITP) is the accelerated destruction or inadequate platelet production mediated by autoantibodies; it is important to consider there are other causes of thrombocytopenia in pregnancy. Other causes include the following: preeclampsia, HELLP syndrome, thrombocytopenic thrombotic purpura, haemolytic uremic syndrome, congenital conditions, drugs (i.e., heparin and quinidine), infections (i.e., human immunodeficiency virus, hepatitis C, cytomegalovirus, and Epstein-Barr virus), lymphoproliferative disorders, bone marrow diseases, and autoimmune diseases (AD) (i.e., systemic lupus erythematosus (SLE) and antiphospholipid syndrome (APS)) [1–5].

In previously healthy women, ITP usually presents as an incidental finding in an asymptomatic woman. There are also a small percentage of cases that present with mucocutaneous bleeding manifestations [4].

2. Case

A 24-year-old woman during week 9.5 of an uncomplicated pregnancy presented to the emergency department with sudden onset of a major epistaxis episode. Her platelet count was 15000 mcL (Figure 1). A multidisciplinary treatment approach was required and the patient was referred to a third-level hospital in December 2013.

The physical examination revealed an active epistaxis that was controlled by anterior nasal packing. The remaining examination was normal. The haemoglobin level was 6.2 g per deciliter (g/dL) and the platelet count was 37,000 platelets per microlitre (mcL). The direct antiglobulin test (Coombs test) was positive; however Evans' syndrome was ruled out based on the laboratory tests which came out negative to detect the presence of haemolysis (i.e., peripheral blood smear, reticulocytes production index, levels of serum lactate dehydrogenase, serum haptoglobin, and indirect bilirubin) and the standard

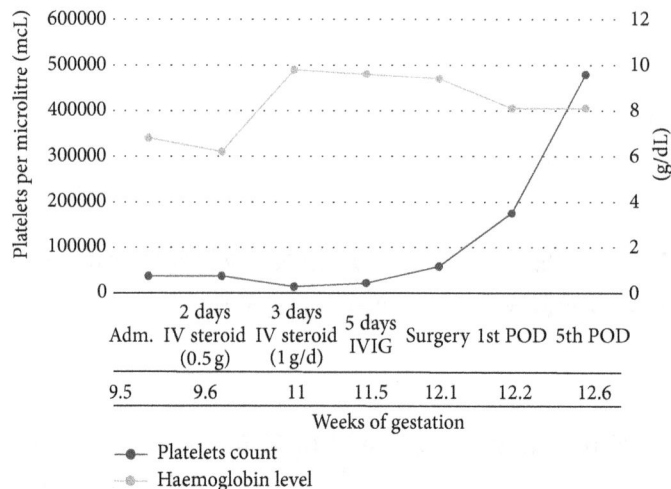

FIGURE 1: Evolution of platelets count and haemoglobin levels during pregnancy on different treatments. Adm.: admission; IV: intravenous; IVIG: intravenous immunoglobulins; POD: postoperative day.

autoimmune profile was negative except for positive IgG anticardiolipin antibodies (aCL) (titer of 47.8 GLP) and moderately positive lupus anticoagulant (LA) (LA1/LA2 ratio: 1.74).

The patient was diagnosed with ITP because she was previously healthy and had no prior history of any thrombosis event, foetal loss, preterm labour, or familiar autoimmunity suggesting APS, SLE, or AD. Consequently, the patient was treated with a transfusion of three units of packed red blood cells and corticosteroids orally and intravenously. The initial treatment included a one-day methylprednisolone bolus of 500 mg and then sustained doses of prednisolone of 50 mg/day.

After six days of treatment, the platelet count dropped to 2,000/mcL. Therefore, it was necessary to add a new course of methylprednisolone bolus of 1 g/day for three days. The patient received a transfusion of 18 units of platelets. The persistence of platelets under 30,000/mcL indicated a failure of corticosteroid treatment. Therefore, a five-day course of intravenous immunoglobulins (IVIG) of 0.4 g/kg/day was used.

Three weeks after disease onset, the patient experienced three additional episodes of epistaxis (all with less than 30,000/mcL platelets; one episode before the first day and two episodes day 0 and day 1 after course of IVIG) that required local control by otolaryngology. Due to the failure of pharmacological treatment, a multidisciplinary consensus between Gynaecology, Internal Medicine, General Surgery, and Rheumatology approved a laparoscopic splenectomy. The surgery was performed the next day and the patient had a platelet count of 18,000/mcL and required transfusion of 12 units of platelets before and during the surgery according with anaesthesiologist. The platelet count in the early postoperative period was 58,000/mcL.

The patient was closely monitored in the intensive care unit (ICU) for 4 days subsequent to the surgery. A rapid increase of platelet count is notorious the following postoperative day (POD), and the patient's count increased to 175,000/mcL on POD 1 and 479,000/mcL by POD 5.

The patient was discharged after 25 days and was in the 13th week of gestation. The pharmacological treatment with prednisolone 40 mg/day was gradually decreased. Additionally, the patient was treated with low molecular weight heparin during the last 8 weeks of gestation as directed by her gynaecologist. As a preventive strategy, the patient was vaccinated for encapsulated bacteria. The patient carried the pregnancy to term without complication and gave birth to a healthy baby girl.

3. Discussion

We here presented an unusual case of ITP associated with positive antiphospholipid antibodies during the first trimester of pregnancy. The patient required splenectomy due to the persistence of low platelet counts and haemorrhagic manifestations despite pharmacological treatment.

The pathogenetic role and the clinical importance of the presence of antiphospholipid antibodies (aPL) in patients with ITP are not clear. Diz-Küçükkaya et al. reported that 37.8% of cases had aPL in a cohort of patients with ITP followed up for 5 years. The authors did not identify any differences in platelet count or response to methylprednisolone [6]. Yang et al. found a similar prevalence of aPL (28.5%) in a cohort of patients with ITP [7] and Stasi et al. demonstrated higher prevalence of aPL (46.3%) in their cohort [8]. However, the series of patients with APS were evaluated for thrombocytopenia risk in the presence of aCL and the results showed that high titre of aCL IgG has a predictive value of 77% for thrombocytopenia [9].

The presence of LA is an important marker of thrombosis in patients with ITP. Thus, Diz-Küçükkaya et al. concluded that the persistent presence of aPL in patients with ITP is an important risk factor for the development of APS [6].

The patient did not fulfill the clinical criteria for APS (thrombotic events, recurrent foetal loss, and preterm birth before 34 weeks of gestation [10]). However, the clinical suspicion of APS alone or with concurrent AD (i.e., polyautoimmunity) is treated according to the APS International Consensus proposed in 2006 [11, 12]. Nevertheless, the presence of aPL and thrombocytopenia without prior thrombosis or foetal loss is not classified as APS [9].

The 2011 American Society of Haematology (ASH) determined there are no studies comparing different treatments or comparing treatment to nontreatment in pregnant women and all data are based on observational studies [5]. Corticosteroids (prednisolone and methylprednisolone: FDA category C) are the most effective and secure pharmacological group to decrease the activity of the disease in pregnant patients. However, side effects can be generated as hypertension, delayed foetal growth, and cleft lip or cleft palate [4, 5, 13, 14].

IVIG is category C according to FDA classification and is administered at 0.4 mg/kg/day for 5 days or 1 mg/kg/day for 2 days and achieves an acceptable response in most cases. However, the high treatment cost does not allow it to be used in all clinics [4, 5, 15].

Splenectomy is a second line of treatment when there is toxicity suspected. This treatment is considered by some authors as third-line treatment because it may induce premature labour. We consider that the spleen is the major area of platelet destruction in autoimmune thrombocytopenia. Thus, splenectomy leads to a high rate of durable complete remissions [1, 13, 16].

According to the ASH, the indication for splenectomy is a platelet count less than 10,000/mcL in the presence of haemorrhage in the second trimester of pregnancy, but there are few reports during the first trimester. During second trimester of pregnancy, the risks of anaesthesia are minimal to the foetus and uterine size does not complicate the procedure [17–19]. Laparoscopic splenectomy is currently recommended because it reduces the stay in bed, avoids other associated complications (i.e., thrombotic manifestations), and decreases the dose, frequency, and duration of analgesic treatment [13].

Alternative therapy such as azathioprine (FDA category D) has been used as an immunosuppressive agent during pregnancy without toxicity. Another option is rituximab (FDA category C), but its use for treating ITP during pregnancy has not been evaluated. However, it has been used for treatment of non-Hodgkin lymphoma during pregnancy [4, 5, 15].

ITP during pregnancy may be a clinical challenge when evidence is limited. Thus, clinicians should consider the risks and benefits of any proposed treatment plans and should obtain a multidisciplinary consensus.

Conflict of Interests

The authors have indicated that they have no conflict of interests regarding the content of this paper.

References

[1] M. Á. Sanz, V. Vicente García, A. Fernández et al., "Guidelines for diagnosis, treatment and monitoring of primary immune thrombocytopenia," *Medicina Clínica*, vol. 138, no. 6, pp. 261.e1–261.e17, 2012.

[2] J. Strong, "Bleeding disorders in pregnancy," *Current Obstetrics & Gynaecology*, vol. 13, pp. 1–6, 2003.

[3] D. B. Cines and V. S. Blanchette, "Medical progress: immune thrombocytopenic purpura," *The New England Journal of Medicine*, vol. 346, no. 13, pp. 995–1008, 2002.

[4] British Committee for Standards in Haematology General Haematology Task Force, "Guidelines for the investigation and management of idiopathic thrombocytopenic purpura in adults, children and in pregnancy," *British Journal of Haematology*, vol. 120, no. 4, pp. 574–596, 2003.

[5] C. Neunert, W. Lim, M. Crowther, A. Cohen, L. Solberg Jr., and M. A. Crowther, "The American Society of Hematology 2011 evidence-based practice guideline for immune thrombocytopenia," *Blood*, vol. 117, no. 16, pp. 4190–4207, 2011.

[6] R. Diz-Küçükkaya, A. Hacihanefioğlu, M. Yenerel et al., "Antiphospholipid antibodies and antiphospholipid syndrome in patients presenting with immune thrombocytopenic purpura: a prospective cohort study," *Blood*, vol. 98, no. 6, pp. 1760–1764, 2001.

[7] Y.-J. Yang, G.-W. Yun, I.-C. Song et al., "Clinical implications of elevated antiphospholipid antibodies in adult patients with primary immune thrombocytopenia," *The Korean Journal of Internal Medicine*, vol. 26, no. 4, pp. 449–454, 2011.

[8] R. Stasi, E. Stipa, M. Masi et al., "Prevalence and clinical significance of elevated antiphospholipid antibodies in patients with idiopathic thrombocytopenic purpura," *Blood*, vol. 84, no. 12, pp. 4203–4208, 1994.

[9] R. Cervera, M. G. Tektonidou, G. Espinosa et al., "Task Force on Catastrophic Antiphospholipid Syndrome (APS) and Non-criteria APS Manifestations (II): thrombocytopenia and skin manifestations," *Lupus*, vol. 20, no. 2, pp. 174–181, 2011.

[10] T. Marchetti, M. Cohen, and P. De Moerloose, "Obstetrical antiphospholipid syndrome: from the pathogenesis to the clinical and therapeutic implications," *Clinical and Developmental Immunology*, vol. 2013, Article ID 159124, 9 pages, 2013.

[11] S. Miyakis, M. D. Lockshin, T. Atsumi et al., "International consensus statement on an update of the classification criteria for definite antiphospholipid syndrome (APS)," *Journal of Thrombosis and Haemostasis*, vol. 4, no. 2, pp. 295–306, 2006.

[12] A. Rojas-Villarraga, J. Amaya-Amaya, A. Rodriguez-Rodriguez, R. D. Mantilla, and J.-M. Anaya, "Introducing polyautoimmunity: secondary autoimmune diseases no longer exist," *Autoimmune Diseases*, vol. 2012, Article ID 254319, 9 pages, 2012.

[13] B. V. Anglin, C. Rutherford, R. Ramus, M. Lieser, and D. B. Jones, "Immune thrombocytopenic purpura during pregnancy: laparoscopic treatment," *Journal of the Society of Laparoendoscopic Surgeons*, vol. 5, no. 1, pp. 63–67, 2001.

[14] W. F. Rayburn, "Glucocorticoid therapy for rheumatic diseases: maternal, fetal, and breast-feeding considerations," *American Journal of Reproductive Immunology*, vol. 28, no. 3-4, pp. 138–140, 1992.

[15] A. Cuker and D. B. Cines, "Immune thrombocytopenia," *Hematology*, vol. 2010, no. 1, pp. 377–384, 2010.

[16] J. R. Stratton, P. J. Ballem, T. Gernsheimer, M. Cerqueira, and S. J. Slichter, "Platelet destruction in autoimmune thrombocytopenic purpura: kinetics and clearance of indium-111-labeled

autologous platelets," *Journal of Nuclear Medicine*, vol. 30, no. 5, pp. 629–637, 1989.

[17] T. Gernsheimer, A. H. James, and R. Stasi, "How I treat thrombocytopenia in pregnancy," *Blood*, vol. 121, no. 1, pp. 38–47, 2013.

[18] R. Mahey, S. D. Kaur, S. Chumber, A. Kriplani, and N. Bhatla, "Splenectomy during pregnancy: treatment of refractory immune thrombocytopenic purpura," *BMJ Case Reports*, vol. 2013, 2013.

[19] T. W. Felbinger, M. Posner, H. K. Eltzschig, and B. S. Kodali, "Laparoscopic splenectomy in a pregnant patient with immune thrombocytopenic purpura," *International Journal of Obstetric Anesthesia*, vol. 16, no. 3, pp. 281–283, 2007.

19

Systemic Lupus Erythematosus with Hepatosplenic Granuloma: A Rare Case

Anju Bharti[1] and Lalit Prashant Meena[2]

[1] *Department of Pathology, King George Medical University, Lucknow 226003, India*
[2] *Department of General Medicine, Institute of Medical Sciences, Banaras Hindu University, Varanasi 221005, India*

Correspondence should be addressed to Lalit Prashant Meena; drlalitmeena@gmail.com

Academic Editor: Maurizio Benucci

Background. Systemic lupus erythematosus (SLE) is an autoimmune disease which is known to present with a wide variety of clinical manifestations. *Case Report.* A 15-year-old male presented with complaints of moderate grade fever and generalized body swelling. There was no history of cough, weight loss, joint pain, oral ulcerations, skin rash, photosensitivity, loss of hair, pain abdomen, jaundice, or any significant illness in the past. Contrast enhanced computerized tomography of the abdomen revealed hypodense lesions in both liver and spleen (without contrast enhancement), suggestive of granulomas along with few retroperitoneal and mesenteric lymph nodes. On the basis of immunological tests and renal biopsy report, SLE with hepatosplenic granulomatosis diagnosis was made. He was given pulse methylprednisolone 500 mg, for 3 days and he showed dramatic improvement clinically. *Conclusion.* Hepatic and splenic granulomas are not common in SLE, but this should be kept in differential diagnosis.

1. Introduction

Systemic lupus erythematosus (SLE) is an autoimmune disease characterized by multisystem involvements. The exact etiology of systemic lupus erythematosus (SLE) is still not clear, although multifactorial interaction with environmental and genetic factors has been associated. Immune complex formation along with activation of complement system has been postulated for various manifestations of systemic lupus erythmatosus [1].

It is uncommon in children and young adolescents, with 0.5-0.6 per 1,00,000 per year being the incidence rate in children younger than 15 years of age. Moreover, it is rarer among male subjects [2]. Only very few reports have described noncaseating epithelioid cell granulomas in necropsy specimens of lymph node, lung, spleen, and serous membranes [3–5].

Although liver dysfunction may be found in SLE (25–50%), but SLE with hepatic and splenic granuloma is very rare. These features may also cause diagnostic confusion with other causes of granulomas. Here, we described a case presented with granulomas in liver and spleen.

2. Case Report

A 15-year-old male presented with complaints of moderate grade fever for 4 months and generalized body swelling with facial puffiness for 2 months. There was no history of cough, weight loss, joint pain, oral ulcerations, skin rash, photosensitivity, loss of hair, pain abdomen, jaundice, or any significant illness in the past. There was no past history of tuberculosis in the patient or in any other family member. General examination revealed moderate pallor and bilateral cervical and axillary lymph nodes, with the largest being of size 1 cm × 1 cm mobile, nontender, and firm. Systemic examination was insignificant except for the presence of palpable spleen, 2 cm below the costal margin. Hemogram was suggestive of bicytopenia (Hb 6.9 g/dL (normal: 12–14 g/dL), TLC 2700/mm^3 (normal: 4000–11000/mm^3), and total platelet count 2,10,000/mm^3 (normal: 150000–400000/mm^3)). Serum amino transferases and alkaline phosphatase were raised (SGOT 316 U/L (normal: 20–40 U/L), SGPT 109 U/L (normal: 20–50 U/L), and S. ALP 2750 IU/L (normal: 44 to 147 IU/L)). Total serum protein (5.1 g/dL, normal: 6.0–8.3 g/dL) and albumin (2.3 g/dL, normal: 3.5–5.5 g/dL) were low. Renal function tests were normal. Mantoux test was negative and ESR was slightly raised. Urine routine and microscopy showed 4-5 RBCs and 8–10 pus cells per high power field and 4+ albuminuria. 24-hour urinary protein was 2.1 gm. Kidney biopsy was done. Chest roentgenogram was normal. Ultrasonography of abdomen revealed mild splenomegaly with a tiny hypoechoic mass in spleen suggestive of splenic granuloma, along with a few subcentimetric retroperitoneal lymph nodes. Bone marrow studies were suggestive of nutritional anemia. Cervical lymph node biopsy showed reactive lymphoid hyperplasia. Barium meal follow through showed jejunoileitis. IgM antibody for Epstein-Barr virus was negative. Serum angiotensin converting enzyme levels were also normal. Based on the clinical picture, the high prevalence of tuberculosis in this part of the world and the investigations, a provisional diagnosis of disseminated tuberculosis was kept. The patient was started on a trial of antituberculous treatment and was asked for review with renal biopsy report. He turned up early with high grade fever, swelling of upper lips, and oral ulceration. On further investigations, his antinuclear and antidouble stranded DNA titers were significantly raised (ANA 7.3 IU/mL, N < 1, and anti-dsDNA 680 IU/mL, N < 40).

Histopathological report of kidney biopsy was suggestive of membranoproliferative (Type) lupus nephritis. Contrast enhanced computerized tomography of the abdomen revealed hypodense lesions in both liver and spleen (without contrast enhancement), suggestive of granulomas along with few retroperitoneal and mesenteric lymph nodes. Consequently, a revised diagnosis of SLE with lupus nephritis and granulomatous hepatitis was now evident, and the child was put on pulse methylprednisolone 500 mg for 3 days. He showed dramatic improvement clinically.

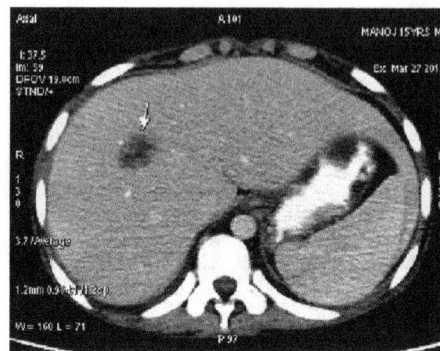

FIGURE 1: Hepatic and splenic granuloma.

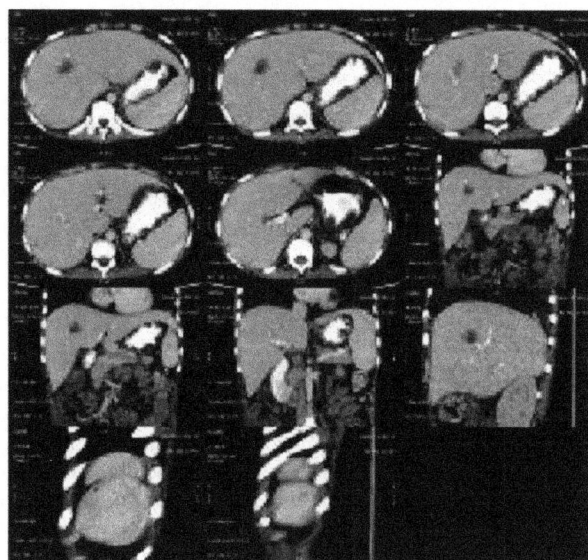

FIGURE 2: Hepatic and splenic granuloma.

3. Discussion

SLE is an autoimmune disease that presents usually with multiorgan manifestations [2]. It is uncommon in children and young adolescents, with 0.5-0.6 per 1,00,000 per year being the incidence rate in children younger than 15 years of age. Moreover, it is rarer among male subjects. This coupled with the initial varied and vague presentation of the disease often leads to missing the diagnosis of the disease at first instance. In patients with SLE, subclinical manifestations or biochemical abnormalities of hepatic involvement are usually described, with overt disease seen rarely. Liver disease is diagnosed usually after one year of diagnosis of SLE. Various forms of hepatic involvement have already been described in SLE. Granulomatous hepatitis in SLE is uncommon, although not rare [6]. It is usually associated with raised hepatic enzymes, especially alkaline phosphatase levels and appears as hypoechoic/hypodense lesions on CT study. Starting the patient on corticosteroid therapy (as the treatment of SLE) is the main concern as the lesions closely mimic a liver abscess [7]. Presence of hepatic and splenic granulomas with generalized lymphadenopathy is well known in tuberculosis and sarcoidosis (Figures 1 and 2).

However, these were ruled out by relevant investigations. Possibility of an autoimmune disease like SLE was not kept initially despite the presence of significant proteinuria and active urinary sediments because of rarity of the disease in a male child, as described earlier. The only viable option was to place the patient on a trial of antituberculous treatment and look for response. However, failure to improve on ATT combined with the reports of renal biopsy, CECT abdomen, and autoimmune markers made the diagnosis of SLE imperative. Pathogenesis of granuloma formation in systemic lupus erythmatosus (SLE) is still not clear. It was postulated as a response to tissue injury and considered as a manifestation of allergic tissue reaction [3]. Although systemic lupus erythmatosus is considered type III hypersensitivity reaction, but type IV mediated mechanism also may play a role in autoimmune nephritis in the pathogenesis granuloma in SLE [8]. Reduced numbers of macrophages and capacity for phagocytosis along with defective clearance of apoptotic bodies by the complement system lead to a high level of apoptotic bodies in patients with SLE [9–11]. Hence, persistence of these apoptotic bodies may stimulate granuloma formation.

Therefore, in patients who present with granulomatous disease along with prolonged fever and constitutional symptoms, though uncommon, noninfectious causes like SLE should also be considered as a diagnostic possibility.

Conflict of Interests

The authors declare that there is no conflict of interests regarding the publication of this paper.

References

[1] C. C. Mok and C. S. Lau, "Pathogenesis of systemic lupus erythematosus," *Journal of Clinical Pathology*, vol. 56, no. 7, pp. 481–490, 2003.

[2] D. Xu, H. Yang, C.-C. Lai et al., "Clinical analysis of systemic lupus erythematosus with gastrointestinal manifestations," *Lupus*, vol. 19, no. 7, pp. 866–869, 2010.

[3] G. Teilum, "Miliary epithelloid-cell granulomas in lupus erythematosus disseminatus," *Acta Pathologica Microbiologica Scandinavica*, vol. 22, no. 1, pp. 73–79, 1945.

[4] G. Teilum and H. E. Poulsen, "Disseminated lupus erythematosus: histopathology, morphogenesis, and relation to allergy," *AMA Archives of Pathology*, vol. 64, no. 4, pp. 414–425, 1957.

[5] S. K. Datta, V. C. Gandhi, H. J. Lee, V. K. Pillay, and G. Dunea, "Granuloma in systemic lupus erythematosus," *South African Medical Journal*, vol. 46, no. 41, pp. 1514–1516, 1972.

[6] V. R. Chowdhary, C. S. Crowson, J. J. Poterucha, and K. G. Moder, "Liver involvement in systemic lupus erythematosus: case review of 40 patients," *The Journal of Rheumatology*, vol. 35, no. 11, pp. 2159–2164, 2008.

[7] B. A. Runyon, D. R. LaBrecque, and S. Anuras, "The spectrum of liver disease in systemic lupus erythematosus. Report of 33 histologically-proved cases and review of the literature," *American Journal of Medicine*, vol. 69, no. 2, pp. 187–194, 1980.

[8] S. Pathak and C. Mohan, "Cellular and molecular pathogenesis of systemic lupus erythematosus: lessons from animal models," *Arthritis Research & Therapy*, vol. 13, no. 5, article 241, 2011.

[9] A. P. Manderson, M. Botto, and M. J. Walport, "The role of complement in the development of systemic lupus erythematosus," *Annual Review of Immunology*, vol. 22, pp. 431–456, 2004.

[10] F. C. Passero and A. R. Myers, "Decreased numbers of monocytes in inflammatory exudates in systemic lupus erythematosus," *Journal of Rheumatology*, vol. 8, no. 1, pp. 62–68, 1981.

[11] M. Herrmann, R. E. Voll, O. M. Zoller, M. Hagenhofer, B. B. Ponner, and J. R. Kalden, "Impaired phagocytosis of apoptotic cell material by monocyte-derived macrophages from patients with systemic lupus erythematosus," *Arthritis & Rheumatology*, vol. 41, no. 7, pp. 1241–1250, 1998.

20

Symptomatic Secondary Selective IgM Immunodeficiency in Adult Man with Undiagnosed Celiac Disease

Eli Magen,[1,2,3] Viktor Feldman,[4] Mishal Joseph,[2] and Hadari Israel[1]

[1] Leumit Health Services, Ashkelon, Israel
[2] Medicine B Department, Barzilai Medical Center, 78306 Ashkelon, Israel
[3] Allergy and Clinical Immunology Unit, Barzilai Medical Center, Barzilai Hospital, Ben Gurion University of Negev, Ashkelon, Israel
[4] Orthopedic Department, Meir Medical Center, Kfar Saba, Israel

Correspondence should be addressed to Eli Magen, allergologycom@gmail.com

Academic Editors: C. Pignata and A. Vojdani

Selective IgM immunodeficiency (SIgMID) is a heterogeneous disorder with no known genetic background and may occur as a primary or a secondary condition. Celiac disease has been reported in association with several humeral immunodeficiencies, including isolated severe selective IgA deficiency, panhypogammaglobulinemia, and isolated combined IgA and IgM deficiency. There are only few reported cases of pediatric and adult patients with SIgMID and celiac disease. In this paper, we describe an adult patient with a symptomatic secondary SIgMID associated with undiagnosed celiac disease, with a resolution of clinical symptoms of immunodeficiency and serum IgM normalization following a gluten-free diet.

1. Introduction

Selective IgM immunodeficiency is a heterogeneous disorder with no known genetic background and may occur as a primary or a secondary condition, with a reported prevalence of 0.03% to 3% [1] Secondary SIgMID is often associated with several neoplasms or autoimmune diseases [2–5]. Primary SIgMID can be asymptomatic or present with a variety of bacterial and viral infections in the pediatric and adult populations [3].

In this paper, we describe an adult patient with a symptomatic secondary SIgMID associated with undiagnosed celiac disease, with a resolution of clinical symptoms of immunodeficiency and serum IgM normalization following a gluten-free diet.

2. Case Report

A 42-year-old previously healthy man, emigrant from Russia, with an unremarkable clinical history presented in April 2011 at our Clinical Immunology Unit with predominant symptoms of fatigue for the past 3 years. He does not smoke and consume alcohol on occasion. A review of systems was significant for chronic fatigue, without deterioration in short term memory or concentration, without sleep disturbances, without weight loss or fever.

Although he was able to continue working, his severe fatigue necessitated frequent time off from work, and eventually he had reduced his work commitment to part time. In September 2009, the patient was admitted into a hospital in Moscow for upper-right lobe pneumonia, and after that he frequently caught colds during 2008-2009. In 2010, the patient was admitted for pneumonia twice. These repeated episodes occurred in different lung fields. No microbiologic source of recurrent pneumonia was identified. Additionally, during 2009-2010 the patient suffered from several episodes of *staphylococcus aureus* associated skin infections.

At presentation in our clinic (January 2011), physical examination was unremarkable. After a systematic evaluation of the patient's history and complaints, comprehensive laboratory work-up of immunodeficiency was performed (Table 1). The blood cell count, biochemistry, liver enzymes, serum iron, ferritin, vitamin B12, zinc, folic acid, TSH, free T4, cortisol, T cells, T cell subsets, B cells, and natural killer cells were within normal limits. Lymphocyte transformation of phytohemagglutinin (PHA), concanavalin A (Con A),

TABLE 1: Immunologic studies.

	Result	Reference range
Innate immunity		
White blood cell count, $10^3/\mu L$	6.9	4.5–10.8
Hemoglobin, g/dL	14.7	13.5–16.9
Absolute neutrophil count, $10^3/\mu L$	4.3	2.0–8.1
Absolute lymphocyte count, $10^3/\mu L$	1.8	0.9–3.3
Absolute monocyte count, $10^3/\mu L$	0.6	0.0–0.8
Absolute eosinophil count, $10^3/\mu L$	0.2	0.0–0.54
Platelets, $10^3/\mu L$	184	150–450
C3, mg/dL	116	90–180
C4, mg/dL	29	10–40
CH50 U/mL	240	101–300
C reactive protein, mg/dL	0.06	0–5
Phagocytosis assay (% phagocytosis)	34.3	25–45
Adaptive immunity		
Lymphocyte subsets, N/μL (%)		
CD3 + T cells	1349 (75)	620–1850 (62–84)
CD3 + CD4 + T cells	1104 (61)	345–1200 (31–61)
CD3 + CD8 + T cells	257 (14)	85–730 (10–38)
CD4/CD8 ratio	4.3	0.9–1.9
CD3 − CD19 + B cells	329 (18)	50–480 (5–26)
CD3 − CD56 + NK cells	134 (7)	15–350 (1–17)
Serum immunoglobulins		
IgM, mg/dL	9	40–230
IgA, mg/dL	172	70–400
IgG, mg/dL	1186	700–1600
IgG1, mg/dL	636	365–941
IgG2, mg/dL	345	165–545
IgG3, mg/dL	52	32–116
IgG4, mg/dL	64	6–121
IgE, mg/dL	11	0–87
Autoantibodies		
ANA	Positive	Negative
Anti-dsDNA antibody	4	Positive: >20
Anti-Smith Ab	11.5	Negative: <15 Positive: >25
ANCA	Negative	Negative
RF	Negative	Negative
IgA-tTG (EU/mL)	14	Negative: <20 Positive: >25
Mitochondrial Ab	Negative	Negative
Serological blood tests		
HIV 1,2 Ab, ELISA	Negative	Negative
HBs-Ag	Negative	Negative
HCV	Negative	Negative
TPHA	Negative	Negative
CMV Ab IgM (AU/mL)	0.13	Nonreactive: <6
CMV Ab IgG (AU/mL)	>250	Positive: >20
EBV EBNA Ab IgG	486	Reactive: >6

Abbreviations: ANA: antinuclear antibodies; ANCA: antineutrophil cytoplasmic antibodies; dsDNA: double-stranded DNA; ELISA: enzyme-linked immunosorbent assay; HIV: human immunodeficiency virus; Ig: immunoglobulin; RF: rheumatoid factor, HCV: hepatitis C Virus; TPHA: treponema pallidum particle agglutination assay; IgA-tTG: IgA anti tissue transglutaminase antibodies; CMV: cytomegalovirus; EBV: epstein barr virus; cpm: counts per minute.

mumps antigen, and purified protein derivative antigen was normal. In vitro lymphocyte proliferative response to *Candida albicans* and tetanus toxoid antigens were also unaffected. Mantoux test was negative. Phagocytic function test using nitroblue tetrazolium and Toll-like receptor 2 (TLR2) on monocytes were normal. The patient had normal quantitative serum IgA, IgG, and IgG subclasses and IgE. However, serum IgM levels were low at 9 mg/dL. The patient was capable of normal antibody responses to pneumococcal polysaccharide antigens following Pneumovax vaccination.

Since antinuclear antibodies were positive, most clinically relevant autoantibodies were checked, but all of them were found to be negative (Table 1).

Serum ANA, anti dsDNA and anti Smith antibodies levels were measured by QUANTA Lite ELISA (Inova, San Diego, CA, USA) using the manufacturer's suggested cut-off of >20 units to define positive results for ANA and anti dsDNA antibodies, >25 IU/mL for anti Smith antibodies. Serologic evaluations of our patients were performed according to the guidelines of European Society for Pediatric Gastroenterology, Hepatology, and Nutrition for the diagnosis of Celiac Disease [6]. According to the guidelines the initial test should be IgA class anti-TG2 from a blood sample. In subjects with either primary or secondary humoral IgA deficiency, at least 1 additional test measuring IgG class CD-specific antibodies should be done (IgG anti-TG2, IgG anti-DGP or IgG EMA, or blended kits for both IgA and IgG antibodies). In our patient the total IgA level was within the normal range. The guidelines recommend tests measuring antibodies against DGP as additional tests in patients who are negative for other CD-specific antibodies but in whom clinical symptoms raise a strong suspicion of CD, but in our patient we had no clinical suspicion for CD until his son had been diagnosed. The guidelines recommend not to perform tests for the detection of IgG or IgA antibodies against native gliadin peptides (conventional gliadin antibody test) for CD diagnosis, so we did not tested the patient for anti gliadin antibodies. It should be mentioned that no genetic testing was done and the HLA type of the patient as well the parents of the patient are not suffering from CD.

Once the diagnosis of symptomatic SIgMID was recognized, the patient was treated aggressively with the courses of several antibiotics using Cephalexin, amoxicillin/clavulanic acid, and trimethoprim/sulfamethoxazole during the five additional episodes of sinusitis and skin infections throughout 13 months.

In March 2011, during the follow-up visit the patient reported that his 7-year-old son underwent colonoscopy with biopsy due to losing weight and iron deficiency, and he had been diagnosed with celiac disease. Consequently, we decided to exclude celiac disease in our patient. Repeated serum immunoglobulin A-class tissue transglutaminase antibodies were within a normal level. The patient was referred to upper endoscopy, and the duodenal biopsy samples showed villous atrophy with crypt hyperplasia. Subsequently, a gluten-free diet was recommenced. Within 4 months, chronic fatigue disappeared and no skin or sinopulmonary infections were observed during the subsequent 9 months of followup. Moreover, repeated laboratory analyses showed

normalization of serum IgM levels (79 mg/dL). In February 2012, the follow-up small bowel mucosal biopsy specimen was normal; the patient was feeling well, there were no signs of any infectious disease and serum IgM level was 128 mg/dL.

3. Discussion

Our patient, who was previously healthy, represents a possible case of celiac disease associated secondary selective IgM deficiency. The main complains of the patient were associated with chronic fatigue and recurrent skin and sinopulmonary infections, without gastrointestinal complains or symptoms. The diagnosis of celiac disease in his son was the main reason for which we performed upper gastrointestinal endoscopy and duodenal biopsy.

Duodenal villous atrophy is not unique for celiac disease and may be observed in several immunodeficiency conditions. This pathology is frequent in symptomatic common variable immunodeficiency (CVID) [6], but our patient did not have clinical and laboratory criteria of CVID. Although the most common pathologic finding in the small intestine in CVID is villous flattening that grossly resembles celiac disease, there are some important differences between the villous flattening of CVID and celiac disease. The absence of plasma cells and the presence of polymorphonuclear infiltrate (PMNI) as well as graft-versus-host disease-like lesions (GVHDL) are thought to be pathologic features that differentiate CVID from untreated CD [7]. In CVID, the villous atrophy is thought to be T-cell mediated, while in celiac disease, there are plasma cell infiltrates with increased amounts of IgM and IgA. Moreover, in celiac disease, removal of gluten from the diet almost always leads to recovery of normal villous architecture. But, in CVID, removal of gluten from the diet improves villous flattening in only approximately 50% of patients [8, 9].

Celiac disease has been reported in association with several humoral immunodeficiencies, including isolated severe selective IgA deficiency [7, 10], panhypogammaglobulinemia, and isolated combined IgA and IgM deficiency [10]. Review of the literature revealed a few reported cases of pediatric and adult patients with SIgMID and celiac disease [3, 7, 10–12] while all reported cases were without unusual risk of infection and in all patients IgM levels returned to normal levels following a gluten-free diet [3, 10, 12] Therefore, our case is the first report of symptomatic secondary SIgMID associated with celiac disease.

The case presented here is in accordance with the previous observations that pediatric CD is very different from adult CD. In children, the classic forms are predominate and usually have positive serology and duodenal biopsies. In contrast, in adults the atypical forms predominate, with fewer positive serology, characterized by common extra-digestive complaints and various accompanying conditions, which makes diagnosis more challenging and greatly accounts for the longer diagnostic delay seen in adults [6, 13].

The pathogenesis of secondary SIgMID associated with celiac disease is unknown. It has been suggested that this secondary SIgMID is related to reduced IgM synthesis due to lymphoreticular dysfunction stimulated by gluten antigen exposure [11, 12] or/and to the defect in B cell differentiation into IgM-immunoglobulin secreting cells [14].

The problem of negative serology in untreated CD patients is becoming increasingly recognized [15]. The common reason of such seronegativity is selective IgA deficiency which may coexist with CD (roughly 2% vs. 0.2% in nonceliac controls) [16]. The reported pooled sensitivities of tTG-IgA in adults and children was 90% and 93% and endomyseal antibodies (IgA-EMA) to monkey esophagus by indirect fluorescent assay (IFA) was close to 96% and 97% in children and adults, respectively [17]. IgG anti-gliadin antibodies (AGA) testing remained the standard diagnostic test for CD in individuals with selective IgA deficiency until recently, but in the past few years, IgG anti-endomysial antibody (EMA), and anti-deamidated gliadin peptide (anti-DGP) assays have been developed that are superior to IgG AGA for this population [17]. Moreover there has been an ongoing discussion on whether AGA-positive individuals without CD (i.e., with negative antibodies against tTG and/or EMA and normal intestinal histology) may represent the mild end of the "gluten sensitivity" spectrum [18].

In conclusion, this case report should alert clinicians to the possibility that celiac disease can be associated with a symptomatic secondary SIgMID. Although rare, this condition may be associated with recurrent respiratory infections.

References

[1] J. T. Cassidy and G. L. Nordby, "Human serum immunoglobulin concentrations: prevalence of immunoglobulin deficiencies," *The Journal of Allergy and Clinical Immunology*, vol. 55, no. 1, pp. 35–48, 1975.

[2] T. Inoue, Y. Okumura, M. Shirahama, H. Ishibashi, S. Kashiwagi, and H. Okubo, "Selective partial IgM deficiency: functional assessment of T and B lymphocytes in vitro," *Journal of Clinical Immunology*, vol. 6, no. 2, pp. 130–135, 1986.

[3] M. F. Goldstein, A. L. Goldstein, E. H. Dunsky, D. J. Dvorin, G. A. Belecanech, and K. Shamir, "Selective IgM immunodeficiency: retrospective analysis of 36 adult patients with review of the literature," *Annals of Allergy, Asthma and Immunology*, vol. 97, no. 6, pp. 717–730, 2006.

[4] T. Takeuchi, T. Nakagawa, Y. Maeda et al., "Functional defect of B lymphocytes in a patient with selective IgM deficiency associated with systemic lupus erythematosus," *Autoimmunity*, vol. 34, no. 2, pp. 115–122, 2001.

[5] N. J. Vogelzang, H. Corwin, and J. L. Finlay, "Clear cell sarcoma and selective IgM deficiency. A case report," *Cancer*, vol. 49, no. 2, pp. 234–238, 1982.

[6] L. Yel, S. Ramanuja, and S. Gupta, "Clinical and immunological features in igm deficiency," *International Archives of Allergy and Immunology*, vol. 150, no. 3, pp. 291–298, 2009.

[7] F. Biagi, "The significance of duodenal mucosal atrophy in patients with common variable immunodeficiency," *American Journal of Clinical Pathology*, vol. 138, pp. 185–189, 2012.

[8] A. Lai Ping So and L. Mayer, "Gastrointestinal manifestations of primary immunodeficiency disorders," *Seminars in Gastrointestinal Disease*, vol. 8, pp. 22–32, 1997.

[9] M. A. Heneghan, F. M. Stevens, E. M. Cryan, R. H. Warner, and C. F. McCarthy, "Celiac sprue and immunodeficiency states: a 25-year review," *Journal of Clinical Gastroenterology*, vol. 25, no. 2, pp. 421–425, 1997.

[10] P. Asquith, R. A. Thompson, and W. T. Cooke, "Serum-immunoglobulins in adult coeliac disease," *Lancet*, vol. 2, no. 7612, pp. 129–131, 1969.

[11] T. E. Blecher, A. Brzechwa-Ajdukiewicz, C. F. McCarthy, and A. E. Read, "Serum immunoglobulins and lymphocyte transformation studies in coeliac disease," *Gut*, vol. 10, no. 1, pp. 57–62, 1969.

[12] M. A. Heneghan, F. M. Stevens, E. M. Cryan, R. H. Warner, and C. F. McCarthy, "Celiac sprue and immunodeficiency states: a 25-year review," *Journal of Clinical Gastroenterology*, vol. 25, no. 2, pp. 421–425, 1997.

[13] A. Fernández, L. González, and J. de-la-Fuente, "Coeliac disease: clinical features in adult populations," *Revista Espanola de Enfermedades Digestivas*, vol. 102, no. 8, pp. 466–471, 2010.

[14] T. Yamasaki, "Selective IgM deficiency: functional assessment of peripheral blood lymphocytes in vitro," *Internal Medicine*, vol. 31, no. 7, pp. 866–870, 1992.

[15] A. Dahele, K. Kingstone, J. Bode, D. Anderson, and S. Ghosh, "Anti-endomysial antibody negative celiac disease: does additional serological testing help?" *Digestive Diseases and Sciences*, vol. 46, no. 1, pp. 214–221, 2001.

[16] A. Meini, N. M. Pillan, V. Villanacci, V. Monafo, A. G. Ugazio, and A. Plebani, "Prevalence and diagnosis of celiac disease in IgA-deficient children," *Annals of Allergy, Asthma and Immunology*, vol. 77, no. 4, pp. 333–336, 1996.

[17] A. Rostom, C. Dubé, A. Cranney et al., "The diagnostic accuracy of serologic tests for celiac disease: a systematic review," *Gastroenterology*, vol. 128, no. 4, supplement 1, pp. S38–S46, 2005.

[18] E. F. Verdu, D. Armstrong, and J. A. Murray, "Between celiac disease and irritable bowel syndrome: the "no man's land" of gluten sensitivity," *American Journal of Gastroenterology*, vol. 104, no. 6, pp. 1587–1594, 2009.

21

Angora Wool Asthma in Textile Industry

Pietro Sartorelli, Riccardo Romeo, Giuseppina Coppola, Roberta Nuti, and Valentina Paolucci

Unit of Occupational Medicine and Toxicology, University of Siena, 16 Bracci Avenue, 53100 Siena, Italy

Correspondence should be addressed to Pietro Sartorelli, pietro.sartorelli@unisi.it

Academic Editors: M. T. Siddiqui and A. Vojdani

Up to now the exposures to hair and skin derivatives of animals have not yet been the subject of systematic studies. The observation of a clinical case has provided the opportunity for a review of the literature. The inpatient was a 49-year-old man, a carder in a textile factory, exposed to angora wool. He noticed the appearance of dyspnea during working hours. There was no eosinophilia in blood, and the results of pulmonary function tests were normal. The nonspecific bronchial provocation test with methacholine demonstrated an abnormal bronchial reactivity. The challenge test with angora wool was positive (decrease in FEV1 of more than 40%) as well as total IGE and specific IgE to rabbit epithelium (433 KU/l and 12.1 KUA/l, resp.). Several sources of allergens were found in the rabbit, and the main allergen was represented by proteins from epithelia, urine, and saliva. Most of these proteins belong to the family of lipocalin, they function as carriers for small hydrophobic molecules (vitamins and pheromones). If the diagnosis of occupational asthma caused by animal hair and skin derivatives may be relatively easy by means of the challenge test, defining etiology is complicated because of the lack of in vitro tests.

1. Introduction

Defining the pathogenesis, prevention, and management of occupational asthma is an involved process. Diagnosis of occupational asthma requires the integration of a multiplicity of data such as respiratory function test, nonspecific bronchial hyperreactivity test, occupational challenge test (OCT), and the timing of symptoms in relation to the occupational activities. Cutaneous tests are particularly helpful in IgE-mediated asthma in relation to the inhalation of protein aeroallergens. For haptens, because they require prior coupling to a protein carrier, they cause problems in laboratory tests. The OCT represents the golden standard for etiological diagnosis of occupational asthma. The substances responsible for occupational asthma are mainly animal allergens, vegetable agents, and chemicals. In addition to major inducers of occupational asthma, there are other agents whose importance is still difficult to understand. Among these there are high molecular weight substances such as hair and skin derivatives of animals. The exposed professional categories are mainly farmers and workers in charge of laboratory animals [1]. Up to now these exposures have not yet been the subject to systematic studies as literature only reports cases of laboratory animal allergy and domestic exposures.

There are various types of angora rabbit. Each breed produces different fur. Angora wool harvesting occurs up to three times a year and is collected by shearing or from the molting fur. This type of wool is commonly used in the textile industry for apparel such as sweaters and suits. The observation of a case of angora wool asthma has provided the opportunity for a review of the literature.

2. Case Report

The in-patient was a 49-year-old man, a carder in a textile factory, mainly exposed to angora wool. He noticed the appearance of dyspnea during working hours. There was no eosinophilia in his blood and the results of pulmonary function tests were normal compared to CECA 1971 reference values. The nonspecific bronchial provocation test with methacholine through dosimeter [2] demonstrated an abnormal bronchial reactivity. A prick test of 12 common allergens (grass, composite, pellitory, olives, cypress, alternaria, dermatophagoides farinaceous and pteronyssinus, aspergillus fumigatus, dog, cat and horse, as well as the negative and positive controls; Lofarma Laboratories, Milan, Italy) were positive to pollens. The results of the prick tests were considered positive when they provoked a rash with an average diameter of ≥ 5 mm [3].

Measurement of total and specific IgE (CAP System, Phadia, Uppsala, Sweden) showed a significant positive finding of total IGE (433 KU/l) and a positive IgE to rabbit epithelium (12.1 KUA/l). After the test with a control substance (talc powder) OCT was carried out by tipping angora wool into a 8 m^3 ventilated room and assessing FEV1 for 8 hours (Figure 1). Exposure to angora wool was stopped after 15 minutes due to the onset of coughing and dyspnea with a decrease in FEV1 of more than 40%. The nasal lavage cell counts after OCT showed an increased percentage of neutrophils (96% neutrophils, 4% epithelial cells).

The patient was also suffering from hands dermatitis. Allergens from the standard tray (SIDAPA) and the textile industry tray were used for patch testing (Firma, Florence, Italy) by the Italian public employers' liability insurance (INAIL) showing a skin positivity to balsam of Peru (++), dimethylaminopropylamine (++), benzalkonium chlorure (++), and triethanolamine (+). An occupational allergic contact dermatitis was diagnosed because triethanolamine is used as surface-active agent in textile industry.

3. Literature Analysis

Recently two PubMed search strings determinants (one more specific, the other more sensitive) have been used to retrieve information on the possible association between occupational risk factors and some pathologies [4]. Using *wool asthma, asthma and rabbit, asthma and rabbit hair, rabbit allergens and lipocalin*, 116 papers were found with the specific string (25 pertinent and 1 highly pertinent) and 197 with the sensitive one (3 pertinent and 5 highly pertinent not retrieved by the specific string). Articles mainly regarding workers in charge of laboratory animals were found. Cases of asthma due to hair and skin derivatives of animals which occurred in the textile industry were not reported in literature. In all 1 case of angora wool asthma was only found [5].

Several allergenic proteins from rabbit have been recognized by crossed immunoelectrophoresis but have not been characterized. Understanding of these important occupational allergens will allow the development of a new diagnostic approach for affected workers and others who may be at risk. Baker et al. [6] recognized as allergens 26 protein bands in the three extracts: 12 in saliva, 7 in urine, and 7 in fur. This was the first evidence that allergens from the rabbit are members of the lipocalin superfamily of proteins, suggesting that similar mechanisms may be involved in eliciting the allergic response to rabbits. The 18 kDa allergen from saliva may be the previously named rabbit allergen, Ory c 1. The major laboratory animal allergens are carried on small particles that are both capable of remaining airborne for extended periods and penetrating the lower airways of

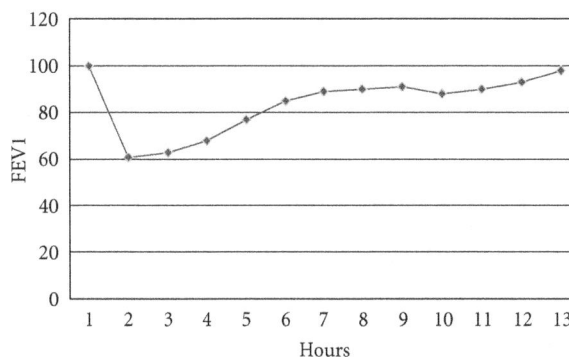

FIGURE 1: Occupational challenge test with angora wool.

exposed workers [7]. Lipocalins share common biological functions, predominantly related to the transport of small hydrophobic molecules, such as vitamins and pheromones. Immune reactivity to lipocalin allergens is not well known. Three of their epitopes were colocalized in their structurally conserved regions. Interestingly, one of the epitopes was recognized by the T cells of all patients and the computer predictions suggested that there would be an epitope in the corresponding parts of human endogenous lipocalins [6, 8]. Experimental studies on sensitizing properties of these molecules were only carried out on laboratory animal allergies [9, 10]. Lipocalins share sequence homology with antigens of the parasitic agent that causes schistosomiasis. The fact that parasite infections also trigger IgE antibody responses may account for the development of laboratory animal allergies in subjects who have never had any previous allergy [9].

4. Discussion

Analysis of the case gives the impression that the detection of specific antigens responsible of asthma in workers exposed to dermal derivatives and skin of animals is quite complex. Even if in the specific case the diagnosis was relatively simple by using OCT, etiology is not easily understandable because of the lack of immunological tests referring asthma to specific occupational compounds. At the moment OCT represents the golden standard for diagnosis and only prick tests can be used in prevention to single out subjects susceptible to developing an allergic respiratory disease to hair and skin derivatives of animals. In textile industry individuals with IgE response to rabbit epithelium should be considered susceptible to developing angora wool asthma.

References

[1] K. Aoyama, A. Ueda, F. Manda, T. Matsushita, T. Ueda, and C. Yamauchi, "Allergy to laboratory animals: an epidemiological study," *British Journal of Industrial Medicine*, vol. 49, no. 1, pp. 41–47, 1992.

[2] S. Amaducci, I. Cerveri, C. Rampulla et al., "Protocollo per l'esecuzione del test di provocazione bronchiale aspecifica," *Fisiop Resp*, vol. 3, pp. 3–15, 1982 (Italian).

[3] P. L. Paggiaro, E. Bacci, D. L. Amram, O. Rossi, and D. Talini, "Skin reactivity and specific IgE levels in the evaluation of allergic sensitivity to common allergens for epidemiological purposes," *Clinical Allergy*, vol. 16, no. 1, pp. 49–55, 1986.

[4] S. Mattioli, F. Zanardi, A. Baldasseroni et al., "Search strings for the study of putative occupational determinants of disease," *Occupational and Environmental Medicine*, vol. 67, no. 7, pp. 436–443, 2010.

[5] M. R. Atazhanov, "Case of bronchial asthma due to increased sensitivity to rabbit wool," *Klinicheskaya Meditsina*, vol. 55, no. 5, p. 133, 1977 (Russian).

[6] J. Baker, A. Berry, L. M. Boscato, S. Gordon, B. J. Walsh, and M. C. Stuart, "Identification of some rabbit allergens as lipocalins," *Clinical and Experimental Allergy*, vol. 31, no. 2, pp. 303–312, 2001.

[7] R. A. Wood, "Laboratory animal allergens," *ILAR Journal*, vol. 42, no. 1, pp. 12–16, 2001.

[8] T. Virtanen, T. Zeiler, and R. Mäntyjärvi, "Important animal allergens are lipocalin proteins: Why are they allergenic?" *International Archives of Allergy and Immunology*, vol. 120, no. 4, pp. 247–258, 1999.

[9] R. K. Bush and G. M. Stave, "Laboratory animal allergy: an update," *ILAR Journal*, vol. 44, no. 1, pp. 28–51, 2003.

[10] J. A. Price and J. L. Longbottom, "Allergy to rabbits. I. Specificity and non-specificity of RAST and crossed-radioimmunoelectrophoresis due to the presence of light chains in rabbit allergenic extracts," *Allergy*, vol. 41, no. 8, pp. 603–612, 1986.

22

Brain Abscess and Keratoacanthoma Suggestive of Hyper IgE Syndrome

Soheyla Alyasin,[1] Reza Amin,[1] Alireza Teymoori,[2] Hamidreza Houshmand,[1] Gholamreza Houshmand,[3] and Mohammad Bahadoram[4]

[1] Department of Pediatrics, Division of Immunology and Allergy, Allergic Research Center, Shiraz University of Medical Science, Shiraz 7134845794, Iran

[2] School of Medicine, Department of Neurosurgery, Ahvaz Jundishapur University of Medical Sciences, Ahvaz 6135715794, Iran

[3] Department of Pharmacology and Toxicology, Pharmacy School, Ahvaz Jundishapur University of Medical Sciences, Ahvaz 6135715794, Iran

[4] Medical Student Research Committee and Social Determinant of Health Research Center, Ahvaz Jundishapur University of Medical Sciences, Ahvaz 6135715794, Iran

Correspondence should be addressed to Hamidreza Houshmand; houshmand_ha@sums.ac.ir

Academic Editor: Alessandro Plebani

Hyper immunoglobulin-E (IgE) syndrome is an autosomal immune deficiency disease. It is characterized by an increase in IgE and eosinophil count with both T-cell and B-cell malfunction. Here, we report an 8-year-old boy whose disease started with an unusual skin manifestation. When 6 months old he developed generalized red, nontender nodules and pathologic report of the skin lesion was unremarkable (inflammatory). Then he developed a painless, cold abscess. At the age of 4 years, he developed a seronegative polyarticular arthritis. Another skin biopsy was taken which was in favor of Keratoacanthoma. Laboratory workup for immune deficiency showed high eosinophil count and high level of immunoglobulin-E, due to some diagnostic criteria (NIH sores: 41 in 9-year-olds), he was suggestive of hyper IgE syndrome. At the age of 8, the patient developed an abscess in the left inguinal region. While in hospital, the patient developed generalized tonic colonic convulsion and fever. Brain computed tomography scan revealed an abscess in the right frontal lobe. Subsequently magnetic resonance imaging (MRI) of the brain indicated expansion of the existing abscess to contralateral frontal lobe (left side). After evacuating the abscesses and administrating intravenous antibiotic, the patient's condition improved dramatically and fever stopped.

1. Introduction

Hyper immunoglobulin-E syndrome (HIES) is a rare primary immunodeficiency disease, characterized by the classical triad of recurrent staphylococcal skin abscesses, pneumonia with pneumatocele formation, and elevated levels of serum IgE, usually over 2,000 IU/mL [1]. HIES is a group of primary immunodeficiencies with overlapping and distinct features most frequently caused by deficiency in STAT3 or DOCK8. New hyper IgE syndrome entities have also been reported [1]. These include impairment of PGM3 function (phosphoglucomutase 3) and an enzyme in the glycosylation pathway (glycosylation defect). Such deficiencies are believed to be the genetic cause of hyper IgE syndrome in patients who do not carry mutations in STAT3 or DOCK8 [2].

DOCK8 hyper IgE syndrome patients present in infancy with severe atopic dermatitis and can later go on to develop severe food allergy with positive skin prick test result and specific IgE to food allergens. T helper 2 cell numbers and cytokines were significantly increased in DOCK8 IgE syndrome and atopic dermatitis patients, compared to STAT3 hyper IgE syndrome patients [3].

Particular progress has been made in deciphering the relevance of STAT3 and DOCK8 for B-cell, T-cell, and natural killer cells immunity as well as in understanding allergic features. Multisystemic features of STAT3 deficient hyper IgE syndrome, for example, are recurrent fractures and osteopenia and high degree of vasculopathy and brain with matter hyper intensities. IgG replacement may add to the clinical care in STAT3-deficient hyper IgE syndrome. In DOCK8-deficient hyper IgE syndrome the high mortality and deaths in early age seem to justify allogenic hematopoietic stem cell transplantation [1].

Both dominant and recessive forms have been reported. Autosomal dominant hyper IgE syndrome is almost always caused by dominant negative heterozygous mutations in the gene encoding STAT3. Specific IgE values, skin prick test, and T-cell subset of STAT3 hyper IgE syndrome patients' properties were analogous to those of healthy individuals except for decreased TH17 cell counts [3]. Patients with autosomal dominant hyper IgE syndrome have a history of staphylococcal abscess. Persistent pneumatoceles develop as a result of recurrent pneumonias. Pruritic dermatitis with eczema like skin lesions occurs. Coarse facial features and high incidence rates for scoliosis and hyperextensible joints also are noticeable. Only one patient had a mutation in the gene encoding Tyk2; all of the other reported patients with autosomal recessive hyper IgE syndrome had mutations in the gene encoding DOCK8. DOCK8 may be important for the formation of the immunologic synapse that leads to T-cell activation. A large majority of patients have severe asthma and food allergies. They also could have recurrent skin viral infections, including severe herpes simplex, herpes zoster, and other viral infections. In addition, patients can have abscesses, candidiasis, upper respiratory infections, and pneumonia. Neurologic problems, including strokes, meningitis, and aneurysms, are prominent. Malignancies are also common [1]. Since many genes and cell types are involved in the pathogenesis of this disease, different clinical manifestations have been reported. Reporting of unusual course and presentation of disease helps improve the knowledge of course of the disease. The following case presented with an unusual skin lesion had multiple episodes of skin abscess formation, keratoacanthoma, and brain abscesses.

2. Case Report

Our patient is an 8-year-old boy whose disease started with an unusual skin manifestation and extraordinary findings were seen during the course of treatment. At 6 months old he developed generalized red, nontender nodules. At the time, the patient had no systemic manifestation of any disease; therefore only biopsy of the lesion was taken. First biopsy was taken when he was 6 months old; the pathologic report of this biopsy was nonspecific inflammatory process. He developed a painless, cold abscess in the medial axis of his thigh at the age of 2. At that time patient had no abnormal findings in the physical examination or laboratory workup. Thus treatment for a simple abscess was done. At the age of 4, he developed a seronegative polyarticular arthritis which included proximal interphalangeal joints of hands, right elbow, both hip joints, and left knee which responded well to usual treatment for juvenile arthritis. The patient was on daily oral prednisolone and folic acid and weekly

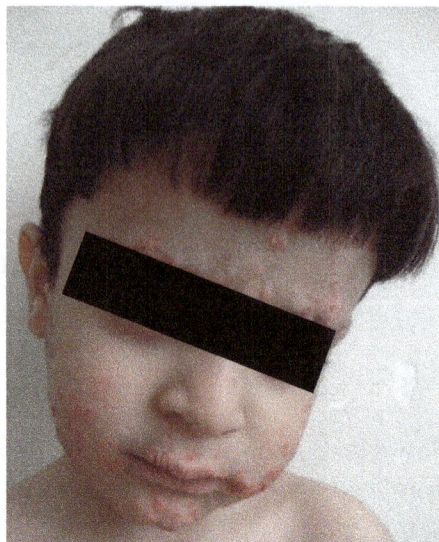

FIGURE 1: Skin manifestations of keratoacanthoma in hyper IgE syndrome (4 years old).

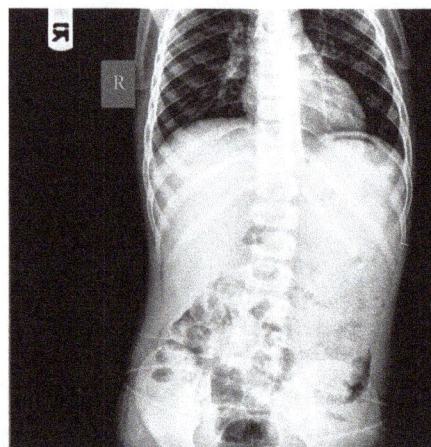

FIGURE 2: Flat upright X-ray that shows normal chest and scoliosis in thoracolumbar region.

oral methotrexate therapy. His ANA level was on normal range. During the same year, another skin biopsy was taken which was in favor of keratoacanthoma (Figure 1), and it also showed wart infection. Multiple eruptive keratoacanthomas of the patient responded well to oral isotretinoin therapy. At this time workup for immune deficiency disease was repeated. A review of family history revealed that the patient's parents were cousins. In addition, workup detected high eosinophil count in complete blood count and high level of immunoglobulin-E but due to financial limitations genetic study was not performed. According to some diagnostic criteria (the National Institute of Health clinical feature scores: 41 in 9-year-olds), he was suggested as hyper IgE syndrome patient (Table 1, Figure 2) [4]. At the age of 8, our patient developed an abscess in the left inguinal region and subsequently he was admitted to the hospital. Complete physical examination was done and nothing except left side

Table 1: Assessment by NIH scoring system with clinical and laboratory tests [4].

Clinical and laboratory finding	Results	Points
Highest serum IgE level (IU/mL)	1,001–2,000	8
Skin abscesses	1-2	2
Pneumonia (episodes over lifetime)	None	0
Parenchymal lung anomalies	Absent	0
Retained primary teeth	>3	8
Scoliosis, maximum curvature	15°–20°	4
Fractures with minor trauma	None	0
Highest eosinophil count (cells/μL)	>800	6
Characteristic face	Mildly present	2
Midline anomaly	Absent	0
Newborn rash	Absent	0
Eczema (worst stage)	Mild	1
Upper respiratory infections per year	1-2	0
Candidiasis	Fingernails	2
Other serious infections	Severe	4
Fatal infection	Absent	4
Hyperextensibility	Absent	0
Lymphoma	Absent	0
Increased nasal width	<1 SD	0
High palate	Absent	0
Young-age correction	>5 years	0
Total		41

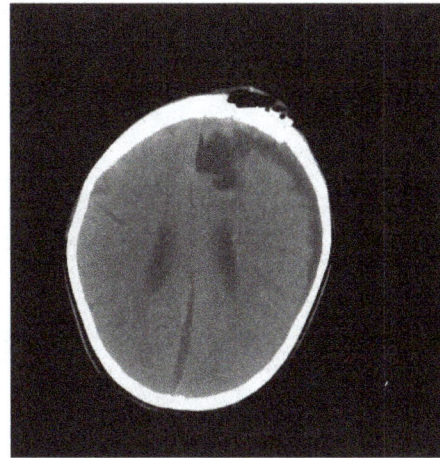

Figure 4: Primary brain CT scan that shows unilateral frontal brain abscess (confined to one hemisphere).

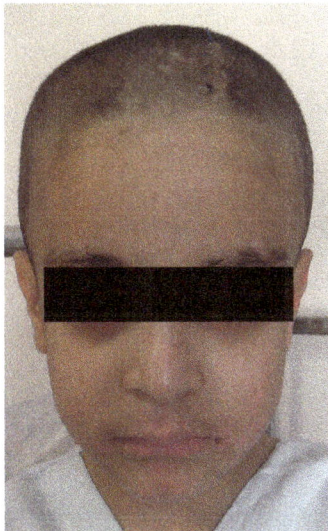

Figure 3: Scars induced after resolution of keratoacanthoma (8 years old).

inguinal abscess, scars of previous skin lesions, and retained primary teeth was detected (Figure 3). In ultrasonography a collection was detected in subcutaneous region. So, treatment was started by draining the abscess and administering broad spectrum intravenous antibiotics. Few days after admission, the patient developed a nonspecific abdominal pain. Abdominal computed tomography showed mild-free fluid with no

abscess formation; also an asymptomatic neural cyst at the root of T10 nerve and outside the spinal canal was seen. The abdominal fluid was not purulent and had no signs of malignancy. During hospitalization, the patient developed generalized tonic colonic convulsion and a fever with no neurologic deficits. Brain computed tomography scan showed an abscess measured 4.6 × 3.3 cm in the right frontal lobe (Figure 4). The abscess was then aspirated. The aspirate showed no evidence of bacterial or fungal infections and pathologic report showed tissue inflammation with inflammatory cells. Gram stain and cultures for bacteria, fungus, and mycobacteria were all negative as well as polymerase chain reaction for mycobacteria and fungus. Patient was febrile for another 2 weeks so we employed broader spectrum antibiotics and IV-IG. After a week passed with no improvement in his condition, a magnetic resonance imaging (MRI) of brain was performed which showed expansion of existing abscess to contralateral frontal lobe (left side) (Figure 5); hence full evacuation of the contents and wall of abscess was done. Repeatedly, diagnostic studies for bacterial, fungal, and mycobacterial infections were negative. After evacuating the abscess, patient's condition improved dramatically and fever stopped. The patient was given intravenous antibiotic for 4 weeks without further complications. In followups, the patient was visited monthly with no neurologic deficits or fever seen.

3. Discussion

Hyper IgE syndrome is a rare, primary, complex immunodeficiency disease which results from dysfunction of both T-lymphocytes and B-lymphocytes [1]. This disease was first named as hyper IgE syndrome by Buckley et al. upon observing an association between recurrent staphylococcal abscess formation, chronic eczema, and high level of IgE in blood circulation [5]. Pathognomonic findings in these patients are the presence of pneumatocele. Other respiratory system associated infections include paranasal sinusitis and otitis media [6–8]. Freeman et al. described a case series of 6

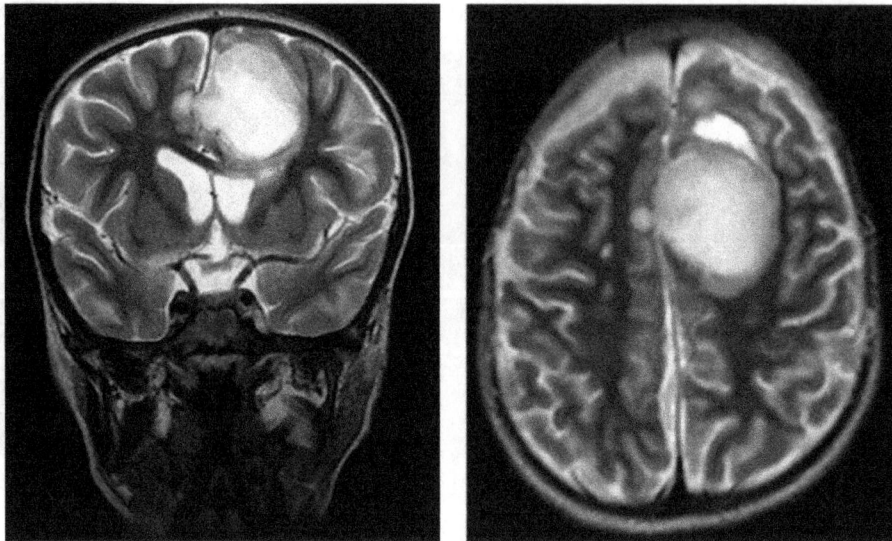

FIGURE 5: Brain MRI showing expansion of aspirated brain abscess to contralateral frontal lobe.

hyper IgE patients who died due to fungal and pseudomonas infection of lung [9].

Autoimmune diseases are another symptom of primary immune deficiency diseases and may invade joints and cause arthralgia and arthritis. Joint involvement is more commonly seen in humoral immunodeficiency diseases other than hyper IgE [10]. Brain abscess is an unusual and lethal infection; it usually presents as a space-occupying lesion and is accompanied by headache, nausea, vomiting, lethargy, stupor, and seizure [11]. Immunodeficiency is a risk factor for brain abscess formation. Gatz SA and colleagues reported brain abscess in girls with hyper IgE syndrome as a complication of bone marrow transplantation [12]. Metin et al. described tuberculous brain abscess in patient with hyper IgE syndrome [13]. Also from Iran Amini and colleagues on Tanaffoss 2010 reported brain abscess in patients with hyper IgE syndrome [14]. Among immune deficiency diseases, common variable immunodeficiency is the most common. Though rare, brain abscess is most commonly seen among CVID patients [15]. Abscess formation is one of the manifestations seen commonly in hyper IgE syndrome and occurs mostly in organs such as skin and deep viscera and predominantly in lungs. Nonetheless, brain abscess in association with hyper IgE syndrome has rarely been reported [16].

Conflict of Interests

The authors declare that there is no conflict of interests regarding the publication of this paper.

References

[1] S. Farmand and M. Sundin, "Hyper-IgE syndromes: recent advances in pathogenesis, diagnostics and clinical care," *Current Opinion in Hematology*, vol. 22, no. 1, pp. 12–22, 2015.

[2] A. Sassi, S. Lazaroski, G. Wu et al., "Hypomorphic homozygous mutations in phosphoglucomutase 3 (PGM3) impair immunity and increase serum IgE levels," *The Journal of Allergy and Clinical Immunology*, vol. 133, no. 5, pp. 1410.e13–1419.e13, 2014.

[3] A. C. Boos, B. Hagl, A. Schlesinger et al., "Atopic dermatitis, STAT3- and DOCK8-hyper-IgE syndromes differ in IgE-based sensitization pattern," *Allergy*, vol. 69, no. 7, pp. 943–953, 2014.

[4] A. P. Hsu, J. Davis, J. M. Puck, S. M. Holland, and A. F. Freeman, "Autosomal dominant hyper IgE syndrome," in *GeneReviews*, University of Washington, Seattle, Wash, USA, 2012, http://www.ncbi.nlm.nih.gov/books/NBK25507/.

[5] R. H. Buckley, B. B. Wray, and E. Z. Belmaker, "Extreme hyper-immunoglobulinemia E and undue susceptibility to infection," *Pediatrics*, vol. 49, no. 1, pp. 59–70, 1972.

[6] K. Görür, C. Özcan, M. Ünal, Y. Akbaş, and Y. Vayisoğlu, "Hyper immunoglobulin-E syndrome: a case with chronic ear draining mimicking polypoid otitis media," *International Journal of Pediatric Otorhinolaryngology*, vol. 67, no. 4, pp. 409–412, 2003.

[7] M. D. S. Erlewyn-Lajeunesse, "Hyperimmunoglobulin-E syndrome with recurrent infection: a review of current opinion and treatment," *Pediatric Allergy and Immunology*, vol. 11, no. 3, pp. 133–141, 2000.

[8] R. C. Shamberger, M. E. Wohl, A. Perez-Atayde, and W. H. Hendren, "Pneumatocele complicating hyperimmunoglobulin E syndrome (Job's syndrome)," *The Annals of Thoracic Surgery*, vol. 54, no. 6, pp. 1206–1208, 1992.

[9] A. F. Freeman, D. E. Kleiner, H. Nadiminti et al., "Causes of death in hyper-IgE syndrome," *The Journal of Allergy and Clinical Immunology*, vol. 119, no. 5, pp. 1234–1240, 2007.

[10] C. Sordet, A. Cantagrel, T. Schaeverbeke, and J. Sibilia, "Bone and joint disease associated with primary immune deficiencies," *Joint, Bone, Spine : Revue du Rhumatisme*, vol. 72, no. 6, pp. 503–514, 2005.

[11] K. A. Ramakrishnan, M. Levin, and S. N. Faust, "Bacterial meningitis and brain abscess," *Medicine*, vol. 37, no. 11, pp. 567–573, 2009.

[12] S. A. Gatz, U. Benninghoff, C. Schütz et al., "Curative treatment of autosomal-recessive hyper-IgE syndrome by hematopoietic cell transplantation," *Bone Marrow Transplantation*, vol. 46, no. 4, pp. 552–556, 2011.

[13] A. Metin, G. Uysal, A. Güven, A. Unlu, and M. H. Öztürk, "Tuberculous brain abscess in a patient with hyper IgE syndrome," *Pediatrics International*, vol. 46, no. 1, pp. 97–100, 2004.

[14] S. Amini, S. Khalilzadeh, and A. A. Velayati, "Pulmonary manifestations of pediatric hyper IgE syndrome," *Medical Sciences Journal of Islamic Azad University—Tehran Medical Branch*, vol. 20, no. 1, pp. 64–67, 2010.

[15] N. C. Patel, I. C. Hanson, and L. M. Noroski, "Methicillin-susceptible Staphylococcus aureus brain abscess in common variable immunodeficiency after an 8-month gap in return to the immunologist," *Journal of Allergy and Clinical Immunology*, vol. 122, no. 5, pp. 1036–1037, 2008.

[16] M. Beitzke, C. Enzinger, C. Windpassinger et al., "Community acquired *Staphylococcus aureus* meningitis and cerebral abscesses in a patient with a Hyper-IgE and a Dubowitz-like syndrome," *Journal of the Neurological Sciences*, vol. 309, no. 1-2, pp. 12–15, 2011.

23

Autoimmune Hepatitis with Anti Centromere Antibodies

Moushumi Lodh,[1] **Debkant Pradhan,**[2] **and Ashok Parida**[3]

[1] *Department of Biochemistry, The Mission Hospital, Durgapur, West Bengal 713212, India*
[2] *Department of Microbiology, The Mission Hospital, Durgapur, West Bengal 713212, India*
[3] *Department of Cardiology, The Mission Hospital, Durgapur, West Bengal 713212, India*

Correspondence should be addressed to Moushumi Lodh; drmoushumilodh@gmail.com

Academic Editors: M. T. Perez-Gracia, C. Pignata, and B. Sarov

We present the case report of a 49-year-old type 2 diabetes mellitus patient presenting with abdominal pain and black stool for 15 days. A proper workup of laboratory investigations helped us diagnose autoimmune hepatitis with anticentromere antibodies. The authors would like to highlight that screening AIH patients for anticentromere antibody is not mandatory but can be considered, especially in the presence of disease-related symptomatology for quicker, more accurate diagnosis and optimum management.

1. Introduction

Autoimmune liver disease is not an uncommon cause of chronic hepatitis in women. Although autoimmune destruction usually occurs without an identifiable trigger, it is generally a progressive hepatitis with increased immunoglobulins and autoantibodies, which primarily responds to immunosuppression.

2. Case Report

A 49-year-old lady presented with history of mild, intermittent abdominal pain of 15 days duration associated with passage of black colored stool, nausea, loss of appetite, and generalized weakness. At admission, she was pale, afebrile, with pulse 110/min, blood pressure 150/90 mm Hg, respiratory rate 26/min, and random plasma glucose 230 mg/dL. There was dyspnea on exertion. Skin was warm with no rash or discoloration. Her abdomen was soft, and bowel sounds were audible. There was a generalized abdominal tenderness with an irregular lump near the epigastrium. The patient was conscious and well oriented with no neurological deficit. She has undergone percutaneous transluminal coronary angioplasty (PTCA) to the right coronary artery 8 years back. The patient had no history of alcohol abuse or received drugs that can idiosyncratically cause hepatitis.

Laboratory investigations were as follows (reference ranges in parentheses): hemoglobin 9.1 g% (12–15), PCV 28.2% (36–46), total count 7000/cumm (4000–10,000), RBC 3.27 million/cumm (4.5–5.5), platelet 1.59 lakhs/cumm (1.5–4), total bilirubin 1.8 mg/dL (upto 1), direct bilirubin 0.8 mg/dL (upto 0.3), glycosylated hemoglobin 10.7% (6–8), total protein 5.7 g/dL (6.5–8.1), albumin 2.4 g/dL (3.5–5), alanine transaminase 257 U/L (0–31), aspartate transaminase 224 U/L (0–32), alkaline phosphatase 793 U/L (30–279), gamma glutamyl transferase 477 U/L (1–94), lipase 96 U/L (upto 160), amylase 48 U/L (25–125), lactic dehydrogenase 1203 U/L (266–500), and prothrombin time 18 seconds (control 11.5) INR 1.58. Urea, creatinine, alpha-1 antitrypsin, serum copper, and electrolytes were within reference range. Viral serologies for antibodies to hepatitis B surface antigen, antihepatitis B surface antigen, antihepatitis B core antigen, antihepatitis C virus, cytomegalovirus, Epstein-Barr virus, herpes simplex virus, and human immunodeficiency virus were all negative. Immunoglobulin G was 1987 mg/dL (700–1600 mg/dL). Antinuclear antibody (ANA) by IFA (1 : 320 titer) on Hep-2 cells (HEp-2000 IgG fluorescent ANA-Ro test system, Immunoconcepts, USA) revealed anticentromere antibodies (Figure 1) showing 40–60 discrete speckles distributed over the nucleus, either dispersed or gathered closely together on the chromosomes of cells undergoing division. Four positive ANA controls (homogeneous, speckled, centromere, and nucleolar) included in the kit were also run for comparison. ANA repeated by enzyme immunoassay was 195.6 units (<20). Immunochromatography showed centromere B and soluble liver antigen/liver-pancreas antigen (SLA/LP) antibodies to be positive. Antithyroid antibodies (antiperoxidase and antithyroglobulin) and antigastric parietal cell antibodies were not detected by line immunoassay. Liver biopsy showed a portal mononuclear cell infiltration, interface hepatitis in the liver tissue, and bridging fibrosis. International autoimmune hepatitis group score was 16. Upper gastrointestinal endoscopy revealed erosive pangastritis with duodenal erosions (D1 and D2). Rapid urease test for *Helicobacter pylori* was negative. Ultrasonography of the whole abdomen was a normal study. Echocardiography revealed severe mitral regurgitation and mild pericardial effusion. Based on all these findings, diagnosis of autoimmune hepatitis with type 2 diabetes mellitus, coagulopathy, and ischemic heart disease was made. The absence of piecemeal necrosis or florid bile duct lesion along with antismooth muscle antibody (ASMA) and antimitochondrial antibody (AMA) negativity ruled out autoimmune hepatitis-primary biliary cirrhosis (AIH/PBC) overlap syndrome. Injection insulin H Mixtard (50:50) 16 units thirty minutes before breakfast, 22 units thirty minutes before lunch, and 14 units before dinner were started. She was put on diabetic diet (1500 kcal/day). Prednisolone 30 mg daily was started in combination with azathioprine 50 mg daily. She was discharged after 7 days in a stable condition with medical advice (pantocid 40 mg once a day (O. D) for 4 weeks, ecosprin 150 mg O. D, cardace 10 mg O. D) and to continue insulin and steroids. At follow up after 4 weeks, her liver enzymes had reduced to within reference range, but ANA still tested positive at 1:160 titer. Random plasma glucose was 140 mg/dL; she did not develop any complication due to steroid therapy.

3. Discussion

Autoimmune hepatitis (AIH) can present as an acute or even an alarmingly fulminant hepatitis or conversely be asymptomatic and recognized only incidentally by routine biochemical tests of liver function. The critical and readily measurable indices reflecting the essence of AIH are a lack of evidence of current viral infection, transferases greater than twice upper normal limit, and immunoglobulin G greater than 1.1 times upper normal limit, interface hepatitis with plasma cell prominence, and positivity to an acceptable titer for SMA, ANA, anti-SLA/LP, or anti-LKM [1]. Our case is noteworthy due to the apparently innocuous presentation and the presence of anticentromere antibody (ACA), which is commonly associated with the limited form of systemic sclerosis, primary biliary cirrhosis, and sometimes with diffuse form of systemic sclerosis.

The immune response that targets the liver in AIH involves cytotoxic T lymphocytes, which damage the hepatocytes via the production of interleukins (IL-2, IL- 12, and tumor necrosis factor-α (TNF-α)). However, the molecular target of the T lymphocyte response has not yet been identified [2]. The Committee for Autoimmune Serology

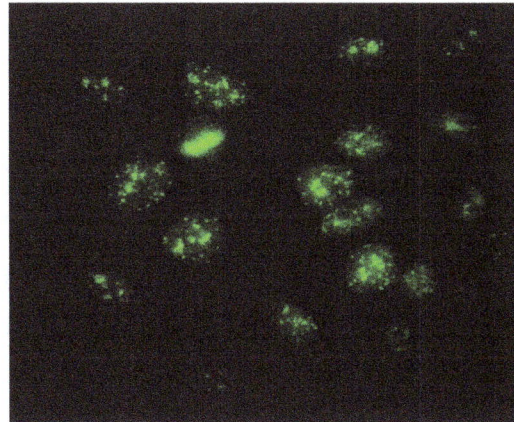

FIGURE 1: Indirect immunofluorescence on HEp-2 cells performed with an autoimmune hepatitis serum and demonstrating centromere staining.

of the International Autoimmune Hepatitis Group (IAIHG) provided guidelines on testing for autoantibodies relevant to AIH and concluded that indirect immunofluorescence assay (IFA) on fresh sections of multiorgan (liver, kidney, and stomach) from rodents (usually rat) should be the first line screening and the use of the three tissues enabling simultaneous detection of virtually all the autoantibodies relevant to liver disease, namely, against smooth muscle antigen (SMA), Antinuclear antibody (ANA), anti-liver-kidney microsome (LKM1), antimitochondrial antibody (AMA), and anticytosolic liver antigen type 1 (LC1) [3]. Despite its limited clinical sensitivity of 7–19%, the testing for anti-SLA antibodies can be considered as pathognomonic markers of AIH, with specificity close to 100% [4]. AIH may be due to dysfunction of cellular and humoral immunity related to systemic sclerosis as anticentromere antibody has been detected in 13% of patients with AIH [5]. Twenty percent of patients of AIH can have other autoimmune diseases such as Hashimotos thyroiditis, type 1 diabetes, rheumatoid arthritis, systemic lupus erythematosus, ulcerative colitis/Crohn's disease, and celiac disease [6]. Our patient had type 2 diabetes mellitus. No significant differences in age, sex, and onset pattern of the disease, progression to hepatic failure, and relapse rate were present between ACA-AIH and other AIH groups [7].

Autoimmune hepatitis is one of the few liver diseases with excellent response to therapy; most patients with AIH have a favorable response to treatment with prednisolone and azathioprine, although some patients with refractory AIH or more aggressive disease require more potent immunesuppressant agents, such as cyclosporine [2]. Patients without cirrhosis who undergo treatment have a 10–20 year survival probability more than 80% [6]. Screening AIH patients for anticentromere antibody is not mandatory but can be considered, especially in the presence of disease-related symptomatology for quicker, more accurate diagnosis and optimum management.

References

[1] I. R. Mackay, "Autoimmune hepatitis: from the clinic to the diagnostics laboratory," *Laboratory Medicine*, vol. 42, no. 4, pp. 224–233, 2011.

[2] H. I. Fallatah and H. O. Akbar, "Elevated serum immunoglobulin G levels in patients with chronic liver disease in comparison to patients with autoimmune hepatitis," *Libyan Journal of Medicine*, vol. 5, no. 1, pp. 1–4, 2010.

[3] D. P. Bogdanos, P. Invernizzi, I. R. Mackay, and D. Vergani, "Autoimmune liver serology: current diagnostic and clinical challenges," *World Journal of Gastroenterology*, vol. 14, no. 21, pp. 3374–3387, 2008.

[4] C. Radzimski, C. Probst, B. Teegen et al., "Development of a recombinant cell-based indirect immunofluorescence assay for the determination of autoantibodies against soluble liver antigen in autoimmune hepatitis," *Clinical and Developmental Immunology*, vol. 2013, Article ID 572815, 7 pages, 2013.

[5] B. C. You, S. W. Jeong, J. Y. Jang et al., "Liver cirrhosis due to autoimmune hepatitis combined with systemic sclerosis," *The Korean Journal of Gastroenterology*, vol. 59, no. 1, pp. 48–52, 2012.

[6] A. Makol, K. D. Watt, and V. R. Chowdhary, "Autoimmune hepatitis: a review of current diagnosis and treatment," *Hepatitis Research and Treatment*, vol. 2011, Article ID 390916, 11 pages, 2011.

[7] T. Himoto, M. Murota, H. Yoneyama et al., "Clinical characteristics of patients with autoimmune hepatitis seropositive for anticentromere antibody," *Hepatology Research*, vol. 40, no. 8, pp. 786–792, 2010.

24

Acute Spontaneously Resolving Pulmonary Vasculitis: A Case Report

James B. Geake[1] and Graeme Maguire[2, 3]

[1] Department of Respiratory and Sleep Medicine, Monash Medical Centre, Melbourne, VIC 3206, Australia
[2] Cairns Clinical School, School of Medicine and Dentistry, Faculty of Medicine, Health and Molecular Sciences, James Cook University, P.O. Box 902, Cairns, QLD 4870, Australia
[3] Baker IDI Central Australia, P.O. Box 1294, Alice Springs, NT 0870, Australia

Correspondence should be addressed to James B. Geake, james.geake@southernhealth.org.au

Academic Editors: A. M. Mansour and A. V. Vanikar

This is the first description that we are aware of describing the spontaneous resolution of an acute pulmonary vasculitis, possibly secondary to microscopic polyangiitis. Haemoptysis is a common symptom for patients presenting to primary and tertiary referral centres, and pulmonary vasculitis is one of a variety of aetiologies that should always be considered. The pulmonary vasculitides are difficult diagnostic and management problems. They are encumbered by a relative paucity of level 1 evidence addressing their diagnosis, classification, and treatment. This is therefore an important paper to publish because it adds to the global breadth of experience with this important clinical condition.

In July 2010 a 43-year-old female presented with a 24-hour history of 30 mL of frank haemoptysis. There were no symptoms suggestive of a respiratory infection. She worked as an office manager and had no relevant occupational or environmental exposures. She had ceased smoking ten years previously having accumulated a ten-pack-year history. She had hypertension treated with amlodipine and perimenstrual migraines. Both parents and her brother were alive without any significant medical diseases.

On presentation peripheral arterial oxygen saturation was 85% on room air, respiratory rate was 24 per minute, blood pressure was 200/100, and temperature was 38.5°C. She remained afebrile thereafter. An ECG demonstrated sinus rhythm, 100 beats per minute. A chest X-ray demonstrated bilateral perihilar infiltrates. A CTPA confirmed diffuse bilateral alveolar infiltrates (Figure 1). No vascular filling defects were identified. Haemoglobin was 99 g/L (115–160). MCV (mean cell volume) was 67 fL (81–96), and the film was suggestive of iron deficiency. White cell count was mildly elevated at 137/nL (3.5–11). Other inflammatory markers were also mildly elevated. ESR (erythrocyte sedimentation rate) was 29 mm (<15).

CRP (C-reactive protein) was 68.1 mgl/L (<8). Creatinine was 65 µmol/L (50–100). Urea was 48 µmol/L (2.7–7.8). Electrolytes were within normal limits. INR (international normalised ratio) was 1.1 (0·9–1.2). APTT (activated partial thromboplastin time) was 28 seconds (25–34). Testing for antiglomerular basement membrane, antinuclear cytoplasmic antibodies (cANCA and pANCA), antinuclear antibodies, and extractable nuclear antigens (ENA) were all negative. Rheumatoid factor was <10 IU/mL (<30). Several sputum samples were sent. No pathogens were identified on standard bacterial and mycobacterial cultures. There was no cytological evidence of malignancy. Urinalysis was normal. Phase contrast microscopy was not performed as the red cell count on several specimens was within normal limits. Albumin/creatinine ratio was 17.7 g/mol creatinine (<3.5). The patient was treated with benzylpenicillin and doxycycline, and there was improved, but persisting haemoptysis. On the third day the patient proceeded to fibre optic bronchoscopy where no source of bleeding or endobronchial abnormality was identified. A surgical lung biopsy was subsequently performed. At the operation blood was noted within the pleural space, the surface of the lung was oozing

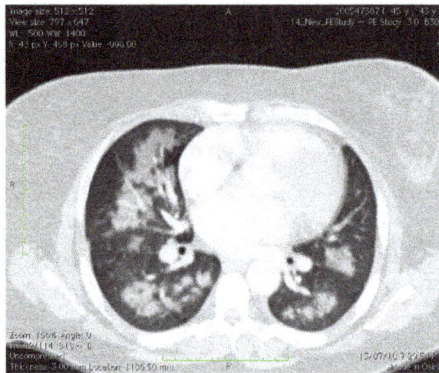

FIGURE 1: Coronal CT chest demonstrating bilateral perihilar pulmonary infiltrates consistent with diffuse alveolar haemorrhage.

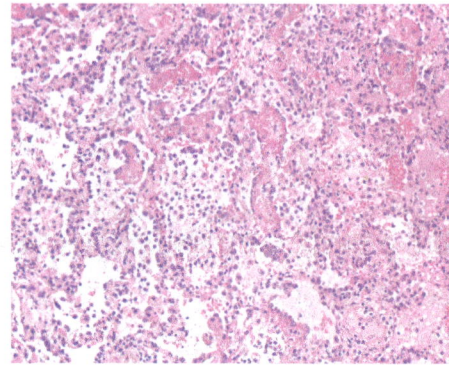

FIGURE 2: Low power magnification of hematoxylin and eosin stained lung biopsy demonstrating a pauci-immune small vessel vasculitis.

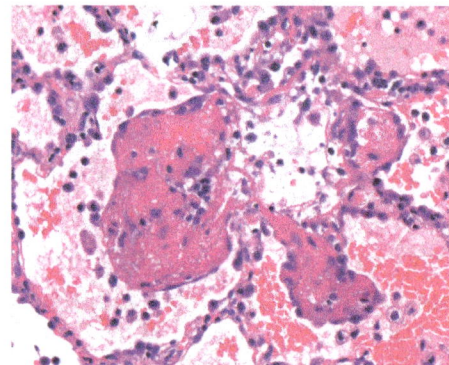

FIGURE 3: High power magnification of hematoxylin and eosin stained lung biopsy demonstrating a pauci-immune small vessel vasculitis.

fresh blood, and the parenchyma was boggy. A wedge biopsy was taken from the right middle lobe. Microscopy demonstrated a widespread interstitial inflammatory process centred on capillary sized vessels. There were associated interstitial haemorrhage and fibrin deposition. Occasional neutrophils and eosinophils were both observed. The disease process was variable in intensity with propensity for different expression on either side of an interlobular septum. No granulomata were identified. Special stains were negative for fungal hyphae and *Pneumocystis* species (Figures 2 and 3). A diagnosis of small vessel pulmonary vasculitis was made, thought to be most consistent with microscopic polyangiitis.

The patient made an uneventful recovery from the surgical procedure and the haemoptysis appeared to rapidly spontaneously settle. Induction immunosuppression with cyclophosphamide and high dose prednisolone was discussed. However, the patient declined. The patient was therefore, discharged three days after the operation with close outpatient surveillance arranged. Repeated clinical reviews with an assessment of lung function, chest radiology, renal function, and urinalysis demonstrated continued complete resolution of pulmonary vasculitis. 12 months after her initial presentation she remained well.

Pulmonary vasculitis should be considered in the differential diagnosis of haemoptysis. Microscopic polyangiitis is a small vessel systemic vasculitis that usually manifests with glomerulonephritis. The lungs are involved in association in approximately 20% to 30% of cases, with diffuse alveolar haemorrhage in approximately 10% to 20% [1, 2]. It is associated with pANCA in 90% of the cases [3]. It is rare for this disease to present with diffuse alveolar haemorrhage in isolation. Treatment recommendations are largely based on historical data demonstrating poor prognosis for patients with pauciimmune glomerulonephritis. No randomised controlled trials have been performed for patients with pulmonary haemorrhage. Many advocate aggressive immunosuppression in this clinical situation with a combination of cyclophosphamide and high dose of prednisolone, with or without plasma exchange [4]. Owing to the toxic effects of this regimen, different strategies have been investigated, and promising disease modifying and biological alternatives continue to emerge, both for induction and maintenance immunosuppression.

Here we described the unusual case of small vessel pulmonary vasculitis with spontaneous remission. Whilst the histology is thought to favour a diagnosis of microscopic polyangiitis, it is possible that an alternate diagnosis was missed, for example, through sampling error. This case highlights the difficulties applying guidelines to rare diseases, particularly when presentations are atypical, as was the case of this patient.

Abbreviations

MCV: Mean cell volume
ESR: Erythrocyte sedimentation rate
CRP: C-reactive protein
INR: International normalised ratio
ENA: Extractable nuclear antigens
ANCA: Antinuclear cytoplasmic antibodies.

Conflict of Interests

Both James Geake and Graeme Maguire confirm there were no financial or other sources of support in the preparation of this paper, and there are no conflicts of interests.

Acknowledgments

There were no internal or external funding sources. J. Geake was responsible for the review of the case data, drafting of the paper, and the review of the literature. G. Maguire was responsible for the supervision and editing of the final paper. Both are guaranators for the final paper. The patient described in this case report was treated by the authors at the Royal Hobart Hospital, in Tasmania, Australia.

References

[1] C. Agard, L. Mouthon, A. Mahr, and L. Guillevin, "Microscopic polyangiitis and polyarteritis nodosa: how and when do they start?" *Arthritis Care and Research*, vol. 49, no. 5, pp. 709–715, 2003.

[2] S. E. Lane, R. A. Watts, L. Shepstone, and D. G. I. Scott, "Primary systemic vasculitis: clinical features and mortality," *QJM*, vol. 98, no. 2, pp. 97–111, 2005.

[3] L. Guillevin, B. Durand-Gasselin, R. Cevallos et al., "Microscopic polyangiitis: clinical and laboratory findings in 85 patients," *Arthritis & Rheumatism*, vol. 42, pp. 421–430, 1999.

[4] P. J. Klemmer, W. Chalermskulrat, M. S. Reif, S. L. Hogan, D. C. Henke, and R. J. Falk, "Plasmapheresis therapy for diffuse alveolar haemorrhage in patients with small-vessel vasculitis," *American Journal of Kidney Diseases*, vol. 42, no. 6, pp. 1149–1153, 2003.

25

Periodic Fever and Neutrophilic Dermatosis: Is It Sweet's Syndrome?

Raheleh Assari,[1] **Vahid Ziaee,**[1,2,3] **Nima Parvaneh,**[3,4] **and Mohammad-Hassan Moradinejad**[1,3]

[1]*Division of Pediatric Rheumatology, Children's Medical Center, Pediatrics Center of Excellence, Tehran 14194, Iran*
[2]*Pediatric Rheumatology Research Group, Rheumatology Research Center, Tehran University of Medical Sciences, Tehran, Iran*
[3]*Department of Pediatrics, Tehran University of Medical Sciences, Tehran, Iran*
[4]*Research Center for Immunodeficiencies, Tehran University of Medical Sciences, Tehran, Iran*

Correspondence should be addressed to Vahid Ziaee; ziaee@tums.ac.ir

Academic Editor: Ahmad M. Mansour

A 7-year-old boy with high grade fever (39°C) and warm, erythematous, and indurated plaque above the left knee was referred. According to the previous records of this patient, these indurated plaques had been changed toward abscesses formation and then spontaneous drainage had occurred after about 6 to 7 days, and finally these lesions healed with scars. In multiple previous admissions, high grade fever, leukocytosis, and a noticeable increase in erythrocyte sedimentation rate and C-reactive protein were noted. After that, until 7th year of age, he had shoulder, gluteal, splenic, kidney, and left thigh lesions and pneumonia. The methylprednisolone pulse (30 mg/kg) was initiated with the diagnosis of Sweet's syndrome. After about 10–14 days, almost all of the laboratory data regressed to nearly normal limits. After about 5 months, he was admitted again with tachypnea and high grade fever and leukocytosis. After infusion of one methylprednisolone pulse, the fever and tachypnea resolved rapidly in about 24 hours. In this admission, colchicine (1 mg/kg) was added to the oral prednisolone after discharge. In the periodic fever and neutrophilic dermatosis, the rheumatologist should search for sterile abscesses in other organs.

1. Introduction

Neutrophilic dermatosis (ND) is a group of disorders with intense neutrophilic infiltration in the skin and extracutaneous involvement. Recently, these disorders have been known as neutrophilic diseases [1]. ND is presented as dermal neutrophilic dermatosis (such as Sweet's syndrome), dermal and hypodermal neutrophilic dermatosis (pyoderma gangrenosum, neutrophilic panniculitis, and skin aseptic abscesses), and epidermal neutrophilic dermatosis [1]. ND may be associated with other systemic disorders such as myeloproliferative disorders, inflammatory bowel disease, and rheumatoid arthritis [1]. In the children, ND may precede the other manifestations of underlying disease for many years [2]. Familial Mediterranean fever and ND have similar clinical manifestations that suggest the possibility of similar mechanism to stimulate neutrophils [3].

In this paper, a case of periodic fever associated with ND (dermal, dermal and hypodermal neutrophilic dermatoses) and hyperleukocytosis, initiated from the neonatal period, was reported.

2. Case Report

A 7-year-old boy was referred to the rheumatology clinic with high grade fever ($T = 39°C$) and warm, erythematous, and indurated plaque above the left knee with the size of about 8×10 cm diameters (Figure 1). According to the previous records of this patient, these indurated plaques had been changed toward abscesses formation and then spontaneous drainage had occurred after about 6 to 7 days, and finally these lesions healed with scars. He had two scars of previous lesions on the outer side of the left thigh and the outer side of right shoulder.

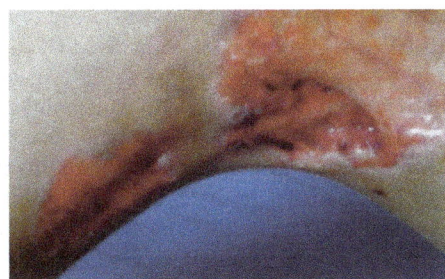

(a)

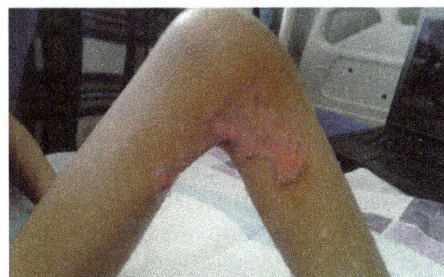

(b)

FIGURE 1: Skin lesion in the left knee in our patients with Sweet's syndrome: (a) acute phase, (b) after 7 days.

He was born at 33rd week of gestational age, with about 2130 g birth weight. He had low Apgar scores at the first and fifth minutes of the birth time. He received surfactant due to prematurity of the lungs. He stayed in hospital for about one month. During the admission he had fever and plantar cellulitis, cellulitis of the right testis, and abscess and necrosis of the root of umbilical cord. So, he received a combination of meropenem and vancomycin antibiotics. The smears and cultures of these lesions were negative. The histopathology of plantar cellulitis represented granulation tissues with nonspecific inflammation. The umbilical cord had delay in seperation for about 45 days. So, the clinicians decided to cut it off. The first complete blood count of his life revealed white blood cell count (WBC) of 9700 per mm^3, with 26% neutrophils and 61% lymphocytes, hemoglobin (Hb) of 13.4 g/dL, and the platelet (PLT) count of 443000 per mm^3. During the first year of life, he had seven admissions for recurrent respiratory infections.

After the first year, he had repetitive admissions due to fever and leukocytosis. He had history of splenic lesions with left lobar pneumonia in second year. About 2 months later, a lung lesion appeared in the left upper lobe with about 10×10 cm size. After that, until 7th year of age, he had shoulder lesion, gluteal lesion, splenic lesions, kidney lesions (enlargement of both kidneys with multiple low-density areas in ultrasonography), left thigh lesion, and pneumonia. In one of these admissions, he presented with pyoderma gangrenosum (PG) and chest wall lesion. In another admission, the erythema nodosum-like lesions on the feet appeared. These recurrences were usually preceded by upper respiratory tract or gastrointestinal infections.

The laboratory data in one admission with abscesses-like formation in upper lobe of right lung revealed white blood cell count 68300 per mm^3, with 82% neutrophils and 10% lymphocytes, hemoglobin 7 g/dL, platelet count 694000 per mm^3, ESR 103 mm/hour, and CRP 78 mg/dL. After treatment with broad spectrum antibiotics for about 10–14 days, the laboratory data demonstrated WBC 10100 per mm^3, with 25% neutrophils, and 65% lymphocytes, Hb 8.9 g/dL, PLT 724000 per mm^3, ESR 41 mm/hour, and CRP 6.1 mg/dL. In all admissions, high grade fever, leukocytosis, and a noticeable increase in erythrocyte sedimentation rate and C-reactive protein were noted. After about 10–14 days, almost all of the laboratory data regressed to nearly normal limits.

In these seven years, all of the cultures and smears for infections were negative. Smears of the lesions showed many white blood cells with 95% neutrophils and 5% lymphocytes. In evaluation for immunodeficiency disorders, CD3, CD4, CD8, CD16, CD19, and CD56 were within the normal limits. The nitroblue tetrazolium (NBT) test was 100 percent. The genetic evaluations for the leukocyte adhesion deficiency (LAD) were negative. In the bone marrow aspiration, the proportion of the myeloid to erythroid increased to 30–40/1, with no evidence of malignancy. The autoantibodies [antinuclear antibodies, rheumatoid factor, and antimyeloperoxidase-antineutrophil cytoplasmic antibody (ANCA)] were negative. The serum levels of immunoglobulins IgG, IgM, IgA, C3, C4, CH50, and angiotensin-converting enzyme (ACE) were normal.

In spite of these results, at the end of 3rd year of life, with suspicion of the immunodeficiency disorders, intravenous immune globulin (IVIG) was initiated monthly. Also, trimethoprim-sulfamethoxazole was added for the prophylaxis. With this treatment, the intervals between the recurrences were prolonged.

The methylprednisolone pulse (30 mg/kg) was initiated with the diagnosis of Sweet's syndrome (SS). Then, all of the signs and symptoms improved rapidly: the fever resolved in less than 24 hours, the lesions did not progress to abscess and resolved without any scars. After discharge, prednisolone with the dose of 0.5–0.75 mg/kg/day was prescribed.

After about 5 months, he was admitted again with tachypnea and high grade fever and leukocytosis. In this admission, he did not have any skin lesion. Chest X-ray showed pleural effusion in both sides especially in the right side (Figure 2). After infusion of one methylprednisolone pulse, the fever and tachypnea resolved rapidly in about 24 hours. The leukocytosis improved in less than 7 days. In this admission, the colchicine (1 mg/kg) was added to the oral prednisolone after discharge. The prednisolone was tapered slowly (0.25 mg/kg/d every 2 months). Fortunately, our patient had no flare-up after 6 months.

3. Discussion

Neutrophilic dermatosis (ND) is a sterile inflammation of skin with normal polymorphonuclear leukocytes [1]. Other organs such as lung, heart, blood vessels, liver, spleen, pancreas, and central nervous system may be affected by the sterile infiltration [4]. Furthermore, this infiltration can present as sterile abscess in other organs [5]. So, neutrophilic

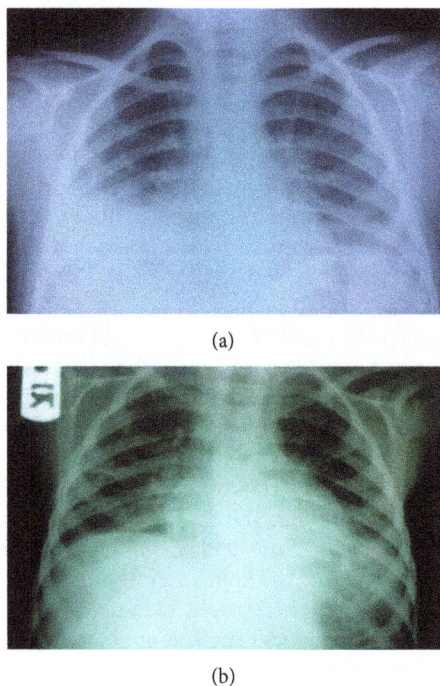

(a)

(b)

FIGURE 2: Chest X-ray in our patients with Sweet's syndrome: (a) pleural effusion in acute phase before treatment, (b) after methylprednisolone pulse therapy.

dermatosis should be proposed as a neutrophilic systemic disease [1]. Histological lesions, the associated peripheral neutrophilia, and the possible reaction to drugs that disturb the neutrophils function supported the potential role of neutrophils in these disorders [6]. Exogenous granulocyte colony stimulating factor (G-CSF) that is used in the treatment of low-neutrophil count disorders suppresses apoptosis and increases survival of neutrophils. Thus, despite low absolute neutrophil counts, the accumulation of neutrophils in skin lesion increased rapidly and the ND manifestations may develop [7]. Increased tyrosine phosphorylation of the proteins in the neutrophils of ND suggests that the possible defect in the tyrosine phosphatase function can prolong the survival of neutrophils [8, 9]. Our patient had high levels of leukocytosis during attacks. So, the numbers of neutrophils might also play a role in the manifestations.

Nowadays, the ND has been proposed as an autoinflammatory disorder [10, 11]. In the autoinflammatory diseases, a number of genetic defects in the innate immune system [12] cause recurrent episodes of sterile inflammation in the skin and other organs without high titers of autoantibodies or autoreactive T cells [13]. Alternatively, overproduction of the IL-1β can release cytokines and chemokines, causing neutrophilic stimulation [14].

On the other hand, IL-1 antagonist has been used in the treatment of autoinflammatory diseases (such as cryopyrin-related periodic disease). Moreover, other than corticosteroids (the main part of treatment in ND), IL-1 antagonist (anakinra) has recently been used in the treatment of SS [15]. So, the response to the IL-1 antagonist could be a diagnostic criterion for autoinflammatory diseases [1].

Autoinflammatory diseases were considered monogenic, such as PAPA (pyogenic sterile arthritis, PG, and acne) syndrome in which a mutation in the *PSTPIP1* gene causes overproduction of IL1 and resultant neutrophil-mediated reactions in skin and organs [16]. Neutrophilic diseases share some clinical features with monogenic autoinflammatory disorders such as periodic fever and neutrophil infiltration in the skin and other organs. The SS was reported in monogenic disorders, such as Majeed syndrome [17]. But the differences in clinical manifestations, even within one group of ND, diversity in the subtypes of ND, and differences in the response to therapy [8] support the concept that neutrophilic diseases may be a new category named polygenic autoinflammatory diseases [1].

According to the von den Driesch diagnostic criteria in Sweet's syndrome [18], our patient had all minor criteria (fever about 39°C, history of upper respiratory tract infections in some recurrences, gastrointestinal infection in one episode, good response to corticosteroid after 36–48 hours, high levels of white blood cells, neutrophils, ESR, and C-reactive protein). The characteristic feature of our patient in laboratory data was high levels of leukocytosis (above 50,000 per mm^3) in each episode. When the WBC count exceeds 50000 per mm^3, the term of leukemoid reaction is used (due to the similarity to leukemia). Most frequently, this term was associated with septicemia and severe bacterial infections such as shigellosis, salmonellosis, and meningococcemia [19]. There was only one report of leukemoid reaction and PG in two middle-aged women [20]. As we know, our report is the first description of the ND and periodic fever associated with leukemoid reaction. Some factors other than cytokines may stimulate neutrophil productions in this disorder and cause leukemoid reaction.

According to the von den Driesch major criteria, our patient had dense neutrophilic infiltration without any vasculitis in the histopathology and tender erythematous plaques or atypical bullous lesions. Furthermore, in one episode, our patient had pyoderma gangrenosum on the lower extremities. In the malignancy-associated SS, the lesions similar to PG were reported [21]. In the other episode, erythema nodosum-like lesions were observed. The subcutaneous neutrophil infiltration with tender dermal nodules similar to EN was also reported in SS [22]. Some episodes were concurrent with skin aseptic abscesses that were not characteristic of SS.

The SS in children is often classified in the classic category, which is idiopathic and triggered by the upper respiratory tract or gastrointestinal infections [23]. In the neonatal SS, the workup for immunodeficiency diseases (neutrophil dysfunction and antibody testing), viral infections (especially HIV), and hematologic diseases should be performed [2]. In addition, the evidences of monogenic autoinflammatory disorders such as CANDLE syndrome (chronic atypical neutrophilic dermatosis, lipodystrophy, and elevated temperature) and familial Sweet's syndrome should be sought in a case with neonatal SS [2].

Aseptic abscesses were reported in some cases with neutrophilic dermatosis or inflammatory bowel disease. The aseptic abscess (AA) syndrome was also described, when organ involvements with sterile abscesses were prominent [23]. These two categories may represent one autoinflammatory disease with different features. Most cases of AA syndrome were young adults and had a rapid response to corticosteroid therapy [24]. Recently, TNF-α blockade [25, 26] has been used in the treatment of AA syndrome. The effectiveness of these treatments is still unclear and should be evaluated with more studies.

Although corticosteroids have rapid responses in ND, the recurrences occur in the course of tapering [2]. Colchicine was proposed for the treatment of ND or SS with no relapses in follow-up [26, 27] (like our patient).

To our knowledge, our report was the first report of ND with multiple skin presentations from the neonatal period. Evaluation of all reported cases and further genetic investigations may lead to the diagnosis of a new autoinflammatory syndrome.

In conclusion, the rheumatologists should be aware of this condition when encountering periodic fever and neutrophilic dermatosis and should search for sterile abscesses in other organs. Moreover, in neonatal leukemoid reaction, when infections, malignancies, and immunodeficiencies are ruled out, the neutrophilic dermatosis and other autoinflammatory diseases should be considered.

Conflict of Interests

The authors declare that there is no conflict of interests regarding the publication of this paper.

References

[1] L. Prat, J. D. Bouaziz, D. Wallach, M. D. Vignon-Pennamen, and M. Bagot, "Neutrophilic dermatoses as systemic diseases," *Clinics in Dermatology*, vol. 32, no. 3, pp. 376–388, 2014.

[2] P. E. A. Gray, V. Bock, D. S. Ziegler, and O. Wargon, "Neonatal sweet syndrome: a potential marker of serious systemic illness," *Pediatrics*, vol. 129, no. 5, pp. e1353–e1359, 2012.

[3] T. Oskay and R. Anadolu, "Sweet's syndrome in familial Mediterranean fever: possible continuum of the neutrophilic reaction as a new cutaneous feature of FMF," *Journal of Cutaneous Pathology*, vol. 36, no. 8, pp. 901–905, 2009.

[4] M.-D. Vignon-Pennamen and D. Wallach, "Neutrophilic disease: a review of extracutaneous neutrophilic manifestations," *European Journal of Dermatology*, vol. 5, no. 6, pp. 449–455, 1995.

[5] M. F. J. André, J.-C. Piette, J.-L. Kémény et al., "Aseptic abscesses: a study of 30 patients with or without inflammatory bowel disease and review of the literature," *Medicine*, vol. 86, no. 3, pp. 145–161, 2007.

[6] P. R. Cohen and R. Kurzrock, "Sweet's syndrome revisited: a review of disease concepts," *International Journal of Dermatology*, vol. 42, no. 10, pp. 761–778, 2003.

[7] T. Kawakami, S. Ohashi, Y. Kawa et al., "Elevated serum granulocyte colony-stimulating factor levels in patients with active phase of sweet syndrome and patients with active Behcet disease: implication in neutrophil apoptosis dysfunction," *Archives of Dermatology*, vol. 140, no. 5, pp. 570–574, 2004.

[8] A. B. Nesterovitch, Z. Gyorfy, M. D. Hoffman et al., "Alteration in the gene encoding Protein Tyrosine Phosphatase Nonreceptor type 6 (*PTPN6/SHP1*) may contribute to neutrophilic dermatoses," *The American Journal of Pathology*, vol. 178, no. 4, pp. 1434–1441, 2011.

[9] H. J. Song, J. Parodo, A. Kapus, O. D. Rotstein, and J. C. Marshall, "Dynamic regulation of neutrophil survival through tyrosine phosphorylation or dephosphorylation of caspase-8," *Journal of Biological Chemistry*, vol. 283, no. 9, pp. 5402–5413, 2008.

[10] I. Ahronowitz, J. Harp, and K. Shinkai, "Etiology and management of pyoderma gangrenosum: a comprehensive review," *American Journal of Clinical Dermatology*, vol. 13, no. 3, pp. 191–211, 2012.

[11] A. B. Nesterovitch, Z. Gyorfy, M. D. Hoffman et al., "Alteration in the gene encoding protein tyrosine phosphatase nonreceptor type 6 (PTPN6/SHP1) may contribute to neutrophilic dermatoses," *The American Journal of Pathology*, vol. 178, no. 4, pp. 1434–1441, 2011.

[12] I. Aksentijevich and D. L. Kastner, "Genetics of monogenic autoinflammatory diseases: past successes, future challenges," *Nature Reviews Rheumatology*, vol. 7, no. 8, pp. 469–478, 2011.

[13] A. Doria, M. Zen, S. Bettio et al., "Autoinflammation and autoimmunity: bridging the divide," *Autoimmunity Reviews*, vol. 12, no. 1, pp. 22–30, 2012.

[14] A. V. Marzano, R. S. Ishak, S. Saibeni, C. Crosti, P. L. Meroni, and M. Cugno, "Autoinflammatory skin disorders in inflammatory bowel diseases, pyoderma gangrenosum and sweet's syndrome: a comprehensive review and disease classification criteria," *Clinical Reviews in Allergy and Immunology*, vol. 45, no. 2, pp. 202–210, 2013.

[15] N. Kluger, D. Gil-Bistes, B. Guillot, and D. Bessis, "Efficacy of anti-interleukin-1 receptor antagonist anakinra (Kineret) in a case of refractory sweet's syndrome," *Dermatology*, vol. 222, no. 2, pp. 123–127, 2011.

[16] C. A. Wise, J. D. Gillum, C. E. Seidman et al., "Mutations in CD2BP1 disrupt binding to PTP PEST and are responsible for PAPA syndrome, an autoinflammatory disorder," *Human Molecular Genetics*, vol. 11, no. 8, pp. 961–969, 2002.

[17] P. J. Ferguson, S. Chen, M. K. Tayeh et al., "Homozygous mutations in LPIN2 are responsible for the syndrome of chronic recurrent multifocal osteomyelitis and congenital dyserythropoietic anaemia (Majeed syndrome)," *Journal of Medical Genetics*, vol. 42, no. 7, pp. 551–557, 2005.

[18] P. von den Driesch, "Sweet's syndrome (acute febrile neutrophilic dermatosis)," *Journal of the American Academy of Dermatology*, vol. 31, no. 4, pp. 535–560, 1994.

[19] L. A. Boxer and P. E. Newburger, "Leukocytosis," in *Nelson Textbook of Pediatrics*, R. M. Kliegman, B. F. Stanton, S. T. Geme, N. F. Schor, and R. E. Behrman, Eds., p. 752, Elsevier, 19th edition, 2011.

[20] J. Ryu, J. Naik, F. C. Yang, and L. Winterfield, "Pyoderma gangrenosum presenting with leukemoid reaction: a report of 2 cases," *Archives of Dermatology*, vol. 146, no. 5, pp. 568–569, 2010.

[21] C. Y. Neoh, A. W. H. Tan, and S. K. Ng, "Sweet's syndrome: a spectrum of unusual clinical presentations and associations," *British Journal of Dermatology*, vol. 156, no. 3, pp. 480–485, 2007.

[22] P. R. Cohen, "Subcutaneous Sweet's syndrome: a variant of acute febrile neutrophilic dermatosis that is included in

the histopathologic differential diagnosis of neutrophilic pan-niculitis," *Journal of the American Academy of Dermatology*, vol. 52, no. 5, pp. 927–928, 2005.

[23] L. C. Uihlein, H. A. Brandling-Bennett, P. A. Lio, and M. G. Liang, "Sweet syndrome in children," *Pediatric Dermatology*, vol. 29, no. 1, pp. 38–44, 2012.

[24] M. André and O. Aumaître, "Aseptic abscesses syndrome," *Revue de Medecine Interne*, vol. 32, no. 11, pp. 678–688, 2011.

[25] M. F. Andre, J. C. Piette, J. L. Kemeny et al., "Aseptic abscesses: a study of 30 patients with or without inflammatory bowel diseases and review of the literature," *Medicine*, vol. 86, pp. 145–161, 2007.

[26] T. Ito, N. Sato, H. Yamazaki, T. Koike, I. Emura, and T. Saeki, "A case of aseptic abscesses syndrome treated with corticosteroids and TNF-alpha blockade," *Modern Rheumatology*, vol. 23, no. 1, pp. 195–199, 2013.

[27] H. Maillard, C. Leclech, P. Peria, M. Avenel-Audran, and J. L. Verret, "Colchicine for Sweet's syndrome. A study of 20 cases," *British Journal of Dermatology*, vol. 140, no. 3, pp. 565–566, 1999.

26

Chronic Granulomatous Disease Presenting as Aseptic Ascites in a 2-Year-Old Child

J. F. Moreau,[1] John A. Ozolek,[2] P. Ling Lin,[3] Todd D. Green,[4] Elaine A. Cassidy,[5] Veena L. Venkat,[6] and Andrew R. Buchert[7]

[1] *School of Medicine, University of Pittsburgh, Pittsburgh, PA 15261, USA*

[2] *Division of Pathology, Children's Hospital of Pittsburgh of UPMC, One Children's Hospital Drive, 4401 Penn Avenue, Pittsburgh, PA 15224, USA*

[3] *Division of Infectious Disease, Children's Hospital of Pittsburgh of UPMC, One Children's Hospital Drive, 4401 Penn Avenue, Pittsburgh, PA 15224, USA*

[4] *Division of Pulmonary Medicine, Allergy and Immunology, Children's Hospital of Pittsburgh of UPMC, One Children's Hospital Drive, 4401 Penn Avenue, Pittsburgh, PA 15224, USA*

[5] *Division of Rheumatology, Children's Hospital of Pittsburgh of UPMC, One Children's Hospital Drive, 4401 Penn Avenue, Pittsburgh, PA 15224, USA*

[6] *Division of Gastroenterology, Children's Hospital of Pittsburgh of UPMC, One Children's Hospital Drive, 4401 Penn Avenue, Pittsburgh, PA 15224, USA*

[7] *The Paul C. Gaffney Diagnostic Referral Service, Children's Hospital of Pittsburgh of UPMC, One Children's Hospital Drive, 4401 Penn Avenue, Pittsburgh, PA 15224, USA*

Correspondence should be addressed to Andrew R. Buchert; andrew.buchert@chp.edu

Academic Editors: N. Kutukculer, C. Pignata, A. Plebani, and A. Vojdani

Chronic granulomatous disease (CGD) is a rare inherited immunodeficiency syndrome that results from abnormal nicotinamide adenine dinucleotide phosphate (NADPH) oxidase function. This defect leads to recurrent catalase-positive bacterial and fungal infections as well as associated granuloma formation. We review the case of a 2-year-old boy who presented with ascites and fever of an unknown origin as manifestations of CGD. Cultures were negative for infection throughout his course, and CGD was suspected after identification of granulomas on peritoneal biopsy. Genetic testing revealed a novel mutation in the CYBB gene underlying his condition. This paper highlights the importance of considering CGD in the differential diagnosis of fever of unknown origin and ascites in children.

1. Introduction

Chronic granulomatous disease (CGD) results from the inability of neutrophils to complete the first step of the respiratory burst pathway, generation of superoxide, with the downstream consequence of impaired microbe killing. CGD leads to recurrent and potentially lethal infections. Pneumonia is the most common infection before diagnosis (47%) [1] and occurs in the majority (79%) of patients within four years of diagnosis [2]. Lymphadenitis is the second most common infection before diagnosis (45%) [1], and subcutaneous abscess is the second most common infection

that occurs within 4 years of diagnosis (43%) [2]. Other presenting infections include osteomyelitis, liver and perirectal abscesses, enteritis, and septicemia [1]. CGD can, in very rare circumstances, present with ascites [3].

The incidence of CGD is estimated to be between 1/200,000 and 1/250,000 US births [2]. Most affected individuals are male because approximately 70% of mutations are X-linked recessive; the remaining 30% of cases are autosomal recessive [1, 2, 4]. In normal individuals, inflammatory stimuli prompt nicotinamide adenine dinucleotide phosphate (NADPH) oxidase (a lysosomal enzyme encoded on chromosome 22) to produce superoxide. Superoxide is converted to hydrogen peroxide via superoxide dismutase and then to hypochlorous acid (by myeloperoxidase), which is lethal to bacteria [5]. Individuals with CGD are able to utilize hydrogen peroxide made by microbes and convert it to hypochlorous acid to preserve microbe killing, yet catalase-positive bacteria can prevent this step by degrading the hydrogen peroxide. Thus, catalase-positive organisms such as *Staphylococcus aureus* are the most common microbial sources of infection; other common pathogenic organisms in patients with CGD are *Burkholderia cepacia*, *Nocardia*, *Serratia*, and *Klebsiella* [2, 6]. Approximately 70% of CGD cases are associated with mutations in the CYBB gene on the X chromosome, but well over 300 different CYBB mutations have been reported in association with the disease [7]. In this paper, we describe an unusual case of CGD in a child with a novel mutation in exon 13 of the CYBB gene who presented with an isolated lymphadenitis and months later developed ascites and culture-negative, granulomatous peritonitis.

2. Case Report

The patient is a 2-year-old male born to a G1P1 mother who had an uncomplicated pregnancy and delivery. His only significant past medical history was an isolated infection one and a half years earlier. His parents noticed a swollen area on his neck near his left ear and took him to our tertiary care children's hospital for evaluation. On admission, he was febrile to 39.3°C and had a leukocytosis of 20×10^9/L. A diagnosis of lymphadenitis was made. A culture of the fluid drained from the abscess grew methicillin-sensitive *S. aureus*, but the blood culture was negative. He was discharged home on amoxicillin/clavulanate. The neck swelling returned after a few days despite oral antibiotics, prompting his parents to bring him back to the hospital. The abscess was drained for the second time, and he was administered intravenous ampicillin/sulbactam. With subsidence of the swelling, the patient was discharged home to complete a 10-day course of antibiotics and had no recurrence of the abscess.

In September 2011, he was admitted with nearly one month of daily fevers up to 39.4°C. His only other symptoms were intermittent dysuria and slightly loose stools at normal frequency (1-2 times daily). Family history of immunological, hematological, and oncological diseases was negative. There was no recent travel. Physical exam was within normal limits except for poor weight gain (decline from 36th to 7th percentile from 12 months of age to admission (28 months)). Abnormal laboratory values included albumin 2.8 g/dL (3.8–5.4 g/dL), alkaline phosphatase 509 IU/L (<290 IU/L), C-reactive protein (CRP) 10.69 mg/dL (0.08–1.2 mg/dL), erythrocyte sedimentation rate (ESR) 131 mm/hr (0–20 mm/hr), ferritin 178.1 ng/mL (10–60 ng/mL), hemoglobin (Hgb) 10.7 g/dL (11.5–13.5 g/dL), hematocrit 30.5% (34.0–40.0%), lactate dehydrogenase 258 IU/L (<171 IU/L), platelets 399×10^9/L ($156–369 \times 10^9$/L), and neutrophils 57% (12–34%). All other laboratory values were within normal limits. The differential diagnoses included Kawasaki disease, hematological malignancy, early juvenile idiopathic arthritis or other rheumatologic process, and intestinal infection.

Lyme disease, toxoplasmosis, Bartonella, cytomegalovirus, and tuberculosis were also considered. Subsequent testing excluded these infectious entities.

After a few days, he defervesced and was discharged home with presumptive diagnosis of a likely, yet to be diagnosed, rheumatological disease. One month later, he developed persistent fever and abdominal distension. Exam was now significant for increased abdominal girth, and a fluid wave was present on physical examination. Laboratory studies revealed an increased platelet count (457×10^9/L) and ESR (74 mm/hr) as well as decreased ferritin (79.2 ng/mL) and Hgb (9.9 g/dL). His albumin also remained low, prompting testing for prealbumin (low at 5.6 mg/dL), proteinuria (negative), and protein losing enteropathy (alpha-1-antitrypsin normal (<20)). An abdominal CT scan showed contour irregularity of the colon, ascites, and diffuse peritoneal enhancement with fat stranding consistent with peritonitis. Paracentesis was done, and cytological evaluation demonstrated purulent fluid with large numbers of neutrophils and macrophages but no malignant cells. Bacterial and fungal cultures were sterile. The serum-to-ascites albumin gradient was 1 g/L, likely excluding portal hypertension as an etiology of the ascites. Gastrointestinal evaluation included esophagogastro-duodenoscopy and colonoscopy with biopsies, endomysial antibody, amylase, and lipase. Duodenal, terminal ileal, and colonic biopsies were unremarkable and without villous abnormalities, inflammatory lymphoid cells, or accumulation of pigmented macrophages; the other studies were likewise normal. Bone marrow biopsy was unremarkable, and a tagged WBC scan demonstrated no specific abnormal foci of uptake. His abdomen remained distended, but the girth was stable. He defervesced on ampicillin/sulbactam and metronidazole and was discharged home to complete an empiric course of antibiotics for peritonitis.

One week later, he again developed persistent fever and increasing abdominal distension and pain, resulting in his refusal to walk. An exploratory laparoscopy revealed massive ascites and an inflamed and friable peritoneum studded with yellow and white nodules. The ascitic fluid was sent for culture, and biopsies of the peritoneum were taken. The ascitic fluid had 1500 WBCs but was sterile. Pathology of the peritoneal biopsies revealed acute and organizing peritonitis with granulomatous features but no evidence of fungal, acid-fast, or bacterial microorganisms (Figure 1). The granulomatous nature of the peritonitis prompted evaluation for CGD. A dihydrorhodamine (DHR) test was performed to assess oxidase burst capability and resulted in negligible fluorescence, consistent with CGD. Genetic testing revealed hemizygosity for the c.1683dupG mutation in exon 13 of the CYBB gene.

3. Discussion

CGD was first described in 1957 independently by Berendes et al. [8] and by Landing and Shirkey [9] as a lethal disease in males associated with increased susceptibility to infection and pigment-containing macrophages in the visceral organs. The pigment forms as macrophages clear

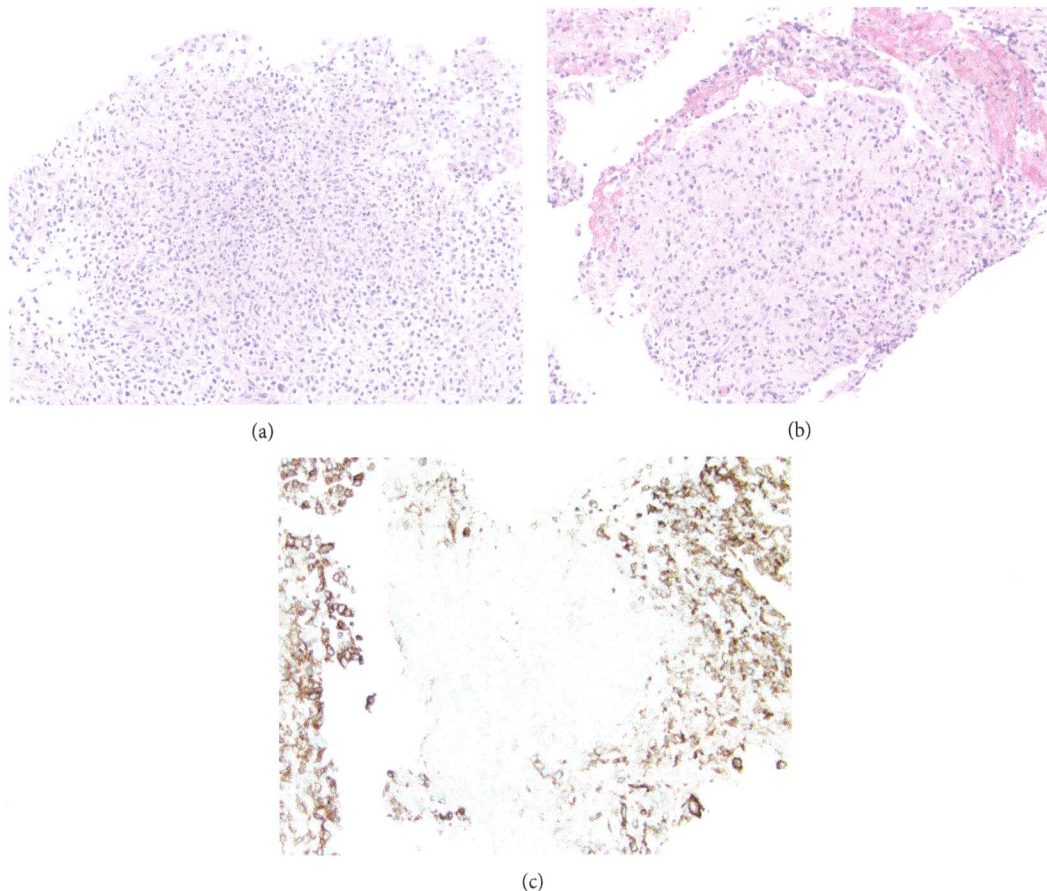

FIGURE 1: (a) Biopsy of peritoneal nodules demonstrated a cellular and organizing peritonitis including neutrophils, mesothelial cells, and abundant macrophages some with epithelioid features (HE, 200x). Focal areas had relatively well-organized granulomas (b) with macrophages that did not express the activated macrophage marker CD163 (c) ((b); HE, 200x, (c); CD163, 200x).

neutrophils that have undergone apoptosis, with subsequent cytoplasmic accumulation of ceroid pigment, hence their golden or orange-brown color by light microscopy [10]. In the 1960s and 1970s, defective NADPH oxidase was found to be the cause of CGD, leading to development of the nitroblue tetrazolium (NBT) test for diagnosis [11, 12]. A few decades later, the DHR was developed as more quantitative measure of oxidative burst, and it is now the preferred test for CGD [12]. Since then, over 400 mutations coding for the NADPH oxidase enzyme have been discovered, and genetic testing for CGD has become available.

Cases of CGD have been associated with defects in genes encoding 4 of the 6 NADPH oxidase subunits, named with reference to their molecular mass (kd) and "phox" for phagocyte oxidase. Flavocytochrome b558 is the redox center of NADPH oxidase and is composed of gp91phox and p22phox. Defects in the X-linked gene encoding gp-91 (CYBB) account for about 70% of known mutations causing CGD, and autosomal recessive p22phox mutations (CYBA gene on chromosome 16) account for an additional 5%. P47-phox (NCF1 gene on chromosome 7) and p67phox (NCF2 gene on chromosome 1) are both regulatory proteins that have also been associated with autosomal recessive defects (about

20% and 5%, resp.) [1, 2, 4, 13]. Rac2 (on chromosome 22) and p40phox (NCF4 gene on chromosome 22) are the other 2 NADPH oxidase subunits, and mutations have thus far not been associated with CGD.

We describe a child with CGD who presents with a rare constellation of fever of an unknown origin, ascites, and culture-negative peritonitis. To our knowledge, this is the first reported case of CGD associated with a c.1683dupG mutation in the CYBB gene [14, 15]. The c.1683dupG mutation in the CYBB gene causes a frameshift mutation that results in formation of a stop codon and thus loss of normal protein function. Ascites has rarely been reported as a presenting sign of chronic granulomatous disease, and, in all of the previously reported cases, bacterial cultures were positive [3, 16, 17]. Our patient did have nonspecific findings that are often present in patients with CGD (fever, microcytic anemia, failure to thrive). While he had a somewhat complicated lymphadenitis in the past, he lacked other infections and the chronicity typical of patients with CGD.

This paper highlights the importance of considering chronic granulomatous disease in the differential diagnosis of fever of unknown origin and ascites. With a broad differential diagnosis and little direct evidence of CGD before peritoneal biopsy, our patient reflects the challenge of making this diagnosis. The previously unreported mutation discovered in this patient may have been responsible for his unique clinical presentation. Past research has found that specific genetic polymorphisms are associated with development of gastrointestinal inflammation and rheumatologic disorders in CGD patients [18]. Other work has shown that the quantity of residual neutrophil reactive oxygen intermediates produced in CGD patients is mutation related and correlates with clinical outcomes [19]. In this context, knowing patient genotype may enable clinicians to provide improved care and is an area that we feel deserves further investigation.

Abbreviations

CGD: Chronic granulomatous disease
NADPH: Nicotinamide adenine dinucleotide phosphate
CRP: C-reactive protein
ESR: Sedimentation rate
Hgb: Hemoglobin
WBC: White blood cell
DHR: Dihydrorhodamine
NBT: Nitroblue tetrazolium.

Disclosure

The authors have no financial relationships relevant to this article to disclose.

Conflict of Interests

No authors have potential conflict of interests.

Authors' Contribution

J. F. Moreau (B.A.) was the primary medical student who provided care to the subject of this paper. She drafted the initial paper and approved the final paper as submitted. J. A. Ozolek (M.D.) was the Pathologist who reviewed the biopsies of the subject of this paper while he was an inpatient. He provided the pathological images included within this paper and both edited and approved the final paper as submitted. P. L. Lin (M.D. and M.S.) has been the primary subspecialist for the subject of this paper since he was diagnosed with chronic granulomatous disease. She edited and approved the final paper as submitted. T. D. Green (M.D.) was the Immunologist who consulted on this case while the subject of this paper was an inpatient. He edited and approved the final paper as submitted. E. A. Cassidy (M.D.) was the Rheumatologist who consulted on this case while the subject of this paper was an inpatient. She edited and approved the final paper as submitted. V. L. Venkat (M.D.) was the Gastroenterologist who consulted on this case while the patient was an inpatient. She edited and approved the final case report as submitted. A. R. Buchert (M.D.) was the primary Inpatient Medical Provider for the subject of this paper and also followed this patient in diagnostic referral clinic until he was diagnosed with chronic granulomatous disease. He edited and approved the final paper as submitted.

References

[1] B. Martire, R. Rondelli, A. Soresina et al., "Clinical features, long-term follow-up and outcome of a large cohort of patients with chronic granulomatous disease: an Italian multicenter study," *Clinical Immunology*, vol. 126, no. 2, pp. 155–164, 2008.

[2] J. A. Winkelstein, M. C. Marino, R. B. Johnston et al., "Chronic granulomatous disease: report on a national registry of 368 patients," *Medicine*, vol. 79, no. 3, pp. 155–169, 2000.

[3] M. Castro, L. Balducci, C. Ciuffetti, V. Lucidi, A. Torre, and S. Bella, "Ascites as an unusual manifestation of chronic granulomatous disease in childhood," *Pediatria Medica e Chirurgica*, vol. 14, no. 3, pp. 317–319, 1992.

[4] C. Casimir, M. Chetty, M. C. Bohler et al., "Identification of the defective NADPH-oxidase component in chronic granulomatous disease: a study of 57 European families," *European Journal of Clinical Investigation*, vol. 22, no. 6, pp. 403–406, 1992.

[5] "Chronic granulomatous disease," in *Hematology: Basic Principles and Practice*, R. Hoffman, Ed., Churchill Livingstone, Philadelphia, Pa, USA, 2009.

[6] S. M. Holland, "Chronic granulomatous disease," *Clinical Reviews in Allergy and Immunology*, vol. 38, no. 1, pp. 3–10, 2010.

[7] D. Roos, D. B. Kuhns, A. Maddalena et al., "Hematologically important mutations: X-linked chronic granulomatous disease (third update)," *Blood Cells Molecules and Diseases*, vol. 45, no. 3, pp. 246–265, 2010.

[8] H. Berendes, R. A. Bridges, and R. A. Good, "A fatal granulomatosus of childhood: the clinical study of a new syndrome," *Minnesota Medicine*, vol. 40, no. 5, pp. 309–312, 1957.

[9] B. H. Landing and H. S. Shirkey, "A syndrome of recurrent infection and infiltration of viscera by pigmented lipid histiocytes," *Pediatrics*, vol. 20, no. 3, pp. 431–438, 1957.

[10] "Chronic granulomatous disease," in *Nelson Textbook of Pediatrics*, R. Kliegman, Ed., Elsevier, Philadelphia, Pa, USA, 2011.

[11] R. L. Baehner and D. G. Nathan, "Quantitative nitroblue tetrazolium test in chronic granulomatous disease," *The New England Journal of Medicine*, vol. 278, no. 18, pp. 971–976, 1968.

[12] C. L. Epling, D. P. Stites, T. M. McHugh, H. O. Chong, L. L. Blackwood, and D. W. Wara, "Neutrophil function screening in patients with chronic granulomatous disease by a flow cytometric method," *Cytometry*, vol. 13, no. 6, pp. 615–620, 1992.

[13] F. Morel, "Molecular aspects of chronic granulomatous disease. 'the NADPH oxidase complex'," *Bulletin de l'Academie Nationale de Medecine*, vol. 191, no. 2, pp. 377–392, 2007.

[14] F. Defendi, E. Decleva, C. Martel, P. Dri, and M. J. Stasia, "A novel point mutation in the *CYBB* gene promoter leading to a rare X minus chronic granulomatous disease variant—impact on the microbicidal activity of neutrophils," *Biochimica et Biophysica Acta*, vol. 1792, no. 3, pp. 201–210, 2009.

[15] J. Rae, P. E. Newburger, M. C. Dinauer et al., "X-linked chronic granulomatous disease: mutations in the *CYBB* gene encoding the gp91-*phox* component of respiratory-burst oxidase," *The American Journal of Human Genetics*, vol. 62, no. 6, pp. 1320–1331, 1998.

[16] T. M. Rossi, J. Cumella, D. Baswell, and B. Park, "Ascites as a presenting sign of peritonitis in chronic granulomatous disease of childhood," *Clinical Pediatrics*, vol. 26, no. 10, pp. 544–545, 1987.

[17] S. Subramaniam, D. Tuman, A. R. Rausen, and S. D. Douglas, "'Ascites' and inguinal hernias: unusual presentation for chronic granulomatous disease of childhood," *The Mount Sinai Journal of Medicine*, vol. 41, no. 4, pp. 566–569, 1974.

[18] C. B. Foster, T. Lehrnbecher, F. Mol et al., "Host defense molecule polymorphisms influence the risk for immune-mediated complications in chronic granulomatous disease," *Journal of Clinical Investigation*, vol. 102, no. 12, pp. 2146–2155, 1998.

[19] D. B. Kuhns, W. G. Alvord, T. Heller et al., "Residual NADPH oxidase and survival in chronic granulomatous disease douglas," *The New England Journal of Medicine*, vol. 363, no. 27, pp. 2600–2610, 2010.

27

Atypical Omenn Syndrome due to Adenosine Deaminase Deficiency

Avni Y. Joshi,[1, 2] **Erin K. Ham,**[2] **Neel B. Shah,**[3] **Xiangyang Dong,**[4]
Shakila P. Khan,[5] **and Roshini S. Abraham**[4]

[1] Division of Pediatric and Adult Allergy and Immunology, Department of Pediatric and Adolescent Medicine,
 Mayo Clinic, Rochester, MN 55905, USA
[2] Department of Internal Medicine, Mayo Clinic, Rochester, MN 55905, USA
[3] Department of Medical Genetics, Mayo Clinic, Rochester, MN 55905, USA
[4] Department of Laboratory Medicine and Pathology, Mayo Clinic, Rochester, MN 55905, USA
[5] Division of Pediatric Hematology and Oncology, Department of Pediatric and Adolescent Medicine, Mayo Clinic,
 Rochester, MN 55905, USA

Correspondence should be addressed to Avni Y. Joshi, joshi.avni@mayo.edu

Academic Editors: I. A. Hagel and A. Plebani

We present here a novel case of an atypical Omenn syndrome (OS) phenotype due to mutations in the *ADA* gene encoding adenosine deaminase. This case is noteworthy for a significant increase in circulating CD56[bright]CD16- cytokine-producing NK cells after treatment with steroids for skin rash.

1. Introduction

Omenn syndrome (OS) is a distinct manifestation of Severe Combined Immunodeficiency (SCID) characterized by erythroderma, hepatosplenomegaly, lymphadenopathy, eosinophilia, and elevated IgE and alopecia [1–3]. Patients with OS usually present in infancy with viral or fungal pneumonitis, chronic diarrhea, and failure to thrive, but in contrast to classic SCID patients also have the above-mentioned characteristics.

Here we present a case of atypical OS in an infant with adenosine deaminase (ADA) deficiency.

2. Case Report

A 2-month-old Somali boy, born to consanguineous parents, presented to our hospital with concerns for immunodeficiency. The initial symptoms included cough, diffuse skin rash (Figure 1), hepatosplenomegaly, and a sepsis-like syndrome. A complete sepsis workup was negative, except for an absolute lymphocyte count (ALC) of 0, which triggered evaluation for an underlying primary immunodeficiency. T-, B- and NK-cell quantitation in blood revealed a T-B-NK- phenotype consistent with Severe Combined Immunodeficiency (SCID). The molecular defect was likely thought to be in the *ADA* gene due to the ethnicity of the patient and the lymphocyte phenotype, therefore, ADA levels were tested and found to be 0 (reference range: 0.3–1.5/g Hb).

Broad-spectrum antibiotics were initiated, but with negative cultures, were maintained on prophylactic antibiotics (Bactrim for Pneumocystis, initial Fluconazole followed by Caspofungin for antifungal, IVIG and Palivizumab for RSV).

His skin rash was extensively evaluated and the pathology was initially regarded as possible graft versus host disease due to maternal engraftment [4], due to the presence of apoptotic keratinocytes. However, the absence of circulating T cells argued against that possibility and chimerism [5] studies on a skin biopsy revealed all cells to be XY in origin, confirming absence of maternal engraftment. Treatment was initiated with steroids and PEG-ADA (biweekly, 60 U/kg/week due to the absence of a matched donor for stem cell transplantation and unsuitability at the time for

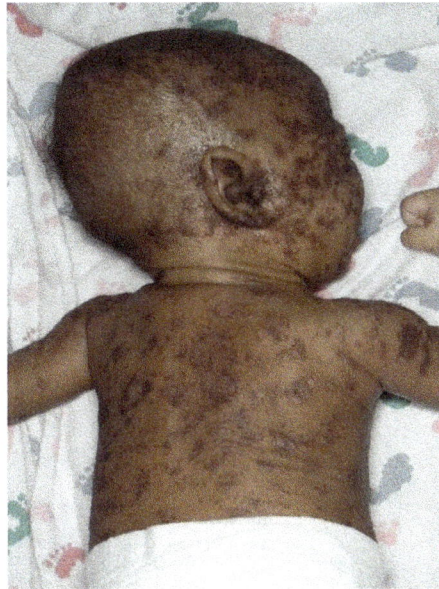

FIGURE 1: Diffuse rash in an infant with ADA deficiency.

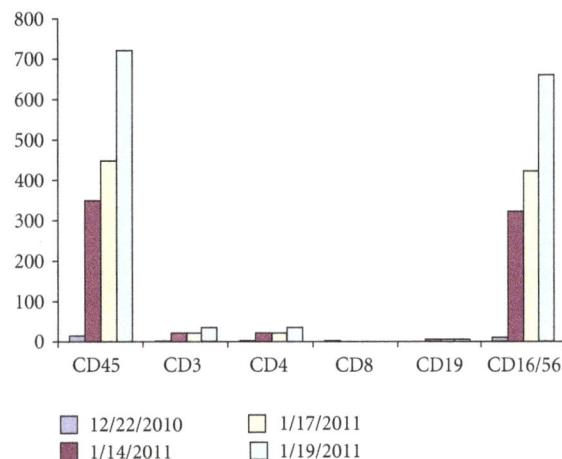

FIGURE 2: Serial T, B, and NK lymphocyte measurements.

gene therapy [6]; trough plasma ADA levels were monitored while on PEG-ADA treatment-range of 30–40 mmol/hr/mL (target levels > 12 mmol/hr/mL), but shortly thereafter, there was a remarkable increase in circulating lymphocyte counts with doubling in a span of 5 days. Lymphocyte immunophenotyping revealed these to be primarily NK cells (CD16/56), with a small number of T cells (Figure 2, PEG ADA started on 01/03/2011).

Analysis of thymic function (CD4 recent thymic emigrants: CD4+ CD45RA+ CD31+) revealed an almost complete lack of naive T cells, contrary to what would typically be expected for age, and T cells that were present had the memory, CD45RO+ phenotype, as often seen in OS. Flow cytometric analysis of the NK-cell population revealed an unusual expansion of cytokine-producing NK cells, CD56^{bright}CD16−, which is typically only 10% of

circulating NK cells (Figure 3). The appearance of this unusually expanded NK cell subset and small numbers of CD45RO+CD4+ T cells in blood was likely related to retrafficking of these cells from the skin lesions rather than *de novo* generation due to ADA treatment due to the short time-interval posttreatment in which the cells were detected. There has previously been one report of skin-infiltrating CD56^{bright}CD16− NK cells in a patient with X-linked (*IL2RG* mutation) SCID who had OS-like features [7].

The patient reported herein had several characteristics of OS as mentioned but was atypical for the presence of the expanded CD56^{br}CD16− NK cells, normal IgE levels, and lack of eosinophilia.

Molecular analysis of the *ADA* gene in both parents revealed a heterozygous Q3X nonsense mutation (c. 7 C>T; CAG>TAG), which has been previously reported to be

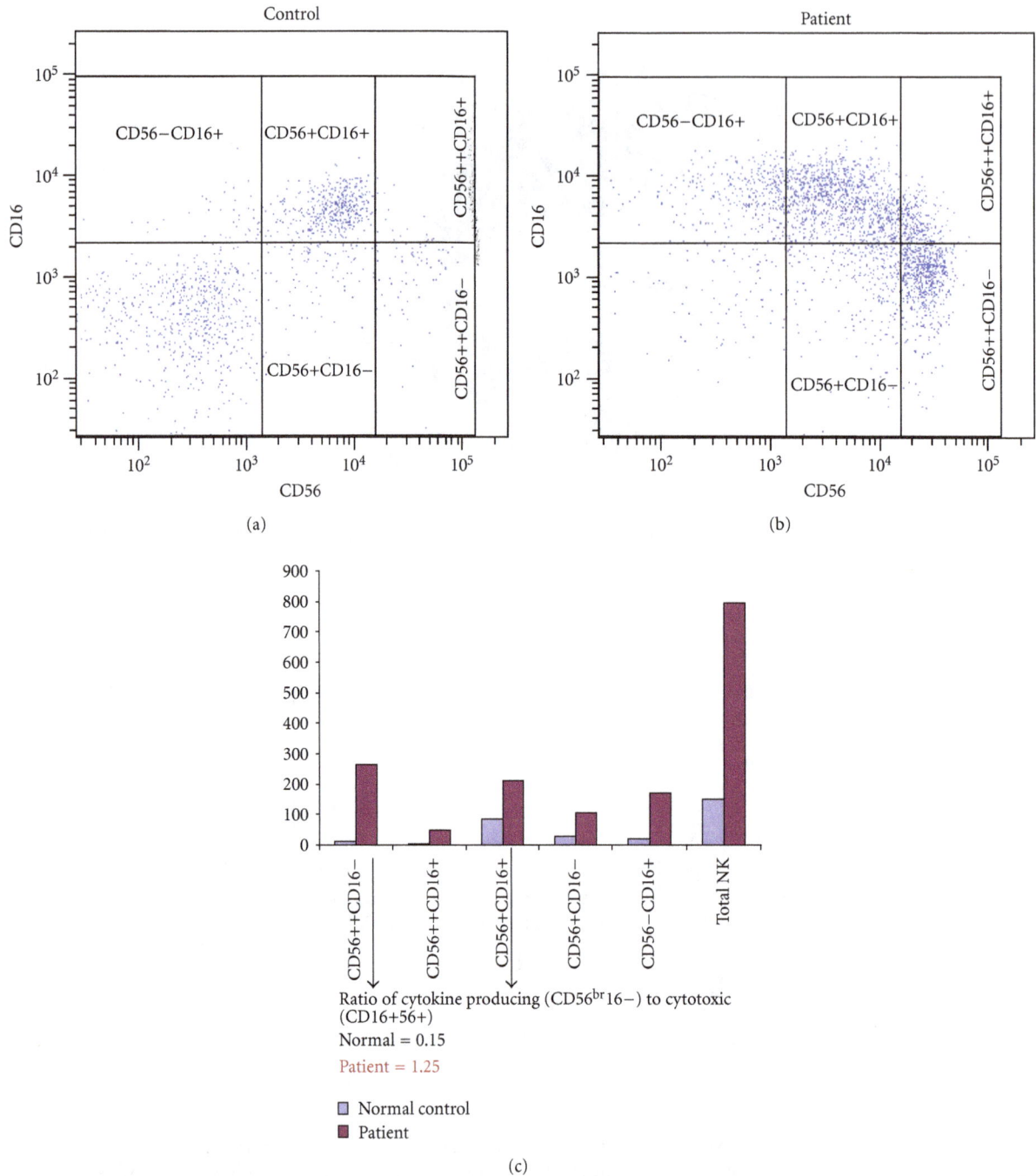

(a)

(b)

(c)

Ratio of cytokine producing (CD56^{br}16−) to cytotoxic (CD16+56+)
Normal = 0.15
Patient = 1.25

□ Normal control
■ Patient

FIGURE 3: Natural Killer (NK) cell phenotyping.

present at a frequency of at least 1 in 5000 to 1 in 10,000 in the Somali population [8].

Despite use of high-dose steroids, his respiratory status worsened and he developed seizures. A spinal tap showed evidence of human herpes virus-6 (HHV 6) via PCR with HHV 6 viremia Bronchial alveolar lavage that revealed *Stenotrophomonas maltophilia* and HHV6. Treatment was initiated with Foscarnet alone followed by combination ganciclovir. Despite aggressive intervention, he continued to be ventilator dependent with worsening pulmonary hypertension due to chronic lung disease. Eventually, the decision to cease supportive care was made in conjunction with the family 40 days after hospitalization.

This is the first report, to the best of our knowledge, of an atypical Omenn syndrome due to ADA deficiency with expansion of CD56^{br}CD16− NK cells. Only 2 other patients with ADA-SCID and features of Omenn syndrome have been reported [9, 10]. The variability in the phenotypic spectrum of classic SCID-associated genes emphasizes the necessity of genotype-phenotype correlations.

Acknowledgment

The authors would like to thank Dr. Michael Hershfield, MD, Duke University Medical Center for his kind assistance in evaluating ADA levels pre- and posttreatment.

References

[1] G. S. Omenin, "Familial reticuloendotheliosis with eosinophilia," *The New England journal of medicine*, vol. 273, pp. 427–432, 1965.

[2] M. Kato, H. Kimura, M. Seki et al., "Omenn syndrome—review of several phenotypes of Omenn syndrome and RAG1/RAG2 mutations in Japan," *Allergology international*, vol. 55, no. 2, pp. 115–119, 2006.

[3] A. Villa, L. D. Notarangelo, and C. M. Roifman, "Omenn syndrome: inflammation in leaky severe combined immunodeficiency," *Journal of Allergy and Clinical Immunology*, vol. 122, no. 6, pp. 1082–1086, 2008.

[4] A. Sottini, E. Quiros-Roldan, L. D. Notarangelo, A. Malagoli, D. Primi, and L. Imberti, "Engrafted maternal T cells in a severe combined immunodeficiency patient express T-cell receptor variable beta segments characterized by a restricted V-D-J junctional diversity," *Blood*, vol. 85, no. 8, pp. 2105–2113, 1995.

[5] A. J. Sieverkropp, R. G. A. Andrews, L. Gaur, and L. E. Shields, "Chimerism analysis by sex determining region Y (SRY) and major histocompatibility complex markers in non-human primates using quantitative real-time polymerase chain reaction," *Tissue Antigens*, vol. 66, no. 1, pp. 19–25, 2005.

[6] M. S. Hershfield, S. Chaffee, R. U. Sorensen, R. Hirschhorn, and E. W. Gelfand, "Enzyme replacement therapy with polyethylene glycol-adenosine deaminase in adenosine deaminase deficiency: overview and case reports of three patients, including two now receiving gene therapy," *Pediatric Research*, vol. 33, no. 1, pp. S42–S48, 1993.

[7] F. Shibata, T. Toma, T. Wada et al., "Skin infiltration of CD56bright CD16- natural killer cells in a case of X-SCID with Omenn syndrome-like manifestations," *European Journal of Haematology*, vol. 79, no. 1, pp. 81–85, 2007.

[8] J. J. Sanchez, G. Monaghan, C. Børsting, G. Norbury, N. Morling, and H. B. Gaspar, "Carrier frequency of a nonsense mutation in the Adenosine Deaminase (ADA) gene implies a high incidence of ADA-deficient Severe combined immunodeficiency (SCID) in Somalia and a single, common haplotype indicates common ancestry," *Annals of Human Genetics*, vol. 71, no. 3, pp. 336–347, 2007.

[9] I. Dalal, D. Tasher, R. Somech et al., "Novel mutations in RAG1/2 and ADA genes in Israeli patients presenting with T-B- SCID or Omenn syndrome," *Clinical Immunology*, 2011.

[10] C. M. Roifman, J. Zhang, A. Atkinson, E. Grunebaum, and K. Mandel, "Adenosine deaminase deficiency can present with features of Omenn syndrome," *Journal of Allergy and Clinical Immunology*, vol. 121, no. 4, pp. 1056–1058, 2008.

28

Bilateral Lung Transplantation in a Patient with Humoral Immune Deficiency: A Case Report with Review of the Literature

Jocelyn R. Farmer,[1] Caroline L. Sokol,[2] Francisco A. Bonilla,[3] Mandakolathur R. Murali,[2] Richard L. Kradin,[4] Todd L. Astor,[5] and Jolan E. Walter[6]

[1] Department of Medicine, Massachusetts General Hospital, Harvard Medical School, Boston, MA 02114, USA
[2] Division of Allergy & Immunology, Massachusetts General Hospital, Harvard Medical School, Boston, MA 02114, USA
[3] Division of Allergy & Immunology, Boston Children's Hospital, Harvard Medical School, Boston, MA 02115, USA
[4] Department of Pathology, Massachusetts General Hospital, Harvard Medical School, Boston, MA 02114, USA
[5] Division of Pulmonary & Critical Care Medicine, Massachusetts General Hospital, Harvard Medical School, Boston, MA 02114, USA
[6] Pediatric Allergy & Immunology and the Center for Immunology and Inflammatory Diseases, Massachusetts General Hospital, Harvard Medical School, Boston, MA 02114, USA

Correspondence should be addressed to Jocelyn R. Farmer; jrfarmer@partners.org

Academic Editor: Jiri Litzman

Humoral immune deficiencies have been associated with noninfectious disease complications including autoimmune cytopenias and pulmonary disease. Herein we present a patient who underwent splenectomy for autoimmune cytopenias and subsequently was diagnosed with humoral immune deficiency in the context of recurrent infections. Immunoglobulin analysis prior to initiation of intravenous immunoglobulin (IVIG) therapy was notable for low age-matched serum levels of IgA (11 mg/dL), IgG2 (14 mg/L), and IgG4 (5 mg/L) with a preserved total level of IgG. Flow cytometry was remarkable for B cell maturation arrest at the IgM+/IgD+ stage. Selective screening for known primary immune deficiency-causing genetic defects was negative. The disease course was uniquely complicated by the development of pulmonary arteriovenous malformations (AVMs), ultimately requiring bilateral lung transplantation in 2012. This is a patient with humoral immune deficiency that became apparent only after splenectomy, which argues for routine immunologic evaluation prior to vaccination and splenectomy. Lung transplantation is a rare therapeutic endpoint and to our knowledge has never before been described in a patient with humoral immune deficiency for the indication of pulmonary AVMs.

1. Introduction

Humoral immune deficiencies as a group are the most common type of primary immune disorder. The underlying etiology is extremely varied, and a growing number of diverse genetic mutations have been described [1]. The defect in antibody production can range from isolated IgA deficiency, which can be clinically silent, to complete IgG deficiency, which has been associated with severe infection, requiring life-long maintenance therapy with IVIG [2]. Combined IgG subclass deficiencies have also been described. Specifically, IgA deficiency has been linked to subclass deficiencies in both IgG2 and IgG4 [3, 4]. Decreased serum levels of IgG2

and IgG4 are sufficient to confer increased susceptibility to pathogens, particularly those requiring opsonization [4]. IgG2 deficiency has also been independently associated with the development of lymphoproliferative autoimmune disease [5].

The epidemiology of humoral immune deficiency is best characterized for common variable immune deficiency (CVID) due to its prevalence in the general population. Outcomes analysis in a cohort of 473 patients with CVID [6] recently demonstrated noninfectious disease complications in 68% of patients, which included autoimmune-mediated cytopenias (thrombocytopenia (14.2%), hemolytic anemia (7%), and neutropenia (<1%)) and chronic lung disease

TABLE 1: The patient had confirmed deficiencies in IgA, IgG2, and IgG4. Immunoglobulin levels are expressed in mg/dL with age-matched reference ranges provided.

	2005	2011	2012
On IVIG	No	Yes	Yes
Trough level	No	Yes	Yes
Low albumin	No	Yes	No
IgG	1240 (639–1344 mg/dL)	2540** (767–1590 mg/dL)	1230 (614–1295 mg/dL)
IgG1	960 (422–1292 mg/dL)	1730** (341–894 mg/dL)	
IgG2	14* (117–747 mg/dL)	171 (171–632 mg/dL)	
IgG3	275** (41–129 mg/dL)	299** (18–106 mg/dL)	
IgG4	5* (10–67 mg/dL)	13 (2–121 mg/dL)	
IgA	11* (70–312 mg/dL)	<7* (69–309 mg/dL)	<7* (69–309 mg/dL)
IgM	151 (34–210 mg/dL)	591** (53–334 mg/dL)	125 (53–334 mg/dL)
IgE		6 (0–100 mg/dL)	

*Abnormally low levels. **Abnormally high levels. Data are presented from 2005 (before IVIG therapy), 2011 (trough level during IVIG therapy at a time of hypoalbuminemia), and 2012 (trough level during IVIG therapy at a time of normal serum albumin).

(28.5%). In patients with chronic lung disease bronchiectasis, granuloma formation, and requirement for oxygen were frequently observed. In contrast, pulmonary AVMs were not described, and progression to lung transplant was a rare clinical endpoint (observed in only 3 out of the total 473 patients).

Here we describe a patient with humoral immune deficiencies in IgA and the IgG subclasses IgG2 and IgG4 who has been followed up at our institution over the past five years. His initial presentation was pancytopenia, for which he underwent splenectomy at the age of 18 and subsequent to which he developed recurrent infections. He was diagnosed with a "CVID-spectrum disease" elsewhere and started on IVIG therapy at the age of 20. His course was further complicated by pulmonary granulomatosis and small pulmonary AVMs, ultimately requiring bilateral lung transplantation at the age of 25. The patient is alive and continues to be followed at 21 months after transplantation.

2. Case Report

The patient was born prematurely at 32 weeks, yet he did not require neonatal intensive care. In childhood, he experienced recurrent acute otitis media and mild asthma; however, he was never hospitalized for a severe pulmonary disease or infection. In 2002 at the age of 15, he developed splenomegaly and cytopenias as follows: neutropenia (granulocyte antibody positive), anemia (direct antiglobulin test positive for IgG), and intermittent thrombocytopenia. In 2005 at the age of 18, he underwent splenectomy to therapeutically manage his cytopenias after a brief trial of steroids, on which he developed shingles. Subsequent to his splenectomy, the patient developed recurrent sinus (requiring hospitalization in 2007), pulmonary (requiring hospitalization in 2009—cultured positive for *H. influenzae*, methicillin-sensitive *S. aureus*, and *C. albicans*), skin (hospitalized in 2007 for abscess—cultured positive for methicillin-resistant *S. aureus*), and central nervous system (hospitalized in 2009—diagnosed with aseptic meningitis that was presumed viral)

infections. In 2007 at the age of 20, the patient was diagnosed with "CVID-spectrum disease" at an outside hospital and started on IVIG infusions (40 g every four weeks). His immunologic workup was fragmented prior to 2009 when he started to follow up at the Massachusetts General Hospital for routine care.

Chart review of immunoglobulin levels in 2005, prior to initiation of IVIG therapy, was notable for low age-matched serum levels of IgA (11 mg/dL), IgG2 (14 mg/dL), and IgG4 (5 mg/dL) with normal serum levels of total IgG (1240 mg/dL) and IgM (151 mg/dL) (Table 1, "2005"). Postinitiation of IVIG therapy in 2007, trough levels of IgG2 and IgG4 normalized (Table 1, "2011"). Of note, intermittent elevations in IgG and IgM trough levels were observed between 2009 and 2012, which correlated with times of hypoalbuminemia (Table 1, comparing "2011" to "2012"). Despite preserved total IgG, the patient had pronounced clinical response to IVIG and was ultimately maintained on 40 g every three weeks to prevent breakthrough infections. Response to pneumococcal antigen prior to documented Pneumovax in 2005 was negative per report. Repeat testing was not accomplished until 2009, at which time 11/23 serotypes remained negative (1.3 mcg/mL being the accepted lower limit reference range at the Massachusetts General Hospital). Complete blood cell counts in 2009 were notable for a persistent anemia and neutropenia, with an otherwise preserved differential (Table 2). Flow cytometry of peripheral blood cells in 2009 (Table 3) demonstrated a normal number of total T cells (CD3+) and T cell subsets (CD4+ and CD8+) with CD4−/CD8− cells accounting for 5% of total lymphocytes and 6% of CD3+ cells, a finding that could suggest an increase in double-negative T cells; however, gamma delta T cells cannot be excluded in the absence of direct TCRαβ staining. Flow cytometry was also notable for a normal number of total (CD19+) and memory (CD27+) B cells. However, immunoglobulin staining on the B cell surface was positive for IgM/IgD and IgM only without evidence of further class switch, suggesting a B cell maturation arrest at the IgM+/IgD+ stage. T cell function was also tested in 2009, with notable decreased proliferative response

TABLE 2: The patient had confirmed anemia and neutropenia. Complete blood counts from 2009 expressed as a range and a median with reference ranges provided.

	Range	Median	Reference
WBC	3.7–9.8	5.2	4.5–11.0 th/μL
HGB	9.7–12.0*	10.2*	13.5–17.5 g/dL
HCT	30.6–37.3*	32.2*	41.0–53.0%
PLT	259–385	308	150–400 th/μL
Neutrophils	0.00–1.48*	0.69*	1.80–7.70 th/μL
Lymphocytes	1.48–5.78	2.20	1.00–4.80 th/μL
Monocytes	1.03–3.63	1.32	0.20–1.20 th/μL
Eosinophils	0.00–0.77	0.40	0.00–0.90 th/μL
Basophils	0.00–0.42	0.10	0.00–0.30 th/μL

*Abnormally low levels. White blood cells (WBC), hemoglobin (HGB), hematocrit (HCT), and platelets (PLT) are shown.

to phytohemagglutinin, pokeweed mitogen, tetanus toxoid, and Candida antigen. In terms of a malignancy workup, bone marrow biopsy in 2004 demonstrated a normocellular marrow with trilineage hematopoiesis; lymph node biopsies in 2005 and 2011 were benign, and serum electrophoresis in 2009 demonstrated minimally elevated levels of free kappa (31.9 to 95.7 mg/L—reference range < 19.4 mg/L) and lambda (40.3 to 62.6 mg/L—reference range < 26.3 mg/L) light chains with a largely preserved ratio (0.8 to 2—reference range < 1.7). Finally, the patient underwent DNA sequencing and analysis to screen for genetic mutations that have been linked to primary immune deficiencies, including those associated with hyper-IgM syndrome (*UNG*, *AICDA*, *CD40*, and *CD40LG*), CVID (*TNFRSF13B* (*TACI*)), X-linked lymphoproliferative disease (*XIAP*), and autoimmune lymphoproliferative syndrome (ALPS) (*CASP8*, *CASP10*, *FADD*, *FAS*, *FASLG*, *KRAS*, *MAGT1*, and *NRAS*). This screening was negative apart from a hemizygous G-to-A transition at position 655 that was detected in *CD40LG*, which is predicted to lead to a missense mutation and is of unknown significance for hyper-IgM syndrome type 1 [9].

In 2009, his course was complicated by severe hypoxemia (requiring 6 to 10 liters of supplemental oxygen at baseline with an arterial partial pressure of oxygen (PaO$_2$) of 64 mm Hg and an arterial partial pressure of carbon dioxide (PaCO$_2$) of 32 mm Hg on room air). Noncontrast computed tomography (CT) imaging of the chest demonstrated multiple nodules in the bilateral lung fields and significant mediastinal lymphadenopathy. Bronchoalveolar lavages (2009 and 2011) demonstrated rare bacteria and yeast without a consistent or predominant viral, bacterial, or fungal etiology, and cytology was without suggestion of malignancy. Quantitative ventilation/perfusion scanning demonstrated technetium-99 localization consistent with right to left pulmonary shunting, and right heart catheterization was highly suggestive of small pulmonary AVMs. Follow-up genetic testing for hereditary hemorrhagic telangiectasia (HHT) by *ACVRL1* and *ENG* gene sequencing and duplication/deletion analysis was negative. Of note, *SMAD4* was never tested; however, he underwent endoscopy and colonoscopy in 2009 and again in 2011 that

was without demonstration of gastrointestinal polyps or gastrointestinal AVMs. Vascular endothelial growth factor (VEGF) levels were found to be elevated (530 pg/mL—reference range 31 to 86 pg/mL), and the patient was started on a course of suppressive doxycycline therapy.

In July of 2011, the decision was made to pursue diagnostic and therapeutic pulmonary wedge resection. Biopsies of the right upper and middle lobes demonstrated peribronchiolar lymphoid hyperplasia that was consistent with humoral immune deficiency but without clear evidence of vasculitis or AVMs. By April of 2012, he met criteria for NYHA Class III-IV functional level and underwent transplantation evaluation. Considerations for lung transplantation included a recent history of biopsy-confirmed (2009 and 2011) hepatitis that included a broad differential of autoimmune, viral, and drug-induced disease etiologies on histopathology. Repeat liver biopsy in 2012, however, was most suggestive of autoimmune hepatitis given the substantial reduction in lobular lymphoid hyperplasia observed between 2011 and 2012 in response to a course of suppressive prednisone and azathioprine therapy. Of note, his pulmonary function continued to worsen during this time despite the immunosuppression.

The patient received bilateral cadaveric donor lung transplantation without requirement for cardiopulmonary bypass on November 21, 2012, at the age of 25. Following surgery, he received standard of care immunosuppression with three doses of antithymocyte globulin and two doses of high-dose methylprednisolone. He was subsequently placed on a steroid taper and started on tacrolimus (titrated to daily levels) and azathioprine (150 mg daily) with appropriate antiviral (donor CMV negative, recipient CMV positive), antibacterial, and antifungal prophylaxis. He was successfully extubated by postoperative day three. Repeat pulmonary function tests and ventilation/perfusion scan demonstrated excellent function of the transplanted organs without early concern for mechanical failure. He was discharged home on postoperative day 15. Subsequent analysis of explanted lung tissue confirmed the diagnosis of small pulmonary AVMs with peripherally localizing lymphoid nodules (Figure 1).

At the 21-month follow-up from transplantation, the patient continues on tacrolimus, prednisone, and sirolimus for immune suppression (switched from mycophenolate mofetil secondary to leukopenia). His posttransplantation course has been complicated by lymphocytic small airway inflammation and minimal acute rejection on serial graft biopsies. More recently (June of 2014), he began to develop accelerated bronchiolitis obliterans syndrome that is currently being managed with extracorporeal photopheresis. He additionally continues on IVIG infusions (40 g every three weeks), which are anticipated to continue life-long for immune protection.

3. Discussion

This is a case of confirmed autoimmune-mediated cytopenias and confirmed humoral immune deficiency, which does not meet criteria for CVID given the preserved level of

TABLE 3: The patient had preserved populations of total T cells, T cell subsets, total B cells, and memory B cells. There was question of an elevated double-negative T cell population that was not confirmed on direct TCR$\alpha\beta$ staining. Flow cytometry analysis of peripheral blood cells in 2009.

	Major antigen	Minor antigen	Measured (cells/mm^3)	Reference range (cells/mm^3)	% of total	% of CD3+	% of CD19+
T cells	CD3+		4092	690–2540	86%	100%	
	CD3+	CD4+	3072	419–1590	64%	75%	
	CD3+	CD8+	785	190–1140	16%	19%	
	CD3+	CD4−/CD8−	235		5%	6%	
B cells	CD19+		352	90–660	7%		100%
	CD19+	CD27+	107		2%		30%
	CD19+	CD27−	245		5%		70%
NK cells	CD16+/56+		335	90–590	7%		

Data are presented in cells/mm^3 or % with reference ranges provided (note that reference ranges for CD4−/CD8− cells, CD27+ cells, and CD27− cells are not established at the Massachusetts General Hospital, and thus normal was defined according to percentages previously described [7, 8]).

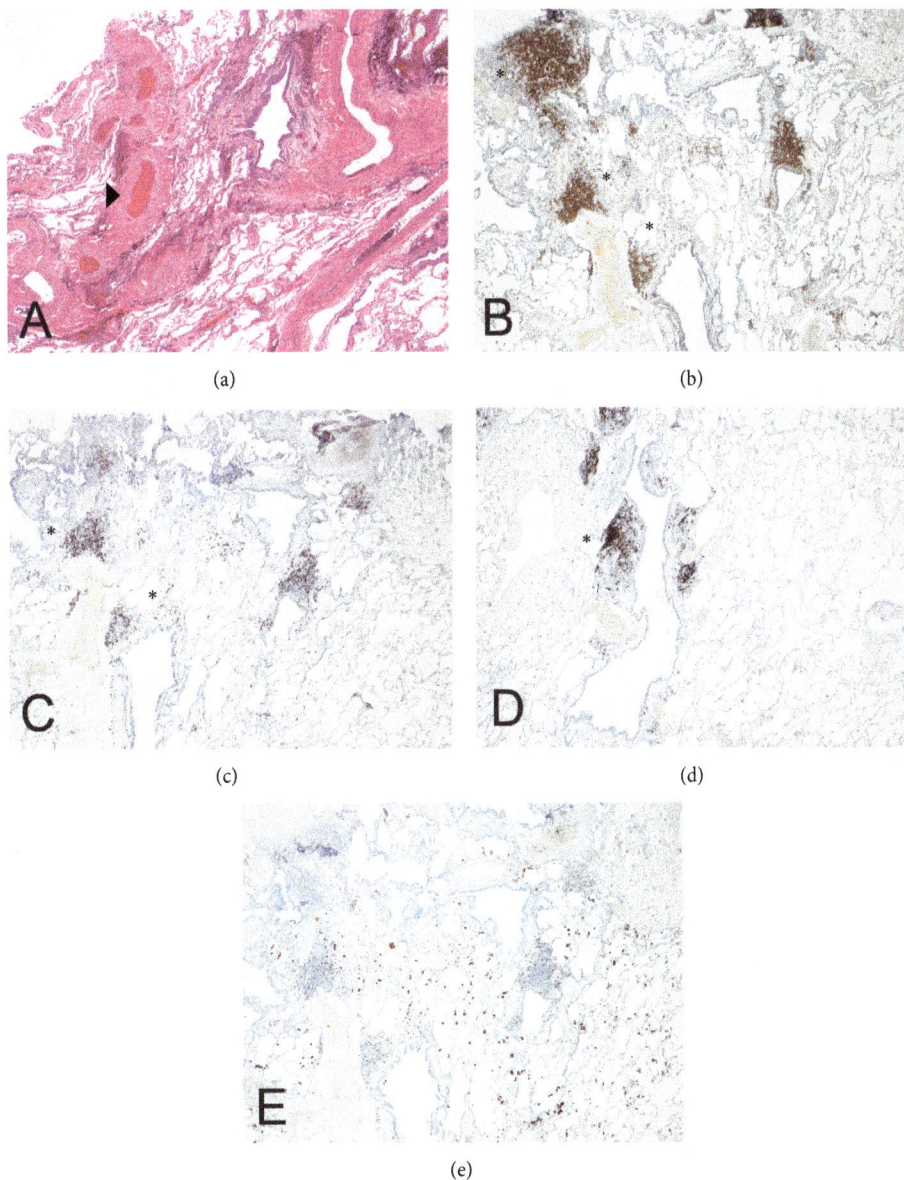

(a)

(b)

(c)

(d)

(e)

FIGURE 1: Small pulmonary AVMs (►) with peripherally localizing lymphoid aggregates (∗) were confirmed on explanted lung pathology. Immunohistochemical staining directed against (a) H/E, (b) CD4, (c) CD8, (d) CD20, and (e) CD68.

total IgG (Table 1). Despite the splenomegaly, autoimmune-mediated cytopenias, and question of an elevated double-negative T cell population (Table 3), the patient screened negative for ALPS on gene sequencing and analysis and otherwise does not fit the full ALPS presentation given the preserved population of memory B cells, the defect in T cell proliferation, and the normal levels of total IgG and IgM in this case [7]. Therefore, we are left with a diagnosis of humoral immune deficiency, specific to IgA, IgG2, and IgG4. While the noted humoral deficits could certainly have predated the patient's splenectomy in 2005, this hypothesis was never validated on laboratory testing and certainly a description of recurrent infections is not clearly documented at this time in the patient's history. Alternatively, the humoral deficits could have developed subsequent to the patient's splenectomy. Overall, humoral immune deficiency is known to be associated with autoimmune-mediated cytopenias. In a retrospective chart review of 326 CVID patients [10], 11% had a history of autoimmune-mediated cytopenias, 54% of which had the first episode of thrombocytopenia or hemolytic anemia prior to the diagnosis of CVID. However, postsplenectomy immune deficiency has also been described. In an analysis of 12 patients who underwent traumatic splenectomy [11], decreased B cell activation was observed in response to polyclonal activator pokeweed mitogen at two days to seven years postoperatively. Coculture analysis further confirmed that the defect was associated with both the T helper cell and the intrinsic B cell compartment of the splenectomized patient. In a more recent comparative analysis of 209 asplenic or hyposplenic adults compared to 140 healthy controls [12], similar total levels of B cells were described. In comparison to the healthy controls, however, the splenectomized patients had a significant reduction ($P < 0.001$) in memory B cells, including both IgM memory B cells and switched memory B cells. Consistent with these data, here we describe preservation of total B cell counts, but with maturation arrest at the IgM+/IgD+ stage of development. Furthermore, genetic testing for known mutations linked to B cell maturation arrest was negative. Therefore, it remains uncertain as to whether the patient had a humoral immune deficiency prior to splenectomy or whether the splenectomy itself initiated a B cell dysregulation. Together these data highlight the importance of screening for humoral immune deficiencies concurrent with the diagnosis of autoimmune-mediated cytopenia and prior to splenectomy and initiation of the perisplenectomy vaccination series.

Pulmonary complications including granulomas, bronchiectasis, and emphysema are known to be associated with primary humoral immune deficiencies [6]. However, pulmonary AVMs are not a frequent complication of humoral immune deficiency, as described in chart [6] or even direct radiographic [13] review. To our knowledge, there are only two case reports linking humoral immune deficiency to pulmonary AVMs, described in a patient with hypogammaglobulinemia [14] as well as IgA and IgG subclass deficiency [15]. We also entertained the possibility that splenectomy itself could have driven the pulmonary pathology in this case. While postsplenectomy pulmonary hypertension driven by chronic thromboemboli has been described [16], our patient had no evidence of pulmonary hypertension on right heart catheterization in 2009, and furthermore pulmonary AVMs are not a known complication after splenectomy [17, 18]. Alternative diagnoses were entertained in consultation with the medical genetics team at Massachusetts General Hospital. However, the patient screened negative for the genetic mutations most frequently associated with HHT (ACVRL1 and ENG). Furthermore, HHT is not commonly associated with the humoral immune deficiencies otherwise described in this case [19]. Given that the pulmonary AVMs were diffuse and small in nature, the patient was not an appropriate candidate for embolization, and he did not clinically benefit from the pulmonary wedge resection. Ultimately the explanted lung pathology confirmed prominent and diffuse AVMs with small surrounding lymphoid nodules (Figure 1). It is unclear if the lymphocytes were driving the vascular pathology in this case. However, the physiology is clear, remarkable for oxygen-resistant hypoxemia with worsening ventilation/perfusion mismatch as the driving etiology for transplantation.

Lung transplantation in patients with humoral immune deficiency is a rare therapeutic endpoint. Several case reports have been described in patients with panhypogammaglobulinemia for the indications of end-stage bronchiectasis, emphysema, and/or granulomatous disease [20–23]. Lung transplantation has also been described in a single patient with IgG1 subclass deficiency, who was transplanted for the indication of end-stage bronchiectasis and was still alive at the nine-year follow-up [24]. Case reports of lung transplantation for the indication of diffuse pulmonary AVMs have also been described. Of note, these case reports are limited to patients with a confirmed diagnosis of HHT [25–28]. Therefore, while it is unclear whether the immune deficiencies herein described predisposed the patient to pulmonary AVMs, this is a unique case description of bilateral lung transplantation for the indication of pulmonary AVMs in a patient without a confirmed diagnosis of HHT but with a confirmed diagnosis of humoral immune deficiency.

IVIG is an important component of posttransplantation management, as hypogammaglobulinemia can be observed in an immunologically competent patient in the context of immunosuppressive therapy. In solid organ transplantation, a significant reduction in risk for infection was recently described with IVIG replacement of approximately 500 mg/kg monthly [29]. In our patient, this calculates to 32 g of IVIG monthly, which is less than the actual 40 g of IVIG that he has been receiving every three weeks. However, much of the management of humoral immune deficiency, especially in the context of solid organ transplantation, remains elusive. For example, while an anti-infective role for IVIG in transplantation has been described [29], the immune-modulatory effects of IVIG are still only partially understood. Additionally, we lack the long-term follow-up necessary to investigate whether patients with humoral immune deficiency are at risk of developing recurrent disease in their transplanted organs.

A growing body of data demonstrates the benefit of hematopoietic stem cell transplantation for the treatment of primary immune deficiency. Survival and cure after transplantation in the context of a well-matched donor, limited infectious disease complications, and no known end-organ damage has reached 90% [30]. For CVID specifically, allogeneic stem cell transplantation was recently described in a cohort of four patients for the indication of malignancy (two patients) and severe end-organ failure with documented granulomatous disease (two patients) [31]. Three of the four patients had long-term survival (between 4.5 and 7 years). However, only one in four patients demonstrated sustained IgG normalization with adequate vaccine response after transplantation, suggesting a true cure for CVID. In patients with primary immune deficiency and end-stage lung disease, a current clinical trial is underway that will directly address whether bilateral orthotopic lung transplantation followed by cadaveric partially matched hematopoietic stem cell transplantation is safe and effective [32], a proof of principle case report having already been demonstrated in 2011 [33]. These data will play a critical epidemiologic role, furthering our understanding of cotransplantation risk and long-term benefit and ultimately directing superior management of humoral immune deficiency and its pulmonary complications.

Conflict of Interests

The authors declare that there is no conflict of interests regarding the publication of this paper.

References

[1] A. Durandy, S. Kracker, and A. Fischer, "Primary antibody deficiencies," *Nature Reviews Immunology*, vol. 13, no. 7, pp. 519–533, 2013.

[2] L. Hammarström, I. Vorechovsky, and D. Webster, "Selective IgA deficiency (SIgAD) and common variable immunodeficiency (CVID)," *Clinical and Experimental Immunology*, vol. 120, no. 2, pp. 225–231, 2000.

[3] V. A. Oxelius, A. B. Laurell, B. Lindquist et al., "IgG subclasses in selective IgA deficiency: importance of IgG2-IgA deficiency," *The New England Journal of Medicine*, vol. 304, no. 24, pp. 1476–1477, 1981.

[4] J. H. Branconier, B. Nilsson, V. A. Oxelius, and F. Karup-Pedersen, "Recurrent pneumococcal infections in a patient with lack of specific IgG and IgM pneumococcal antibodies and deficiency of serum IgA, IgG2 and IgG4," *Scandinavian Journal of Infectious Diseases*, vol. 16, no. 4, pp. 407–410, 1984.

[5] V. Garg, S. Lipka, K. Rizvon, J. Singh, S. Rashid, and P. Mustacchia, "Diffuse nodular lymphoid hyperplasia of intestine in selective IgG 2 subclass deficiency, autoimmune thyroiditis, and autoimmune hemolytic anemia: case report and literature review," *Journal of Gastrointestinal and Liver Diseases*, vol. 21, no. 4, pp. 431–434, 2012.

[6] E. S. Resnick, E. L. Moshier, J. H. Godbold, and C. Cunningham-Rundles, "Morbidity and mortality in common variable immune deficiency over 4 decades," *Blood*, vol. 119, no. 7, pp. 1650–1657, 2012.

[7] J. B. Oliveira, J. J. Bleesing, U. Dianzani et al., "Revised diagnostic criteria and classification for the autoimmune lymphoproliferative syndrome (ALPS): report from the 2009 NIH International Workshop," *Blood*, vol. 116, no. 14, pp. e35–e40, 2010.

[8] H. Morbach, E. M. Eichhorn, J. G. Liese, and H. J. Girschick, "Reference values for B cell subpopulations from infancy to adulthood," *Clinical and Experimental Immunology*, vol. 162, no. 2, pp. 271–279, 2010.

[9] S. Rigaud, E. Lopez-Granados, S. Sibéril et al., "Human X-linked variable immunodeficiency caused by a hypomorphic mutation in *XIAP* in association with a rare polymorphism in *CD40LG*," *Blood*, vol. 118, no. 2, pp. 252–261, 2011.

[10] J. Wang and C. Cunningham-Rundles, "Treatment and outcome of autoimmune hematologic disease in common variable immunodeficiency (CVID)," *Journal of Autoimmunity*, vol. 25, no. 1, pp. 57–62, 2005.

[11] G. Sieber, H.-G. Breyer, F. Herrmann, and H. Ruhl, "Abnormalities of B-cell activation and immunoregulation in splenectomized patients," *Immunobiology*, vol. 169, no. 3, pp. 263–271, 1985.

[12] P. U. Cameron, P. Jones, M. Gorniak et al., "Splenectomy associated changes in IgM memory B cells in an adult spleen registry cohort," *PLoS ONE*, vol. 6, no. 8, Article ID e23164, 2011.

[13] K. M. Thickett, D. S. Kumararatne, A. K. Banerjee, R. Dudley, and D. E. Stableforth, "Common variable immune deficiency: respiratory manifestations, pulmonary function and high-resolution CT scan findings," *QJM: Monthly Journal of the Association of Physicians*, vol. 95, no. 10, pp. 655–662, 2002.

[14] L. J. Couderc, E. Caubarrere, E. Oksenlendler, and J. P. Clauvel, "Vascular malformations and hypogammaglobulinaemia," *The Lancet*, vol. 1, no. 8529, p. 385, 1987.

[15] K.-C. Tse, G. C. Ooi, A. Wu et al., "Multiple brain abscesses in a patient with bilateral pulmonary arteriovenous malformations and immunoglobulin deficiency," *Postgraduate Medical Journal*, vol. 79, no. 936, pp. 597–599, 2003.

[16] X. Jaïs, V. Ioos, C. Jardim et al., "Splenectomy and chronic thromboembolic pulmonary hypertension," *Thorax*, vol. 60, no. 12, pp. 1031–1034, 2005.

[17] A. di Sabatino, R. Carsetti, and G. R. Corazza, "Post-splenectomy and hyposplenic states," *The Lancet*, vol. 378, no. 9785, pp. 86–97, 2011.

[18] S. Y. Kristinsson, G. Gridley, R. N. Hoover, D. Check, and O. Landgren, "Long-term risks after splenectomy among 8,149 cancer-free American veterans: a cohort study with up to 27 years follow-up," *Haematologica*, vol. 99, no. 2, pp. 392–398, 2014.

[19] F. S. Govani and C. L. Shovlin, "Hereditary haemorrhagic telangiectasia: a clinical and scientific review," *European Journal of Human Genetics*, vol. 17, no. 7, pp. 860–871, 2009.

[20] M. Yeatman, K. NcNeil, J. A. Smith et al., "Lung Transplantation in patients with systemic diseases: an eleven-year experience at Papworth Hospital," *The Journal of Heart and Lung Transplantation*, vol. 15, no. 2, pp. 144–149, 1996.

[21] A. T. Hill, R. A. Thompson, J. Wallwork, and D. E. Stableforth, "Heart lung transplantation in a patient with end stage lung disease due to common variable immunodeficiency," *Thorax*, vol. 53, no. 7, pp. 622–623, 1998.

[22] C. M. Burton, N. Milman, C. B. Andersen, H. Marquart, and M. Iversen, "Common variable immune deficiency and lung transplantation," *Scandinavian Journal of Infectious Diseases*, vol. 39, no. 4, pp. 362–367, 2007.

[23] C. Cunningham-Rundles and C. Bodian, "Common variable immunodeficiency: clinical and immunological features of 248 patients," *Clinical Immunology*, vol. 92, no. 1, pp. 34–48, 1999.

[24] P. A. Beirne, N. R. Banner, A. Khaghani, M. E. Hodson, and M. H. Yacoub, "Lung transplantation for non-cystic fibrosis bronchiectasis: Analysis of a 13-year experience," *Journal of Heart and Lung Transplantation*, vol. 24, no. 10, pp. 1530–1535, 2005.

[25] M. Reynaud-Gaubert, P. Thomas, J.-Y. Gaubert et al., "Pulmonary arteriovenous malformations: lung transplantation as a therapeutic option," *European Respiratory Journal*, vol. 14, no. 6, pp. 1425–1428, 1999.

[26] G. Svetliza, A. De La Canal, E. Beveraggi et al., "Lung transplantation in a patient with arteriovenous malformations," *Journal of Heart and Lung Transplantation*, vol. 21, no. 4, pp. 506–508, 2002.

[27] M. V. Misra, M. P. Mullen, S. O. Vargas, H. B. Kim, and D. Boyer, "Bilateral lung transplant for hereditary hemorrhagic telangiectasia in a pediatric patient," *Pediatric Transplantation*, vol. 16, no. 8, pp. E364–E367, 2012.

[28] H. Fukushima, T. Mitsuhashi, T. Oto et al., "Successful lung transplantation in a case with diffuse pulmonary arteriovenous malformations and hereditary hemorrhagic telangiectasia," *The American Journal of Transplantation*, vol. 13, no. 12, pp. 3278–3281, 2013.

[29] S. Mawhorter and M. H. Yamani, "Hypogammaglobulinemia and infection risk in solid organ transplant recipients," *Current Opinion in Organ Transplantation*, vol. 13, no. 6, pp. 581–585, 2008.

[30] M. A. Slatter and A. R. Gennery, "Advances in hematopoietic stem cell transplantation for primary immunodeficiency," *Expert Review of Clinical Immunology*, vol. 9, no. 10, pp. 991–999, 2013.

[31] M. Rizzi, C. Neumann, A. K. Fielding et al., "Outcome of allogeneic stem cell transplantation in adults with common variable immunodeficiency," *Journal of Allergy and Clinical Immunology*, vol. 128, no. 6, pp. 1371.e2–1374.e2, 2011.

[32] P. Szabolcs, "Sequential cadaveric lung and bone marrow transplant for immune deficiency disease (BOLT+BMT)," National Library of Medicine (US), Bethesda, Md, USA, 2013, http://clinicaltrials.gov/show/ NCT01852370 NLM Identifier:NCT01852370.

[33] P. Szabolcs, R. Buckley, R. D. Davis et al., "Tandem HLA-mismatches cadaveric unrelated donor lung transplant followed by CD3- and CD19-depleted bone marrow transplant from the same donor permits withdrawal of systemic immunosuppression with graft acceptance and functional immune reconstitution," in *Proceedings of the 53rd American Society of Hematology Annual Meeting and Exposition*, abstract 1006, San Diego, Calif, USA, 2011.

29

Hereditary Angioedema and Gastrointestinal Complications: An Extensive Review of the Literature

Napoleon Patel,[1] Lisbet D. Suarez,[1] Sakshi Kapur,[1] and Leonard Bielory[2]

[1]*Department of Internal Medicine, Atlantic Health System, Overlook Medical Center, 99 Beauvoir Avenue, Summit, NJ 07902, USA*
[2]*Division of Allergy and Immunology, Rutgers University Robert Wood Johnson University Hospital, New Brunswick, NJ 07103, USA*

Correspondence should be addressed to Napoleon Patel; napoleonpatel@gmail.com

Academic Editor: Jiri Litzman

Hereditary Angioedema (HAE) is a rare autosomal dominant (AD) disease characterized by deficient (type 1) or nonfunctional (type 2) C1 inhibitor protein. The disorder is associated with episodes of angioedema of the face, larynx, lips, abdomen, or extremities. The angioedema is caused by the activation of the kallikrein-kinin system that leads to the release of vasoactive peptides, followed by edema, which in severe cases can be life threatening. The disease is usually not diagnosed until late adolescence and patients tend to have frequent episodes that can be severely impairing and have a high incidence of morbidity. Gastrointestinal involvement represents up to 80% of clinical presentations that are commonly confused with other gastrointestinal disorders such as appendicitis, cholecystitis, pancreatitis, and ischemic bower. We present a case of an HAE attack presenting as colonic intussusception managed conservatively with a C1 esterase inhibitor. Very few cases have been reported in the literature of HAE presentation in this manner, and there are no reports of any nonsurgical management of these cases.

1. Introduction

HAE is a condition presenting as recurrent attacks of angioedema usually without symptoms of pruritus or urticaria. It is an autosomal dominant condition typically presenting in childhood, characterized by nonpitting edema of subcutaneous and mucosal tissues and usually associated with the upper respiratory and gastrointestinal systems [1, 2]. Patients may experience nausea, vomiting, diarrhea, pain syndromes, and laryngeal swelling that may be life threatening [3]. This topic review will focus on the gastrointestinal complications of HAE as a potential area of misdiagnosis leading to surgical morbidity. It has been estimated that 1 in 10,000–50,000 persons is affected by HAE across any ethnic group. Although a recent study from Norway proposed that 1 per 100,000 of the population may be affected, the exact prevalence of the disease is not known [2, 4]. The age of onset of HAE is variable and can present in children less than one year old, with laryngeal attacks developing usually after the age of three and increasing in frequency after puberty [3].

2. Case Presentation

A 19-year-old female presented to the Emergency Department (ED) with complaints of abdominal pain. The patient was in her usual state of health when she experienced an acute onset of abdominal pain, localized to the right upper quadrant. The pain was described as cramp-like in character, accompanied by numerous bouts of vomiting and diarrhea, both of which were nonbloody. Her past medical history was significant for low complement C4 performed at the time of diagnosis. The patient's father has a known history of type 1 HAE. Her medications include an intravenous (IV) C1 esterase inhibitor (Cinryze) taken every 3 days for HAE symptom prophylaxis and subcutaneous (SC) icatibant (Firazyr) to be used during an acute attack. The patient was on a clinical trial of Cinryze for prophylaxis as instructed by her allergy specialist. She had experienced similar episodes in the past which resolved with immediate treatment with Cinryze and Firazyr. The patient's symptoms were well controlled on this regimen until 1 month ago when her symptoms increased

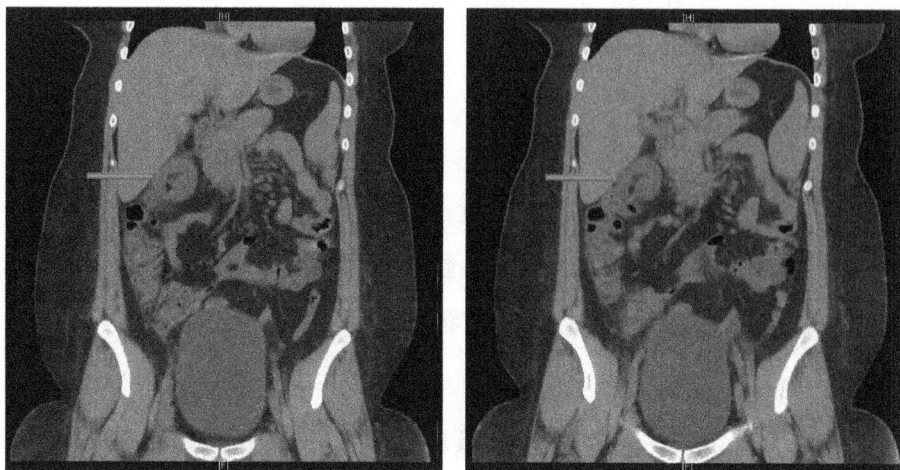

FIGURE 1: CT abdomen demonstrating colocolic intussusception at the hepatic flexure (arrow).

in frequency to 1 episode a week. She denied any change in her daily activities but did admit increased stress due to college final exams. Within an hour of her current symptom onset the patient used one application of Cinryze and Firazyr, but the pain was unrelenting and she decided to go to the nearest ED. In the ED the patient was found to have an elevated blood pressure of 148/100 mmHg. Her physical exam revealed tenderness in the umbilical and right upper quadrant upon light palpation. There was no guarding, rigidity, or rebound tenderness, and Murphy's sign was not elicited. Her head, neck, chest, extremities, and skin exam did not reveal any significant findings.

Laboratory work-up revealed a normal complete blood count and comprehensive metabolic panel. Serum amylase, lipase, and urinalysis were all within normal limits. Her C-reactive peptide was not obtained at the time of evaluation. Abdominal CT scan demonstrated a 2.4 cm segment of colocolic intussusception in the region of the hepatic flexure with a normal appearance of the appendix (Figure 1).

The patient was admitted to the hospital and was given supportive care with IV fluids and pain medications and kept nothing per mouth (NPO) while the surgery team was consulted along with her outpatient allergy specialist. Additional diagnosis such as tumor or adhesions causing her abdominal pain was not contemplated given that she had no prior history of abdominal surgeries and the CT findings did not reveal a mass of concern. Her allergist recommended beginning treatment with three 1,000-unit doses of IV Cinryze delivered every 2 hours in an attempt to subside the edema causing the intussusception. The initiation of therapy with IV Cinryze was roughly 4 hours after arrival to the ED. If the treatment failed, then the patient would be scheduled to undergo air-contrast enema for decompression. Overnight the patient's abdominal pain resolved, and repeat CT imaging demonstrated resolution of the intussusception and a normal appearance of the bowel wall with no evidence of obstruction (Figure 2). The patient was able to tolerate advancement in her diet and was discharged home later

that day with a follow-up appointment with her allergy specialist.

3. Discussion

The angioedema in HAE develops secondary to excess bradykinin production due to low levels of functionally active C1 inhibitor (C1 INH). This leads to the activation of the kallikrein-kinin system causing the release of vasoactive peptides and ultimately angioedema formation [5]. Several types of HAE resulting from a genetic disorder have been identified that are not related to acquired C1 inhibitor deficiency or drug induced angioedema. Type 1 HAE is the cause of the disease in about 85% of HAE patients due to deficiency of the C1 INH protein (quantitative defect). Type 2 HAE comprises the majority of the remaining 15% of patients with HAE with a normal or elevated level of the C1 INH protein but with a functional deficiency (qualitative defect). Both types 1 and 2 are a result of a mutation in the C1 INH gene [3, 5]. A third type of HAE has been found, primarily in women, with normal C1 INH protein and the mutation is actually in the coagulation factor XII gene [5].

Characteristic locations for HAE attacks involve the skin, upper respiratory tract, and gastrointestinal system [1, 2]. Symptoms are self-limited, progressing over hours, and can persist from 1 to 4 days and the frequency of attacks can vary from weekly to a few attacks per year [1, 6]. Premonitory symptoms associated with HAE can develop as little as hours or up to days before the start of an attack [7].

Common prodromal symptoms include nausea abdominal pain, rash, fatigue, muscle aches, numbness, and tingling [8]. Prodromal skin changes can be described as a nonurticarial erythematous discoloration on the extremities and trunk with reticulate and serpentine appearance similar to that of erythema marginatum [9]. Cutaneous attacks of HAE typically involve swelling of the skin, which was present in 97% of episodes in one study with 221 patients. Face, genitals, upper more often than lower extremities, and rarely

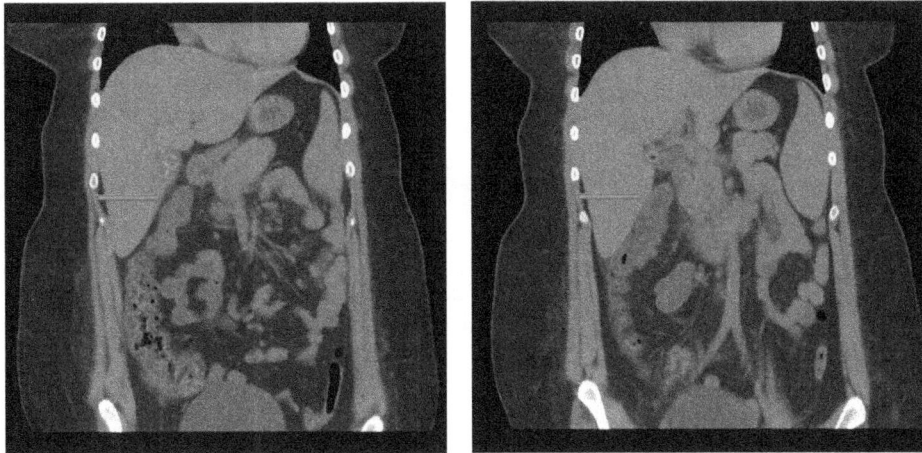

FIGURE 2: CT abdomen after C1 INH treatment, demonstrating resolution of intussusception (arrow).

the neck and trunk were the most notable locations of swelling. Laryngeal edema is the most serious complication that can become life threatening but is a relatively rare event. Only 0.9% of all edema episodes involved laryngeal edema. However, 51% of patients did admit to experiencing some sensation of tightness in the throat, hoarseness, and aphonia/dysphonia in their lifetime. Laryngeal edema can occur alone or with simultaneous swelling of the soft palate, tongue, and uvula [10]. There have also been reports of attacks manifesting as headaches, temporary neurologic deficits, swelling and spasms of the urethra and bladder, joint swelling, chest tightness and pain, and renal colic [10, 11].

Gastrointestinal tract involvement is an important feature and one of the most common in HAE. The difficulty in recognizing gastrointestinal symptoms as being related to HAE often leads to a delay in diagnosis and to unnecessary surgical procedures [1, 12, 13]. The most common symptoms include varying degrees of nausea, vomiting, diarrhea, and abdominal pain, which are the result of intestinal edema [1, 12–14]. The abdominal pain can present acutely or as recurrent pain and is described by patients to be cramping and colicky in nature [14]. The pain patients experience can be moderate to severe in intensity and is usually present in 43–93% of all HAE attacks [12]. Many of these abdominal pain symptoms can occur for many years without any associated respiratory or cutaneous involvement. Not only does the transient edema of the bowel wall cause the aforementioned symptoms, but it may also lead to intestinal pseudoobstruction [13, 14]. The entire gastrointestinal tract can be involved in HAE attacks leading to a wide range of clinical manifestations (Table 1). The oropharynx and esophagus can be involved which leads to feeling of dysphagia. Stomach and small intestinal involvement cause nonspecific findings of abdominal pain, vomiting, and diarrhea. Liver involvement can lead to elevated transaminases, exudative ascites, and reversible parenchymal changes. Pancreatic edema can cause partial duct obstruction, which can present as recurrent episodes of pancreatitis [13, 14]. Constipation was a common finding when there was colonic involvement, with only a few reported cases of intussusception [13–15]. Severe consequences such

TABLE 1: Gastrointestinal manifestations of Hereditary Angioedema.

Site	Clinical manifestation	Frequency (%)
Skin	Swelling and edema	97% [10]
Oropharynx	Laryngeal edema	0.9% [10]
	Tongue swelling	0.3% [10]
	Dysphagia	16% [34]
Abdomen	Nausea and vomiting	88% [34]
	Crampy and colicky abdominal pain	43–93% [12]
	Abdominal distention	72.8% [15]
	Ascites	30% [15] 80% [35]
	Diarrhea	15% [36] 65% [14]
Circulatory system	Hypovolemic shock	4.4% [15]
Less frequent presentation	Pancreatitis	Rare [13, 14, 37]
	Intussusception	Rare [13–15, 38]
	Tetany	Rare [15]
	Dysuria	Rare [39]

as circulatory collapse may occur due to a combination of vasodilation, fluid loss from emesis and diarrhea, and fluid extravasation from bowel wall edema and ascites. This can lead to considerable hypovolemia and hemoconcentration. According to one observation study of 33,000 gastrointestinal attacks in 153 HAE patients, circulatory collapse occurred in 4.4% of all attacks [15]. In the same study, there was only one case of intussusception, and the patient underwent surgical resection without reported complications. The majority of abdominal attacks last 2–4 days with preceding symptoms of irritability, fatigue, hunger, aggressiveness, and erythema marginatum [15].

TABLE 2: Key findings of an international Internet based survey of HAE patients in relation to surgical interventions.

Population group	Number of patients who underwent unnecessary surgery due to misdiagnosis (n)
Patients in the United States with HAE	24 out of 125 (19%)
Patients in the United Kingdom with HAE	12 out of 52 (24%)

The nonspecific character of HAE symptoms can lead to an extensive work-up and unless there is a high index of clinical suspicion, the diagnosis can be delayed leading to inappropriate surgical interventions. Nationwide surveys in Denmark and Spain found mean delays in diagnosis of 13–16 years, with an international Internet based survey finding of 8.3-year delay in diagnosis [16]. This delay often leads to misdiagnosis and one study of 235 patients found that 1/3 of patients experiencing abdominal symptoms underwent appendectomies and exploratory laparotomies [17]. Table 2 represents key results of the international Internet based survey of HAE patients revealing the unnecessary surgical interventions patients may endure before their disease is identified.

Obtaining a detailed patient history and performing a thorough physical exam are crucial to help direct the medical team to appropriate diagnostic testing. Questions pertaining to time of onset, duration, age at first attack, intervals between attacks, triggering medication and events, family history of similar symptoms, and a thorough review of systems are areas of interest that should be investigated [12]. The physical exam should include skin inspection for cutaneous angioedema, typically nonpitting with no associated pruritus. Tongue, lip, and oral airway swelling may be present as well as stridor on respiratory auscultation. The abdominal exam may be nonspecific and the patient may exhibit diffuse abdominal tenderness on palpation with bowel sounds hyper- or hypoactive and shifting dullness if ascites is present. The physical exam is mostly helpful during the acute attacks [12, 14].

To confirm the diagnosis of HAE it is important to correlate the history and physical exam findings with laboratory and radiographic evidence. The recommended initial screening laboratory testing for HAE includes serum C4 level, C1 INH antigenic protein, C1 INH function/activity, and serum C1q levels which is the result from C1 INH breakdown [3, 14]. The C4 level is typically low in most cases of HAE and is the quickest and most readily available screening test [14, 18]. However, there is one case in the literature of a patient with consistent normal complement C4 levels [19]. The findings of a low C4 along with low C1 INH level and activity and a normal C1q level are confirmatory tests for HAE type 1, while type 2 HAE laboratory findings would reveal a normal C1 INH and C1q levels, but low C1 INH functional activity. Complement studies should be repeated after one month to confirm the results and diagnosis [3, 14].

Most abdominal attacks are not associated with elevations in the white blood cell count, but patients experiencing severe exacerbation may present with elevated neutrophils without bands. An increase in hematocrit was also notable, likely secondary to hemoconcentration from dehydration and fluid translocation to the intestinal wall [13, 20, 21]. A recent study did find a correlation between C-reactive protein levels in HAE patients. Asymptomatic patients with HAE were found to have elevated C-reactive protein levels at baseline. The C-reactive protein levels increased during attacks and were more likely to be elevated in abdominal attacks as compared to other locations [22]. Table 3 lists the most common gastrointestinal disorders and their distinguishing features in comparison with abdominal attacks of HAE.

Radiologic tests may be helpful during initial investigations of abdominal pain episodes but not necessary to confirm a diagnosis of HAE. Abdominal X-ray during an acute attack may show dilated small bowel loops, thickened mucosal folds, air fluid levels, and a "thumbprint" sign representing an area of mucosal edema [14, 23]. An ultrasound of the abdomen can identify ascites and bowel wall edema better than X-ray. Computed tomography (CT) with contrast may be the most sensitive of the three imaging modalities mentioned because of its ability to identify milder degrees of intestinal edema, ascites, and dilated loops of bowel. A CT is also useful in helping to eliminate other potential etiologies for the patient's abdominal pain [14, 23, 24]. Findings on imaging are transient and bowel wall edema and ascites may quickly resolve after the attack subsides and appear normal if studies are delayed [14, 23]. Imaging is generally not required if a patient with a known diagnosis of HAE is having symptoms similar to episodes in the past.

The literature on endoscopic procedures in HAE episodes is minimal, and it is generally not a recommended step during diagnosis. Upper endoscopy reports described the mucosa to appear erythematous and edematous with findings of small nodules and raised erosions [13, 14]. Colonoscopy has revealed areas of extensive mucosal edema leading to almost total occlusion of the colonic lumen, with biopsies showing normal histology [13]. The scarcity of reports about endoscopic evaluation may be due to self-limiting course of HAE and because of the high risk of precipitating an oropharyngeal attack with endoscopic manipulation [13, 14].

The treatment options for HAE patients involve supportive care, individualized action plans, pharmacological treatment, and prophylactic measures. This combination can prevent or minimize future attacks and save the patient from unnecessary exploratory laparotomies, appendectomies, or other invasive procedures. These treatment guidelines are based on the World Allergy Organization (WAO) 2012 and practice parameters developed by a Joint Task Force of American College of Allergy, Asthma and Immunology and American Academy of Allergy, Asthma and Immunology in 2013 [25, 26]. During an acute attack the initial steps in every case should be to assess hemodynamic stability and target therapy to achieve stability. Airway patency and protection should be the first priority because edema in the oropharynx can lead to fatal asphyxiation [14, 25]. Those in severe respiratory distress may need intubation until medical therapy gains

TABLE 3: Clinical presentation of HAE abdominal attacks in comparison to other gastrointestinal disorders.

Disorder	Sign/symptom	Laboratory data	Distinguishing features
HAE abdominal attacks	Nausea, vomiting, diarrhea, crampy abdominal pain	Type 1 HAE: low C4 and C1 inhibitor level/activity, normal C1q level [3]; Type 2 HAE: normal C1 inhibitor level, low activity, normal C1q level [3]	History of HAE, colonoscopy: massive segmental mucosal edema [13]; CT abdomen: intestinal edema, ascites, dilated loops; Attacks usually begin in childhood, but they can occur at any age [34]
Acute diverticulitis	Acute LLQ abdominal pain and tenderness, fever, anorexia, nausea, vomiting, constipation or loose stools	Mild to moderate leukocytosis	LLQ palpable abdominal mass; CT abdomen: evidence of colonic diverticula, wall thickening, pericolic fat infiltration, abscess formation or extraluminal air or contrast. At age of 40 less than 5% are affected, at age of 60 that number is 30%, and by age of 80 50–65% of adults are affected [40]
Acute appendicitis	Periumbilical abdominal pain that migrates to RLQ with noted rebound tenderness, anorexia, nausea, vomiting, fever	Leukocytosis with neutrophils >70%, elevated levels of CRP, SAA, ProCT [41]	Peak incidence occurs at age 10–19 years [42], Alvarado Score >7 meets criteria for surgical appendectomy; CT abdomen: enlarged appendix diameter >6 mm, appendiceal wall >2 mm thick, inflammatory compression of adjoining adipose tissue, RLQ abscess formation, calcified appendicolith [43]
Small bowel obstruction (SBO)	Diffuse abdominal pain, colicky with waxing/waning characteristic, nausea, vomiting, abdominal distention and tenderness, hyperactive or hypoactive bowel sounds, feculent emesis; Peritonitis should be suspected when rigidity, rebound tenderness, or guarding presents [44]	Leukocytosis, hemoconcentration, electrolyte imbalance	Most common in adults with history of abdominal surgery raising suspicion for peritoneal adhesions (75% cases); the second most common cause is hernias; Plain film of abdomen displays air-fluid levels, small bowel distention and paucity of air in rectal vault [44]; Passage of stool and flatus do not rule out SBO [44]; CT abdomen with contrast is diagnostic method of choice
Pancreatitis	Acute onset of abdominal pain, located in epigastrium with radiation to back, nausea and vomiting, low grade fever, tachypnea, epigastric tenderness to palpation	Leukocytosis, hemoconcentration with elevated hematocrit, elevated serum amylase and lipase	Most common occurrence in childhood between ages of 15 and 19 years; History of gallstones or alcohol abuse; CT abdomen with IV contrast is recommended when suspecting pancreatic necrosis, worsening response to therapy, or questionable diagnosis [44]
Inflammatory bowel disease-ulcerative colitis (UC) and Crohn's disease (CD)	UC: bloody diarrhea, with symptoms of urgency and tenesmus [45]; CD: chronic or nocturnal abdominal pain, diarrhea; Weight loss, fever; rectal bleeding may or may not be present; extraintestinal manifestations including inflammation of eyes, skin, or joints [46]	Elevated acute phase reactants CRP, ESR; UC: p-ANCA positive; CD: ASCA positive, p-ANCA negative	Both: most frequently diagnosed in the second decade of life. Stool examination to rule out infectious etiology; UC: disease limited to colon. Sigmoidoscopy or colonoscopy: loss of vascular pattern, friability and ulceration; Biopsy: crypt atrophy, increase presence of lymphocytes and plasma cells at crypt bases [45]; CD: primarily involving distal ileum, though any part of alimentary tract may be involved in a transmural inflammatory pattern; Endoscopy: deep serpiginous ulcers and "cobblestone" appearance; Biopsy: granulomas noted on specimen [47]
Intussusception	Abdominal pain, nausea, vomiting, diarrhea, hematochezia [48]	Similar to bowel obstruction: leukocytosis, hemoconcentration, electrolyte imbalance	Peak age at presentation is 4–8 months; History of tumor or prior abdominal surgery [49]; CT abdomen: "target sign" indicative of intussusception [49]
Celiac disease	Abdominal discomfort, weight loss, diarrhea, increased flatus	Iron and folate deficiency, steatorrhea, hypoalbuminemia, hypocalcemia, elevated serum transaminases	May manifest as early as childhood after introduction of gluten in diet; Positive serologic testing serum IgA anti-tissue transglutaminase and IgA anti-endomysial antibody have sensitivities of 80–95% and specificities of 95–99%. Mucosal intestinal biopsy showing blunted villi, hyperplastic crypts with increased number of mitotic figures [50]

HAE: Hereditary Angioedema, LLQ: left lower quadrant, RLQ: right lower quadrant, CRP: C-reactive protein, ESR: Erythrocyte Sedimentation Rate, SAA: Serum Amyloid A, ProCT: serum procalcitonin, p-ANCA: perinuclear antineutrophil cytoplasmic antibodies, and ASCA: anti-Saccharomyces cerevisiae.

levels of efficacy [25, 26]. The patient should have intravenous IV access placed immediately to administer IV hydration to counter the hypotension a patient may develop secondary to fluid shifts and to administer medications [14]. There are 3 medications that are currently approved for treatment in acute attacks in HAE that include a plasma-derived C1 INH for intravenous administration and bradykinin antagonist and inhibitors icatibant and ecallantide via subcutaneous administration [14, 25, 26]. All these first line options have shown themselves to be safe and effective in acute attacks. It is recommended that all patients with HAE should have access to these on-demand therapeutic agents, which the patient may self-administer, as early treatment has been shown to be advantageous [26]. Plasma-derived C1 INH replacement protein marketed as Berinert is made from pooled human blood and works by replacing the deficient protein thereby inhibiting angioedema pathways. The adverse side effects that have been reported include nausea, vomiting, abdominal pain, muscle spasms, diarrhea, headache, and rash [14]. Some thrombotic events have been noted in premature neonates at extremely high doses; however, this has occurred in off-label use [26].

Icatibant marketed as Firazyr is a bradykinin receptor antagonist that has been approved for on-demand use by the FDA in acute attacks. Bradykinin can cause angioedema by activation of B2 bradykinin receptors. This pathway is blocked by icatibant because the medication competitively binds to these B2 receptors. Efficacy studies have shown that when compared to placebo and tranexamic acid significantly more patients had symptom relief at the 4-hour follow-up period with icatibant [27]. Comparing the icatibant treatment group to placebo, initial symptom relief occurred at 0.8 hours compared to 3.5 hours, and complete symptom relief occurred at 8 hours compared to 36 hours. None of the patients treated with icatibant required any additional rescue medications before symptom resolution [28]. It is recommended in patients 18 years or older. Side effects reported include transient local injection site irritation, but no allergic reactions have been reported [26]. Another option is treatment with a kallikrein inhibitor such as ecallantide, marketed as Kalbitor. By inhibiting kallikrein activity, the cleavage of kininogen to bradykinin is inhibited therefore impeding edema progression [26]. It has been approved by the FDA for on-demand treatment in patients 16 and above for all types of HAE attacks [14, 26]. Some patients may develop nonneutralizing antibodies to the drug after repeated uses, leading to anaphylactoid-type reactions in 2-3% of the patients. This is why the FDA recommends that a trained healthcare provider administer the medication, preferably in a facility with the ability to manage anaphylaxis [25]. Another agent approved for the treatment of acute attacks of HAE is conestat alfa (branded as Ruconest), a human recombinant C1 esterase inhibitor purified from the milk of transgenic (genetically modified) rabbits. It is intended to restore the level of functional C1 esterase inhibitor in the plasma, which will subsequently treat the acute attack of swelling. In comparison to the plasma-derived C1 INH, it demonstrated comparable time to first improvement and to resolution of symptoms, making it a reasonable alternative [29].

Epinephrine, antihistamines, and corticosteroids have been proven to be ineffective and are not recommended as part of the HAE treatment regimen. This is because the swelling caused in HAE is due to bradykinin, and the medications mentioned above do not antagonize the generation of effects of bradykinin. Prior to the research and development of the present approved interventions, fresh frozen plasma FFP had been used to abate acute HAE attacks because it contains high circulating levels of C1 INH protein, but it also contains prekallikrein, kininogen, and coagulation factor XII which may lead to worsening of attacks in some patients. Caution is advised if this treatment option is considered [25].

Novel to our case is the fact that after being treated with Cinryze the patient's intussusception resolved completely, as confirmed by CT scan. This management strategy prevented further invasive interventions, including air-contrast enema. There are only a few reports of intussusception in the literature regarding HAE patients, all of which relied on surgical management as the ultimate treatment of this complication, given the lack of evidence on alternative management, along with the pressing factor of worsening complications if surgery is delayed [15].

A necessary part of the treatment regimen is to prevent future attacks. One method can be achieved through an individualized patient action plan. The action plan can be established between the patient and a healthcare professional in order to educate patients on recognizing an attack, recognizing triggers, learning how to self-administer treatment, and planning routes to facilitate access to healthcare. Patients should be advised to carry an identification card to assist healthcare professionals in delivering care [26]. Patients may need short- to long-term prophylaxis if an invasive procedure or stress event is expected. Prophylaxis in the short term can be achieved with C1 INH replacement and short-term therapy with high dose 17 alpha-alkylated androgens with FFP and plasma reserved for those cases where approved medications are not immediately available [14, 25]. The need for long-term prophylaxis must be individualized based on the patient's frequency and severity of attacks. Low to moderate doses of androgens have been effective in long-term prophylaxis because androgens increase the serum levels of C1 INH and reduce the likelihood of attacks [30]. Antifibrinolytics, such as tranexamic acid and epsilon aminocaproic acid, have also been shown to provide long-term prophylaxis but are less effective than androgens [3, 25]. The use of antifibrinolytics is reported to have higher adverse effect profiles such as coagulation defects with increased bleeding and hypercoagulable conditions, so cautious use is recommended when using these agents [3]. Plasma-derived C1 INH has been effective for long-term prophylaxis because of its long plasma half-life. Reductions in frequency, severity, and duration of attacks have been described in double blind placebo controlled studies with Cinryze, a C1 INH concentrate [31]. It has been FDA-approved for adolescent and adult prophylaxis [25].

The prognosis for patients with HAE before current treatment modalities reached as high as 25–50% in some families with the cause of death almost always secondary to laryngeal edema and fatal asphyxiation [32]. A recent study found that mortality was 29% in patients with undiagnosed HAE compared to 3% in patients with a known diagnosis of HAE [33]. This stresses the importance of early diagnosis and that patient education and access to treatment can greatly reduce mortality.

4. Conclusion

Gastrointestinal symptoms are a common feature of HAE attacks and can present in a wide array of clinical manifestations. Symptoms can be nonspecific and may overlap with other abdominal conditions leading to delay in diagnosis and treatment. Physicians should consider HAE as a differential diagnosis when presented with a cause of unexplained abdominal pain. A combination of an individualized action plan, pharmacologic therapy, and prophylactic measures can help prevent years of patient distress and unnecessary surgeries and decrease mortality.

Conflict of Interests

The authors declare that they have no conflict of interests.

References

[1] M. M. Gompels, R. J. Lock, M. Abinun et al., "C1 inhibitor deficiency: consensus document," *Clinical and Experimental Immunology*, vol. 139, no. 3, pp. 379–394, 2005.

[2] Y.-T. Huang, Y.-Z. Lin, H.-L. Wu et al., "Hereditary angioedema: a family study," *Asian Pacific Journal of Allergy and Immunology*, vol. 23, no. 4, pp. 227–233, 2005.

[3] T. Bowen, M. Cicardi, H. Farkas et al., "2010 international consensus algorithm for the diagnosis, therapy and management of hereditary angioedema," *Allergy, Asthma & Clinical Immunology*, vol. 6, no. 1, article 24, 2010.

[4] O. Roche, A. Blanch, T. Caballero, N. Sastre, D. Callejo, and M. López-Trascasa, "Hereditary angioedema due to C1 inhibitor deficiency: patient registry and approach to the prevalence in Spain," *Annals of Allergy, Asthma and Immunology*, vol. 94, no. 4, pp. 498–503, 2005.

[5] K. Bork, J. Frank, B. Grundt, P. Schlattmann, J. Nussberger, and W. Kreuz, "Treatment of acute edema attacks in hereditary angioedema with a bradykinin receptor-2 antagonist (Icatibant)," *Journal of Allergy and Clinical Immunology*, vol. 119, no. 6, pp. 1497–1503, 2007.

[6] M. Cicardi and A. Agostoni, "Hereditary angioedema," *The New England Journal of Medicine*, vol. 334, no. 25, pp. 1666–1667, 1996.

[7] A. Reshef, M. J. Prematta, and T. J. Craig, "Signs and symptoms preceding acute attacks of hereditary angioedema: results of three recent surveys," *Allergy and Asthma Proceedings*, vol. 34, no. 3, pp. 261–266, 2013.

[8] M. J. Prematta, A. K. Bewtra, R. J. Levy et al., "Per-attack reporting of prodromal symptoms concurrent with C1-inhibitor treatment of hereditary angioedema attacks," *Advances in Therapy*, vol. 29, no. 10, pp. 913–922, 2012.

[9] D. Yucelten and S. Kus, "Chicken-wire erythema, but not urticaria, as the presenting sign of hereditary angioedema," *European Journal of Dermatology*, vol. 16, no. 2, pp. 197–198, 2006.

[10] K. Bork, G. Meng, P. Staubach, and J. Hardt, "Hereditary angioedema: new findings concerning symptoms, affected organs, and course," *The American Journal of Medicine*, vol. 119, no. 3, pp. 267–274, 2006.

[11] U. C. Nzeako, E. Frigas, and W. J. Tremaine, "Hereditary angioedema: a broad review for clinicians," *Archives of Internal Medicine*, vol. 161, no. 20, pp. 2417–2429, 2001.

[12] U. C. Nzeako and H. J. Longhurst, "Many faces of angioedema: focus on the diagnosis and management of abdominal manifestations of hereditary angioedema," *European Journal of Gastroenterology and Hepatology*, vol. 24, no. 4, pp. 353–361, 2012.

[13] J. S. Koruth, A. J. Eckardt, and J. M. Levey, "Hereditary angioedema involving the colon: endoscopic appearance and review of GI manifestations," *Gastrointestinal Endoscopy*, vol. 61, no. 7, pp. 907–911, 2005.

[14] S. Jalaj and J. S. Scolapio, "Gastrointestinal manifestations, diagnosis, and management of hereditary angioedema," *Journal of Clinical Gastroenterology*, vol. 47, no. 10, pp. 817–823, 2013.

[15] K. Bork, P. Staubach, A. J. Eckardt, and J. Hardt, "Symptoms, course, and complications of abdominal attacks in hereditary angioedema due to C1 inhibitor deficiency," *American Journal of Gastroenterology*, vol. 101, no. 3, pp. 619–627, 2006.

[16] A. Zanichelli, M. Magerl, H. Longhurst, V. Fabien, and M. Maurer, "Hereditary angioedema with C1 inhibitor deficiency: delay in diagnosis in Europe," *Allergy, Asthma and Clinical Immunology*, vol. 9, no. 1, article 29, 2013.

[17] A. Agostoni and M. Cicardi, "Hereditary and acquired C1-inhibitor deficiency: biological and clinical characteristics in 235 patients," *Medicine*, vol. 71, no. 4, pp. 206–215, 1992.

[18] M. M. Gompels, R. J. Lock, J. E. Morgan, J. Osborne, A. Brown, and P. F. Virgo, "A multicentre evaluation of the diagnostic efficiency of serological investigations for C1 inhibitor deficiency," *Journal of Clinical Pathology*, vol. 55, no. 2, pp. 145–147, 2002.

[19] Y. Karim, H. Griffiths, and S. Deacock, "Normal complement C4 values do not exclude hereditary angioedema," *Journal of Clinical Pathology*, vol. 57, no. 2, pp. 213–214, 2004.

[20] I. Ohsawa, S. Nagamachi, H. Suzuki et al., "Leukocytosis and high hematocrit levels during abdominal attacks of hereditary angioedema," *BMC Gastroenterology*, vol. 13, article 123, 2013.

[21] N. Cohen, A. Sharon, A. Golik, R. Zaidenstein, and D. Modai, "Hereditary angioneurotic edema with severe hypovolemic shock," *Journal of Clinical Gastroenterology*, vol. 16, no. 3, pp. 237–239, 1993.

[22] Z. L. M. Hofman, A. Relan, and C. E. Hack, "C-reactive protein levels in hereditary angioedema," *Clinical & Experimental Immunology*, vol. 177, no. 1, pp. 280–286, 2014.

[23] A. I. de Backer, A. M. de Schepper, J. E. Vandevenne, P. Schoeters, P. Michielsen, and W. J. Stevens, "CT of angioedema of the small bowel," *American Journal of Roentgenology*, vol. 176, no. 3, pp. 649–652, 2001.

[24] M. Wakisaka, M. Shuto, H. Abe et al., "Computed tomography of the gastrointestinal manifestation of hereditary angioedema," *Radiation Medicine*, vol. 26, no. 10, pp. 618–621, 2008.

[25] B. L. Zuraw, J. A. Bernstein, D. M. Lang et al., "A focused parameter update: hereditary angioedema, acquired C1 inhibitor deficiency, and angiotensin-converting enzyme inhibitor-associated angioedema," *Journal of Allergy and Clinical Immunology*, vol. 131, no. 6, pp. 1491–1493, 2013.

[26] T. Craig, E. A. Pürsün, K. Bork et al., "WAO guideline for the management of hereditary angioedema," *World Allergy Organization Journal*, vol. 5, no. 12, pp. 182–199, 2012.

[27] M. Riedl, "Icatibant, a selective bradykinin B_2 receptor antagonist, proves effective and safe in treating the symptoms of hereditary angioedema (HAE) attacks," *The Journal of Allergy and Clinical Immunology*, vol. 121, no. 2, supplement 1, p. S103, 2008.

[28] W. R. Lumry, H. H. Li, R. J. Levy et al., "Randomized placebo-controlled trial of the bradykinin B2 receptor antagonist icatibant for the treatment of acute attacks of hereditary angioedema: the FAST-3 trial," *Annals of Allergy, Asthma and Immunology*, vol. 107, no. 6, pp. 529–537, 2011.

[29] A. L. Manson, J. Dempster, S. Grigoriadou, M. S. Buckland, and H. J. Longhurst, "Use of recombinant C1 inhibitor in patients with resistant or frequent attacks of hereditary or acquired angioedema," *European Journal of Dermatology*, vol. 24, no. 1, pp. 28–34, 2014.

[30] M. A. Riedl, "Critical appraisal of androgen use in hereditary angioedema. a systematic review," *Annals of Allergy, Asthma and Immunology*, vol. 114, no. 4, pp. 281.e7–288.e7, 2014.

[31] B. L. Zuraw, P. J. Busse, M. White et al., "Nanofiltered C1 inhibitor concentrate for treatment of hereditary angioedema," *The New England Journal of Medicine*, vol. 363, no. 6, pp. 513–522, 2010.

[32] K. Bork, "Recurrent angioedema and the threat of asphyxiation," *Deutsches Arzteblatt*, vol. 107, no. 23, pp. 408–414, 2010.

[33] K. Bork, J. Hardt, and G. Witzke, "Fatal laryngeal attacks and mortality in hereditary angioedema due to C1-INH deficiency," *Journal of Allergy and Clinical Immunology*, vol. 130, no. 3, pp. 692–697, 2012.

[34] M. M. Frank, "Hereditary angioedema: the clinical syndrome and its management in the United States," *Immunology and Allergy Clinics of North America*, vol. 26, no. 4, pp. 653–668, 2006.

[35] H. Farkas, G. Harmat, P. N. Kaposi et al., "Ultrasonography in the diagnosis and monitoring of ascites in acute abdominal attacks of hereditary angioneurotic oedema," *European Journal of Gastroenterology and Hepatology*, vol. 13, no. 10, pp. 1225–1230, 2001.

[36] A. S. Grumach, S. O. R. Valle, E. Toledo et al., "Hereditary angioedema: first report of the Brazilian registry and challenges," *Journal of the European Academy of Dermatology and Venereology*, vol. 27, no. 3, pp. e338–e344, 2013.

[37] D. M. García, A. C. Torres, A. R. Serrato, and M. Á. G. Ordóñez, "Acute pancreatitis associated with hereditary angioedema," *Gastroenterologia y Hepatologia*, vol. 33, no. 9, pp. 633–637, 2010.

[38] A. Witschi, L. Krähenbühl, E. Frei, J. Saltzman, P. J. Späth, and U. R. Müller, "Colorectal intussusception: an unusual gastrointestinal complication of hereditary angioedema," *International Archives of Allergy and Immunology*, vol. 111, no. 1, pp. 96–98, 1996.

[39] E. W. Nielsen, J. T. Gran, B. Straume, O. J. Mellbye, H. T. Johansen, and T. E. Mollnes, "Hereditary angio-oedema: new clinical observations and autoimmune screening, complement and kallikrein-kinin analyses," *Journal of Internal Medicine*, vol. 239, no. 2, pp. 119–130, 1996.

[40] A. C. Travis and R. S. Blumberg, "Diverticular disease of the colon," in *CURRENT Diagnosis & Treatment: Gastroenterology, Hepatology, & Endoscopy*, N. J. Greenberger, R. S. Blumberg, and R. Burakoff, Eds., chapter 21, McGraw-Hill, New York, NY, USA, 2nd edition, 2012, http://accessmedicine.mhmedical.com/content.aspx?bookid=390&Sectionid=39819254.

[41] M. H. Abbas, M. N. Choudhry, N. Hamza, B. Ali, A. A. Amin, and B. J. Ammori, "Admission levels of serum amyloid a and procalcitonin are more predictive of the diagnosis of acute appendicitis compared with C-reactive protein," *Surgical Laparoscopy, Endoscopy and Percutaneous Techniques*, vol. 24, no. 6, pp. 488–494, 2014.

[42] S. Ozkan, A. Duman, P. Durukan, A. Yildirim, and O. Ozbakan, "The accuracy rate of Alvarado score, ultrasonography, and computerized tomography scan in the diagnosis of acute appendicitis in our center," *Nigerian Journal of Clinical Practice*, vol. 17, no. 4, pp. 413–418, 2014.

[43] M. Karul, C. Berliner, S. Keller, T. Y. Tsui, and J. Yamamura, "Imaging of appendicitis in adults," *RöFo: Fortschritte auf dem Gebiete der Röntgenstrahlen und der Nuklearmedizin*, vol. 186, no. 6, pp. 551–558, 2014.

[44] M. H. Flasar and E. Goldberg, "Acute abdominal pain," *Medical Clinics of North America*, vol. 90, no. 3, pp. 481–503, 2006.

[45] A. Kornbluth and D. B. Sachar, "Ulcerative colitis practice guidelines in adults: American college of gastroenterology, practice parameters committee," *American Journal of Gastroenterology*, vol. 105, no. 3, pp. 501–523, 2010.

[46] G. R. Lichtenstein, S. B. Hanauer, and W. J. Sandborn, "Management of Crohn's disease in adults," *The American Journal of Gastroenterology*, vol. 104, no. 2, pp. 464–484, 2009.

[47] K. M. B. Dunn and D. A. Rothenberger, "Colon, rectum, and anus," in *Schwartz's Principles of Surgery*, chapter 29, McGraw-Hill, 2009.

[48] H. Honjo, M. Mike, H. Kusanagi, and N. Kano, "Adult intussusception: a retrospective review," *World Journal of Surgery*, vol. 39, no. 1, pp. 134–138, 2015.

[49] A. Tavakkoli, S. W. Ashley, M. J. Zinner et al., "Small intestine," in *Schwartz's Principles of Surgery, 10e*, F. Brunicardi, D. K. Andersen, T. R. Billiar, and etal, Eds., McGraw-Hill, New York, NY, USA, 2014, http://accessmedicine.mhmedical.com/content.aspx?bookid=980&Sectionid=59610870.

[50] J. S. Trier, "Intestinal malabsorption," in *CURRENT Diagnosis & Treatment: Gastroenterology, Hepatology, & Endoscopy*, N. J. Greenberger, R. S. Blumberg, and R. Burakoff, Eds., chapter 20, McGraw-Hill, New York, NY, USA, 2nd edition, 2012, http://accessmedicine.mhmedical.com/content.aspx?bookid=390&Sectionid=39819252.

30

A Girl with Autoimmune Cytopenias, Nonmalignant Lymphadenopathy, and Recurrent Infections

Marjolein A. C. Mattheij,[1,2] **Ellen J. H. Schatorjé,**[1,3] **Eugenie F. A. Gemen,**[4]
Lisette van de Corput,[5] **Peet T. G. A. Nooijen,**[6] **Mirjam van der Burg,**[7] **and Esther de Vries**[1]

[1] Department of Pediatrics, Jeroen Bosch Hospital, P.O. Box 90153, 5200 ME 's-Hertogenbosch, The Netherlands
[2] University Medical Centre Antwerp, Antwerp, Belgium
[3] Radboud University Medical Centre Nijmegen, Nijmegen, The Netherlands
[4] Laboratory for Clinical Chemistry and Hematology, Jeroen Bosch Hospital, P.O. Box 90153,
   5200 ME 's-Hertogenbosch, The Netherlands
[5] Department of Medical Immunology, University Medical Center Utrecht, P.O. Box 85500, Utrecht, The Netherlands
[6] Department of Pathology, Jeroen Bosch Hospital, P.O. Box 90153, 5200 ME 's-Hertogenbosch, The Netherlands
[7] Department of Immunology, Erasmus Medical Center, P.O. Box 2040, 3000 CA Rotterdam, The Netherlands

Correspondence should be addressed to Esther de Vries, e.d.vries@jbz.nl

Academic Editors: V. Lougaris and A. Plebani

We describe a girl, now 9 years of age, with chronic idiopathic thrombocytopenic purpura, persistent nonmalignant lymphade-nopathy, splenomegaly, recurrent infections, and autoimmune hemolytic anemia. Her symptoms partly fit the definitions of both autoimmune lymphoproliferative syndrome (ALPS) and common variable immunodeficiency disorders (CVIDs). Genetic analysis showed no abnormalities in the ALPS-genes FAS, FASLG, and CASP10. The CVID-associated TACI gene showed a homozygous polymorphism (Pro251Leu), which is found also in healthy controls.

1. Introduction

Acute idiopathic thrombocytopenic purpura (ITP) is a well-known clinical entity in children. Generally, in children the disease is self-limiting and easily distinguished from a hematological malignancy, even without investigating the bone marrow [1]. However, the case becomes more complicated when the ITP becomes chronic and accom-panying profound lymphadenopathy develops. We describe the diagnostic dilemma in a girl with these problems, who with time also developed recurrent respiratory infections, suffered from a prolonged episode of intractable diarrhea, a severe episode of varicella zoster infection and autoimmune hemolytic anemia.

2. Patient

The girl, now 9 years of age, is the second child of healthy nonconsanguineous Caucasian parents. She was born after an uncomplicated pregnancy and delivery and showed normal growth and development. Her family history reveals allergy on the paternal side and autoimmune disease and malignancies on the maternal side. At the age of 14 months, she developed ITP and showed a partial slow recovery after 3 days of high-dose intravenous immunoglobulins (IVIGs) fol-lowed by prednisolone. One year later, she suffered a relapse during a mild parainfluenza type 3 infection and treatment with 3 days of high-dose IVIG was started again. A few days after receiving this second course of high-dose IVIG she developed cervical, axillary and inguinal lymphadenopathy and enlarged tonsils: this lymphadenopathy never resolved. There was no hepatomegaly, splenomegaly, or mediastinal or abdominal lymph node enlargement at that time. Blood tests showed a mild normocytic anemia (Hb 6.4 mmol/L, MCV 77 fL) and granulocytopenia ($0.7–1.0 \times 10^9$/L) and large unstained cells in the hematology analyzer (8%; 0.4×10^9/L). A bone marrow aspirate and biopsy showed some atypical lymphocytes and specific maturational disturbances, but no malignancy. Bone marrow immunophenotyping was normal. FAS-mediated apoptosis of T-lymphoblasts was normal (two separate tests in two different laboratories). She suffered from recurrent upper respiratory tract infections and two pneumonias in the following years and a prolonged episode of intractable diarrhea. The infection frequency improved on cotrimoxazole prophylaxis. The enlarged tonsils, cervical, axillary and inguinal lymphadenopathy and variable amounts of atypical lymphocytes in her differential remained, splenomegaly developed as well. The parents increasingly felt that she got tired more easily than other children of her age. At the age of 5 years, an adenoidectomy was performed; this procedure was combined with an excision of an inguinal lymph node for histological examination. At the age of 7 years, an episode of severe varicella zoster infection occurred which was treated successfully with 1 week of intravenous aciclovir. Five months later, she acutely developed autoimmune hemolytic anemia, which initially responded well to another course of high-dose IVIG and prednisone, but she relapsed when the prednisone was slowly tapered and stopped. Unexpectedly, her chronic thrombocytopenia improved upon this treatment. At the age of 8 years, she developed pulmonary problems with dyspnea after an (probably viral) airway infection; high resolution CT scan showed a granulomatous lymphocytic interstitial lung disease (GLILD), a form of pulmonary lymphoproliferative disease. Therapy with mycophenolic acid was started, after which she showed a slow but nearly complete pulmonary recovery; she is still slightly dyspneic upon exertion. She also developed a uveitis, which was treated with prednisolone eye drops. Now, at the age of 9 years, she is relatively stable on mycophenolic acid; stem cell transplantation is being considered.

3. Material and Methods

Upon her first presentation at the pediatric immunology clinic in 's-Hertogenbosch at 5 years of age, extensive investigations were performed (Table 1). Four-color immunophenotyping was performed as previously described [2, 3]. One representative paraffin-embedded tissue block of both lymph node (18 mm) and adenoid (20 mm) was selected and immunohistochemical stainings were performed (Table 2). Routine protocols for Benchmark XT Ventana were used. Kappa, lambda, and EBV were assessed using routine in situ hybridisation technique (Kappa, ISH, Ventana; lambda, ISH, Ventana; EBER). Genomic DNA was isolated from peripheral blood granulocytes using the autopure kit (Qiagen, Venlo, the Netherlands). Exon-specific M13-tagged primers were used for amplification by PCR of all coding exons including flanking regions from the genes FAS (NCBI NM_00043), FASLG (NCBI NM_000639), CASP10 (NCBI NM_032974) and TACI (TNFRSF13B, NCBI NM_012452) followed by fluorescent sequencing (Applied Biosystems BigDye Terminator v1.1 Applied Biosystems).

4. Results

Table 1 shows the lymphocyte subpopulations in comparison with age-matched reference values from our laboratory [2].

T-lymphocytes were slightly low to just normal, naive helper-T-lymphocytes and recent thymic emigrants were clearly decreased; double-negative TCR$\alpha\beta^+$ T-lymphocytes (cells without expression of CD4 or CD8 coreceptors) were normal to just increased in subsequent experiments, performed during episodes without immunosuppressive treatment.

Histological examination of lymphoid tissue revealed retention of the architectural features with a combined mild follicular hyperplasia and mild paracortical T zone expansion. In one lymph node a single granuloma was observed without necrosis or eosinophilia. Ziehl-Neelsen and other stainings for microorganisms were negative. The CD20 and CD79 positive B-cells were restricted to the normal B-cell areas. The follicular centres were highlighted by CD21 and CD23 B-cells, which stained the follicular dendritic cell meshwork. T-lymphocytes (CD2$^+$, CD3$^+$) showed mild expansion in the paracortical T zone. BCL2 was negative and the proliferation in MIB1 was mainly restricted to the centrocytes and centroblasts in the reactive follicular centres. Kappa and lambda revealed a polyclonal plasma cell population. ALK staining was negative, there was no pathological CD30 staining. There were no signs of Rosai Dorfman; EBV was negative. Thus, histological examination showed abnormalities, but did not point to a specific diagnosis.

Analysis of the FAS, FASLG, and CASP10 genes revealed no abnormalities. Direct fluorescent sequencing of the TACI gene showed two polymorphisms, a homozygote polymorphism (p.Pro251Leu), and a heterozygote silent polymorphism.

5. Discussion

The girl we describe poses a diagnostic dilemma: there are several clinical entities that can be considered. Firstly, she undoubtedly fits the diagnosis of "Evans syndrome"—which is defined by the presence of at least two autoimmune cytopenias—since she suffers from chronic idiopathic thrombocytopenic purpura and autoimmune hemolytic anemia [4]. However, this is only a descriptive diagnosis that does not encompass all her features. "Evans syndrome" is increasingly being associated with specific diseases, such as autoimmune lymphoproliferative syndrome (ALPS) and common variable immunodeficiency (CVID) and, mainly in adults, lymphoproliferative disorders [4–8].

Since she also suffers from persistent nonmalignant lymphadenopathy and splenomegaly, ALPS is an option for this girl. ALPS is a disorder of lymphocyte apoptosis leading to chronic nonmalignant lymphoproliferation. Affected individuals often suffer from autoimmune cytopenia, splenomegaly and hepatomegaly [9]. Laboratory findings include hypergammaglobulinemia and expansion of a unique population of circulating T-lymphocytes, referred to as TCR$\alpha\beta^+$ double negative T-cells which owe their name to the fact that they do not express CD4 or CD8 coreceptors [10]. These T-cells respond poorly to antigens. The genetic deficit in most patients is a mutation in the FAS gene which encodes a cell surface receptor which, upon stimulation, induces programmed cell death [11]. The diagnostic criteria for ALPS have recently been revised. The two required

TABLE 1: Investigations in peripheral blood.

General investigations	Results	Interpretation
Hemoglobin	7.5–7.9 mmol/L	Low to normal
Neutrophils	$1.3–5.3 \times 10^9$/L	Intermittently low
Lymphocytes	$1.6–3.2 \times 10^9$/L	Low
ACE	73 U/mL	Mildly elevated
ANCA	Negative	Normal
ANA	Negative	Normal
TPO-antibodies	Negative	Normal
Thyreoglobulin antibodies	Negative	Normal
Serology rubella	IgG pos, IgM neg	Normal after vaccination
Serology CMV	IgG and IgM neg	No exposure
Serology EBV	IgG and IgM neg	No exposure
Serology HIV	Negative	No exposure
Serology parvovirus	IgG and IgM neg	No exposure
Serology bartonella henselae	IgM negative	No recent exposure
Serology toxoplasma gondii	IgG and IgM neg	No exposure
PCR blood CMV	Negative	No recent exposure
PCR blood EBV	Negative	No recent exposure
Antibody response to diphtheria and tetanus toxoid antigens	>4-fold increase in titer	Normal
Antibody response to pneumococcal polysaccharides	2-fold increase in titer	Weak response
Mantoux	Negative	Normal
M-proteins	Negative	Normal
IgM (age 7 years)	1.03 g/L	Normal
IgA (age 7 years)	0.19 g/L	Low
IgG (age 7 years)	13.4 g/L	Mildly elevated
IgG1 (age 7 years)	11.6 g/L	Mildly elevated
IgG2 (age 7 years)	0.92 g/L	Normal
IgG3 (age 7 years)	1.55 g/L	Mildly elevated
IgG4 (age 7 years)	0.058	Normal
Blood lymphocyte subpopulations	**Absolute count***	**Age-matched reference****
Leucocytes	4.6	9.3 (4.5–14)
Lymphocytes	1.94	2.4 (1.2–4.7)
T-lymphocytes (T) (CD3$^+$)	1.01	1.80 (0.77–4.0)
Double negative TCR$\alpha\beta^+$ T (CD3$^+$TCR$\alpha\beta^+$CD4$^-$CD8$^-$)	0.08	0.03 (0.01–0.1)
Helper-T-lymphocytes (Th) (CD3$^+$CD4$^+$)	0.58	0.91 (0.36–2.80)
Th naive (CD3$^+$CD4$^+$CD45RA$^+$CD27$^+$)	**0.11**	0.70 (0.20–2.50)
Th terminally differentiated (CD3$^+$CD4$^+$CD45RA$^+$CD27$^-$)	0	0.00 (0.00–0.03)
Th central memory (CD3$^+$CD4$^+$CD45RA$^-$CD27$^+$)	0.45	0.18 (0.00–0.51)
Th effector memory (CD3$^+$CD4$^+$CD45RA$^-$CD27$^-$)	0.02	0.02 (0.00–0.17)
Cytotoxic T-lymphocytes (Tc) (CD3$^+$CD8$^+$)	**0.19**	0.60 (0.20–1.70)
Tc naive (CD8$^+$CD45RA$^+$CD197$^+$CD27$^+$)	0.09	0.24 (0.04–1.30)
Tc terminally differentiated (CD8$^+$CD45RA$^+$CD197$^-$CD27$^-$)	**0**	0.14 (0.06–0.34)
Tc central memory (CD8$^+$CD45RA$^-$CD197$^+$CD27$^+$)	0.08	0.02 (0.01–0.04)
Tc effector memory (CD8$^+$CD45RA$^-$CD197$^-$CD27$^-$)	0.2	0.14 (0.05–0.41)
Recent thymic emigrants (CD3$^+$CD4$^+$CD45RA$^+$CD31$^+$)	**0.1**	0.59 (0.20–1.70)
Regulatory T (CD3$^+$CD4$^+$CD25^{++}CD127$^-$)	**0**	0.07 (0.02–0.27)
B-lymphocytes (B) (CD19$^+$)	0.45	0.29 (0.10–0.80)
Naive B (CD19$^+$CD27$^-$IgM$^+$IgD$^+$)	0.37	0.21 (0.07–0.63)
Natural effector B (CD19$^+$CD27$^+$IgM$^+$IgD$^+$)	0.06	0.03 (0.01–0.09)
Switched memory B (CD19$^+$CD27$^+$IgM$^-$IgD$^-$)	0.01	0.02 (0.01–0.05)
Transitional B (CD19$^+$CD38^{++}IgM^{++})	0.01	0.03 (0.01–0.07)

TABLE 1: Continued.

Blood lymphocyte subpopulations	Absolute count*	Age-matched reference**
CD5$^+$ B (CD19$^+$CD5$^+$)	0.11	0.09 (0.02–0.46)
CD10$^+$ B (CD19$^+$CD10$^+$)	0.08	0.05 (0.01–0.21)
NK-cells (CD3$^-$/CD16 and/or 56$^+$ cells)	0.14	0.20 (0.07–0.59)
	Ratio	Age-matched reference**
TCR-$\alpha\beta$/TCR-$\gamma\delta$	**32.7**	9.4
Th/Tc	**3.1**	1.7
κ/λ	1.14	1.5
	Percentage	Reference
TACI$^+$ cells	10.6	2.6 (1–12.6)***
BAFF-R$^+$ cells	99.5	>95****

All investigations were performed at the age of 5 years, unless otherwise stated. ACE: angiotensin converting enzyme; ANCA: antineutrophil cytoplasmic antibody; ANA: antinuclear antibody; BAFF: B-cell activating factor; CMV: cytomegalovirus; EBV: epstein-barr virus; HIV: human immunodeficiency virus; Ig: immunoglobulin; neg: negative; NK: Natural Killer; R: receptor; pos: positive; SD: standard deviation; TACI: transmembrane activator and calcium-modulator and cyclophilin ligand interactor; Tc: T-cytotoxic; TCR: T-cell receptor; Th: T-helper; TPO-antibodies: thyroid peroxidase antibody. *$\times 10^9$/L, values in bold represent values that fall outside of the normal range. **Mean, 90% range. ***Mean; total range. ****Total range. For T-lymphocyte reference values see [3], for B-lymphocyte reference values see [2].

TABLE 2: Used antibodies.

Antibody	Source*
Determination of blood lymphocyte subpopulations	
CD3, CD4, CD5, CD8, CD10, CD14, CD16, CD19, CD20, CD21, CD24, CD25, CD27, CD31, CD38, CD45, CD45RA, CD45RO, CD56, CD127, CD197, CD268, TCR$\alpha\beta$, TCR$\gamma\delta$, cyIgG1	Becton Dickinson
CD185	Research and Diagnostics Systems
cyCD257	eBioscience
CD267 (biotin)	PeproTech
IgD, IgM, Kappa, Lambda	Dakopatts
Immunohistochemical investigations	
CD2 (AB75, 1:200), CD4 (1H6), CD8 (C8/144B, 1:50), CD23 (1B12), CD56 (123C3.D5), BCL2 (124)	Monosan
CD3 (polyclonal), CD5 (4C7), CD10 (56C6), CD15 (MMA), CD21 (2G9), CD30 (BER-H2), CD45 (RP2/18), CD79a (JCB117), ALK (ALK-01), Mib-1 (30-9)	Ventana
CD20 (L26,1:400)	Dakopatts

*Becton Dickinson Biosciences (California, CA, USA), Research and Diagnostics Systems (Minneapolis, MN, USA), eBioscience (San Diego, CA, USA), PeproTech (Rocky Hill, CT, USA), Dakopatts (Glostrup, Denmark), Monosan (Uden, The Netherlands), and Ventana (Tucson, AZ, USA).

criteria for the diagnosis of ALPS are (1) chronic (>6 months), nonmalignant, noninfectious, lymphadenopathy, or/and splenomegaly, (2) elevated CD3$^+$TCR$\alpha\beta^+$CD4$^-$CD8$^-$ double-negative T-cells [10]. There are also four secondary accessory criteria; for a *definite* ALPS diagnosis a patient has to meet both required criteria and one of the primary accessory criteria. The diagnosis of ALPS is *probable* when two required criteria and any one of the secondary accessory criteria is present [10]. According to these criteria, our patient does not have ALPS, since she does not have consistently elevated CD3$^+$TCR$\alpha\beta^+$CD4$^-$CD8$^-$ double-negative T-cells. There are several well-defined ALPS-related disorders. Of these, RALD (RAS-associated autoimmune lymphoprolipherative disease) could be an option, but our girl shows no characteristic features of this disorder such as elevations in cells of myeloid origin [10].

The girl's recurrent infections could point to possible CVID. This disease is characterized by recurrent infections and hypogammaglobulinemia. Additional clinical manifestations vary, but can include autoimmunity, splenomegaly and nonmalignant lymphoproliferation [9]. CVID is a heterogeneous group of disorders; the age of onset can be in childhood, adolescence, or even adult life. Most patients have no molecular diagnosis as yet; cases can be sporadic, or familial. There is a high incidence of hematological malignancies in CVID [12]. For a definite diagnosis, all of the following criteria need to be present: (1) onset of immunodeficiency at greater than 2–4 years of age, (2) absent isohemagglutinins and/or poor response to vaccines and (3) exclusion of defined causes of hypogammaglobulinemia. Criteria for the diagnosis of *probable* CVID are a marked decrease of IgG (at least 2 SD below the mean for age) and

TABLE 3: Signs of ALPS and CVID definitions in our patient.

ALPS[10]	
Required criteria:	
Chronic nonmalignant noninfectious lymphoproliferation	+
Elevated CD3+TCRαβ+CD4−CD8− double-negative T-cells	±
Accessory criteria:	
Primary:	
Pathogenic mutation in *FAS, FASLG,* or *CASP10* genes	−
Defective lymphocyte apoptosis (in 2 separate assays)	−
Secondary:	
Elevated soluble FASL or serum interleukin-10 or interleukin-18 or serum plasma vit B12 levels	#
Typical immunohistological findings	−
Autoimmune cytopenias and elevated IgG levels	+
Family history of nonmalignant noninfectious lymphoproliferation	−
CVID	
Hypogammaglobulinemia	±(IgA deficiency)
Specific antibody deficiency	±(antipolysaccharide response decreased)
Autoantibodies	−
Malignancy	−
Lymphadenopathy	+
Splenomegaly	+

+ Present in our patient; ± partly or not consistently present in our patient; − not present in our patient; # not tested. ALPS: Autoimmune lymphoproliferative syndrome; CVID: common variable immunodeficiency disorders.

a marked decrease in at least one of the isotypes IgM or IgA and for *possible* CVID a marked decrease (at least 2 SD below the mean for age) in one of the major isotypes (IgM, IgG, and IgA) [11]. Our patient, however, only suffers from IgA deficiency and shows reasonable responses to vaccines.

The girl, therefore, only partly fits ALPS as well as CVID definitions (Table 3) and the diagnosis remains obscure. Even extensive genetic analysis did not help in this case. The ALPS-genes *FAS, FASLG* and *CASP10* revealed no abnormalities; the CVID-associated *TACI*-gene showed one homozygous polymorphism (Pro251Leu). This homozygous polymorphism has been identified in 6 out of 912 healthy controls from Sweden, similar to what is seen in CVID or IgA-deficient patients (Personal communication U. Salzer, Centre of Chronic Immunodeficiency, University Medical Centre, Freiburg, Germany). Moreover, recent work showed that the terminal intracellular part of *TACI* including Pro251Leu is dispensable for *TACI* signaling, which also supports the view that the Pro251Leu variation is not harmful [13].

Now and then, pediatric hematologists and immunologists are confronted with a patient like this without a clear diagnosis where manifestations overlap between these two adjacent fields and the clinical course is different from what is usually seen. As also shown by this girl, not all cases of autoimmune thrombocytopenia in children are self-limiting, nor all persistent profound lymphadenopathies malignant. These "hematological" features can be the first manifestation of a primary immunodeficiency syndrome. Unfortunately, this girl also illustrates that despite recent successes in further classifying primary immunodeficiencies, there are still children with clinical and laboratory features which linger between several diagnostic entities. It is important to share the medical history of these children with other specialists in the field, so that combination of experience may enhance further classification of these diseases in the future.

Authors' Contribution

All the authors meet the following conditions: (1) substantial contributions to conception and design, acquisition of data, or analysis and interpretation of data; (2) drafting the paper or revising it critically for important intellectual content; (3) final approval of the version to be published. E. J. H. Schatorjé provided the information about age-matched reference values for the lymphocytes; E. F. A. Gemen provided the information about the material and methods for the lymphocyte subpopulations and interpretation of these data; L. van de Corput provided information about the material and methods for the *FAS, FASLG,* and *CASP10* mutations; P. T. G. A. Nooijen provided the information about the material and methods for the lymphoid tissue and the interpretation of these data; M. van der Burg provided the information about the material and methods for the genetic analysis and the interpretation of these data. M. A. C. Mattheij is the clinical researcher and E. de Vries is the overall supervisor of this paper.

Conflict of Interests

The authors declare that they have no conflict of interests.

References

[1] V. Blanchette and P. Bolton-Maggs, "Childhood immune thrombocytopenic purpura: diagnosis and management," *Hematology/Oncology Clinics of North America*, vol. 24, no. 1, pp. 249–273, 2010.

[2] E. J. H. Schatorjé, E. F. A. Gemen, G. A. Driessen et al., "Age matched reference values for B-lymphocyte subpopulations and CVID classifications in children," *Scandinavian Journal of Immunology*, vol. 74, no. 5, pp. 502–510, 2011.

[3] E. J. H. Schatorjé, E. F. A. Gemen, G. A. Driessen et al., "Paediatric reference values for peripheral T cell compartment," *Scandinavian Journal of Immunology*, vol. 75, no. 4, pp. 436–444, 2012.

[4] M. Michel, V. Chanet, A. Dechartres et al., "The spectrum of Evans syndrome in adults: new insight into the disease based on the analysis of 68 cases," *Blood*, vol. 114, no. 15, pp. 3167–3172, 2009.

[5] D. T. Teachey, "New advances in the diagnosis and treatment of autoimmune lymphoproliferative syndrome," *Current Opinion in Pediatrics*, vol. 24, no. 1, pp. 1–8, 2012.

[6] A. E. Seif, C. S. Manno, C. Sheen, S. A. Grupp, and D. T. Teachey, "Identifying autoimmune lymphoproliferative syndrome in children with Evans syndrome: a multi-institutional study," *Blood*, vol. 115, no. 11, pp. 2142–2145, 2010.

[7] A. Ramyar, A. Aghamohammadi, K. Moazzami et al., "Presence of idiopathic thrombocytopenic purpura and autoimmune hemolytic anemia in the patients with common variable immunodeficiency," *Iranian Journal of Allergy, Asthma and Immunology*, vol. 7, no. 3, pp. 169–175, 2008.

[8] D. T. Teachey, C. S. Manno, K. M. Axsom et al., "Unmasking Evans syndrome: T-cell phenotype and apoptotic response reveal autoimmune lymphoproliferative syndrome (ALPS)," *Blood*, vol. 105, no. 6, pp. 2443–2448, 2005.

[9] G. Bussone and L. Mouthon, "Autoimmune manifestations in primary immune deficiencies," *Autoimmunity Reviews*, vol. 8, no. 4, pp. 332–336, 2009.

[10] J. B. Oliveira, J. J. Bleesing, U. Dianzani et al., "Revised diagnostic criteria and classification for the autoimmune lymphoproliferative syndrome (ALPS): report from the 2009 NIH International Workshop," *Blood*, vol. 116, no. 14, pp. e35–e40, 2010.

[11] J. Mohammadi, C. Liu, A. Aghamohammadi et al., "Novel mutations in TACI (TNFRSF13B) causing common variable immunodeficiency," *Journal of Clinical Immunology*, vol. 29, no. 6, pp. 777–785, 2009.

[12] M. B. Narra and N. I. Abdou, "Autoimmune lymphoproliferative syndrome in a patient with common variable immunodeficiency: dichotomy of apoptosis," *Annals of Allergy, Asthma and Immunology*, vol. 98, no. 6, pp. 585–588, 2007.

[13] B. He, R. Santamaria, W. Xu et al., "The transmembrane activator TACI triggers immunoglobulin class switching by activating B cells through the adaptor MyD88," *Nature Immunology*, vol. 11, no. 9, pp. 836–845, 2010.

31

An IgG4-Related Salivary Gland Disorder: A Case Series Presenting with a Different Clinical Setting

Masayuki Ishida, Hiroaki Fushiki, and Yukio Watanabe

Department of Otolaryngology, Head & Neck Surgery, University of Toyama, Toyama 930-0194, Japan

Correspondence should be addressed to Hiroaki Fushiki, hfushiki@med.u-toyama.ac.jp

Academic Editors: F. Blanco-Favela, A. Plebani, M.-Y. Shiau, and P. Szodoray

Küttner tumor is a chronic inflammatory disease that presents with a firm swelling of the submandibular gland and often mimics a neoplasm. Recently evidence suggests that Küttner tumor may be a type of disorder characterized by IgG4-related inflammations. Herein, we report 3 cases of submandibular gland swellings with severe fibrosis, inflammation with marked lymphoplasmacytic infiltration; this pathology mimics clinical manifestation of a malignant tumor in 18-fluorodeoxyglucose positron emission tomography (FDG-PET) findings.

1. Introduction

Küttner tumor, commonly known as chronic sclerosing sialadenitis, is a chronic inflammatory disease that presents with firm swelling of the submandibular gland and often mimics a malignant tumor clinically [1]. Recent studies have shown that the pathogenesis of Küttner tumor can be characterized by IgG4-related multifocal inflammations [2, 3]. In the present study, we report 3 cases of an IgG4-related salivary gland disorder that cause bilateral or unilateral swelling of the submandibular gland, each presenting with a different clinical setting. Diagnostic features of the disorder will be discussed together with a literature review.

2. Case Report

Case 1. A 77-year-old male visited our university hospital because of a 2-month history of bilateral swelling of the submandibular region. Bilateral diffused enlargement of the submandibular glands was elastic hard and had good mobility on palpation. A computed tomography (CT) scan showed that the submandibular gland was bilaterally enlarged to approximately 30 mm (Figure 1). There was no significant swelling of lymph nodes in the neck. Laboratory tests were negative for SS-A and SS-B antibodies, with no increase in amylase activity. The swelling could not be resolved by treatment with antibiotics and antiphlogistic agents. A biopsy sample of the left submandibular gland was taken under local anesthesia. The biopsied tissue was white and hard. Histopathological examination revealed extensive fibrosis and diffuse lymphocyte infiltration, with scattering of a small number of eosinophilic leucocytes and lymphoid follicles. The salivary gland tissue was highly atrophied.

Case 2. A 59-year-old female was admitted to our university hospital because of a swelling in the right submandibular gland region for the third time. Swellings in the right submandibular gland region had occurred twice in the previous 2 years, and the biopsy samples showed "reactive lymph node" both times. CT showed that the right submandibular gland was enlarged to 40 mm × 20 mm, with several lymph nodes measuring up to 15 mm in the periphery of the parotid gland and the right upper deep cervical region.

18-fluorodeoxyglucose positron emission tomography (FDG-PET) showed a high and slightly heterogeneous increase in accumulations of FDG in the right submandibular region (standardized uptake value, SUV: 6.24), with a slight increase in accumulations in the upper dorsal to the right submandibular region, the right cervical regions, and the supraclavicular fossa (Figure 2). Laboratory tests were negative for SS-A and SS-B antibodies, with no increase in amylase activity. In order to rule out a possible right

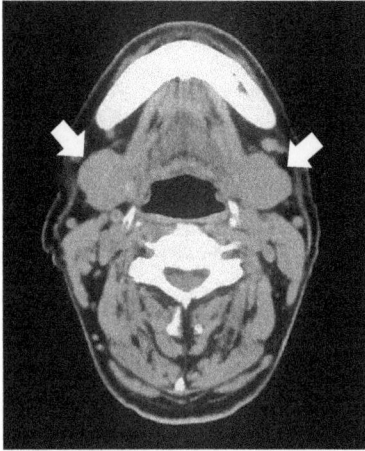

FIGURE 1: Cervical CT images of Case 1. Bilateral swelling of the submandibular glands (arrows).

submandibular gland cancer with lymph node metastases or malignant lymphoma, the right submandibular gland was extirpated under general anesthesia. Histopathological examination revealed diffused, double-layered, small-sized gland ducts accompanied by lymphoid follicles forming a high-degree lymphocyte infiltration. Plasma cell and eosinophilic leukocyte infiltrations, relatively high-degree fibrosis, and many IgG4-positive plasma cells were also observed (Figure 3). Subsequent swelling occurred in the unaffected submandibular gland after a period, which was resolved by steroid treatment.

Case 3. A 61-year-old male was admitted to our university hospital because of a 1-year history of swelling of the right submandibular region. He reported that the swelling enlarged gradually over the year. CT showed a slightly contrast-enhanced mass, measuring 32 mm × 22 mm in the right submandibular region. Salivary gland scintigraphy (Tc-99 m) showed a decrease in accumulations in the right posterior submandibular gland in early images. Laboratory tests were negative for SS-A and SS-B antibodies, with no increase in amylase activity. The right submandibular gland was extirpated under general anesthesia. Histopathological examination revealed that the submandibular glands were enlarged because of marked lymphocyte infiltration and only a few normal submandibular glands were present. There was a remarkably high degree of plasma cell infiltration in the fibroid portion of the glands.

3. Discussion

In 1896, Küttner identified a disorder that causes tumor-like swelling of the submandibular glands, which was named after him [1]. It differs from nonspecific chronic sialadenitis in that the submandibular gland is commonly affected, hard tumor-like mass is present in clinical manifestation, and pathology shows florid lymphoplasmacytic infiltrate

accompanied by prominent and progressive fibrosis. In 108 cases described by Isacsson and Lundquist, the mean age at diagnosis was 42–45 years, with no gender difference [4]. The chief complaint is recurrent pain and/or swelling in one side of the neck [4]. Recent studies have shown that Küttner tumor and Mikulicz's disease are serologically similar disorders that cause IgG4-related inflammations of the salivary gland and they both may produce similar lesions in organs other than the salivary gland [2, 3, 5–7]. Lesions of IgG4-related inflammations include the lacrimal glands, autoimmune pancreatitis, sclerosing cholangitis, interstitial nephritis, and retroperitoneal fibrosis [6, 7].

The 3 cases reported in this study are summarized in Table 1. A definite diagnosis of the disorders in this study was made by histopathological examination of the salivary glands; all cases were diagnosed with IgG4-related chronic sclerosing sialadenitis, on the basis of the presence of high-degree infiltration of IgG4-positive plasma cells in the swollen submandibular gland tissues.

All 3 cases showed swelling of the submandibular region, but each presented with a different clinical manifestation. If the disease affects both sides, as in Case 1, systemic autoimmune disorders such as Küttner tumor, Mikulicz's disease, or Sjögren's syndrome should be considered initially in the differential diagnosis. Mikulicz's disease, first reported by Mikulicz in 1892, is a disorder of unknown cause, showing sustained left-right symmetric swellings of the lacrimal gland as well as the salivary gland [8]. In contrast, Sjögren's syndrome is manifested by xerostomia and keratoconjunctivitis sicca accompanied by the swelling of the salivary glands. Küttner tumor and Mikulicz's disease are serologically characterized by high levels of serum IgG and its subtype IgG4, and it is mostly negative for the antinuclear antibodies (ANA) and anti-SS-A and -SS-B, which are often positive in Sjögren's syndrome [5]. Histological examination showed the presence of IgG4-positive plasma cell infiltration in Mikulicz's disease but not in Sjögren's syndrome [5]. Chronic sclerosing sialadenitis with widespread involvement of the major and minor salivary glands has been reported as a usual presentation [9]. Mikulicz's disease and Küttner tumor may be subtypes of an identical clinical entity with IgG4-related inflammations, with the extent and severity of the lesions within the salivary gland presenting with different clinical manifestations.

In unilateral cases similar to our tumor-like Cases 2 and 3, it may not be easy to diagnose this disorder. If the submandibular swelling occurs unilaterally with abnormal accumulations on FDG-PET (Case 2), malignancy such as a cancer or lymphoma is more likely to be suspected. Measurement of serum IgG4 concentrations is useful for diagnosing Mikulicz's disease: it was significantly greater in Mikulicz's disease than in other salivary gland diseases (a cutoff value of 135 mg/dL) [10]. It may be also useful in differentiating clinically Küttner tumor from neoplasm. If serum IgG4 concentration is within normal range, biopsy sample should be taken for a definite diagnosis (Case 3). Once a definite diagnosis of IgG 4-related chronic sclerosing sialadenitis is made on the basis of pathology, FDG-PET may be useful for characterizing multifocal lesions other

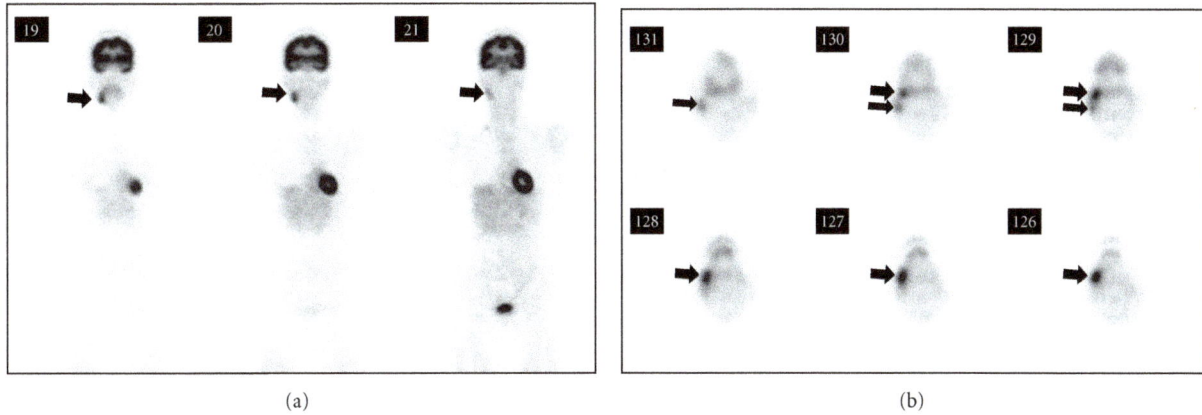

FIGURE 2: FDG-PET images of Case 2. (a) Intense uptake (SUV: 6.24) in the right submandibular gland (arrows). (b) Intense uptake in the right submandibular gland (thick arrows) and the deep interior cervical area (thin arrows).

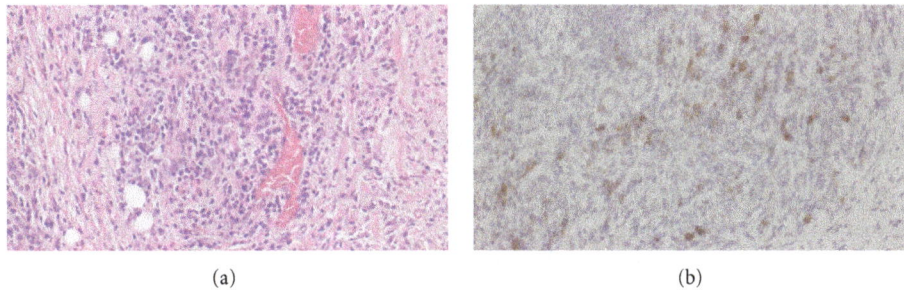

FIGURE 3: Histopathological examination of Case 2. (a) Small-sized gland ducts with plasma cell and eosinophilic leukocyte infiltrations (H&E stain ×40). (b) IgG4-positive plasma cells (stained with IgG4 monoclonal antibody ×40). Mouse monoclonal antibody to human IgG4 (clone, HP6025; dilution, 1 : 100; Zymed Laboratories Inc., Calif, USA).

TABLE 1: Summary of three case reports.

	Case 1	Case 2	Case 3
Age, gender	77 years old, male	59 years old, female	61 years old, male
Swelling of the submandibular gland	Both sides	Initially, on the right side; after a period of time, on the left side	Right side
Serum amylase	Within normal range	Within normal range	Within normal range
Serum SS-A antibody	Negative	Negative	Negative
Serum SS-B antibody	Negative	Negative	Negative
Serum IgG (863–1589 mg/dL)	2441	1313	1196
Serum IgG4 (4–108 mg/dL)	451	241	64
IgG4-positive plasma cells in salivary gland tissue	Positive	Positive	Positive
Histopathological diagnosis	Chronic sclerosing sialadenitis	Chronic sclerosing sialadenitis	Chronic sclerosing sialadenitis
Other organ lesions	No	No	No
Other image findings	none	Intense uptake on PET	Decrease in accumulations on salivary gland scintigraphy

than the salivary gland and/or assessing the therapeutic effects of corticosteroids [7]. Kitagawa et al. [2] found that 5 out of 12 patients with Küttner tumor were associated with sclerosing lesions in the extrasalivary gland tissues. Treatment with steroids shows a good response in Küttner tumor and Mikulicz's disease [3, 5, 11].

In clinical practice, we recommend that Küttner tumor should be treated as a systemic disorder rather than a salivary gland disorder, by otolaryngologists. Clinical whole-body examination and followup is necessary to find simultaneous and/or emerging IgG4-related inflammations of other sites when they did it.

References

[1] H. Küttner, "Über entzündliche tumoren der submaxillarspeicheldrüse," *Beitr Klin Chir*, vol. 15, pp. 815–828, 1896.

[2] S. Kitagawa, Y. Zen, K. Harada et al., "Abundant IgG4-positive plasma cell infiltration characterizes chronic sclerosing sialadenitis (Küttner's tumor)," *American Journal of Surgical Pathology*, vol. 29, no. 6, pp. 783–791, 2005.

[3] T. Kamisawa, H. Nakajima, and T. Hishima, "Close correlation between chronic sclerosing sialadenitis and immunoglobulin G4," *Internal Medicine Journal*, vol. 36, no. 8, pp. 527–529, 2006.

[4] G. Isacsson, B. Ahlner, and P. G. Lundquist, "Chronic sialadenitis of the submandibular gland. A retrospective study of 108 cases," *Archives of Oto-Rhino-Laryngology*, vol. 232, no. 1, pp. 91–100, 1981.

[5] M. Yamamoto, C. Suzuki, Y. Naishiro, H. Takahashi, Y. Shinomura, and K. Imai, "The significance of disease-independence in Mikulicz's disease—revival interests in Mikulicz's disease," *Nihon Rinshō Men'eki Gakkai Kaishi*, vol. 29, no. 1, pp. 1–7, 2006 (Japanese).

[6] H. Hamano, S. Kawa, Y. Ochi et al., "Hydronephrosis associated with retroperitoneal fibrosis and sclerosing pancreatitis," *Lancet*, vol. 359, no. 9315, pp. 1403–1404, 2002.

[7] T. Tanabe, K. Tsushima, M. Yasuo et al., "IgG4-associated multifocal systemic fibrosis complicating sclerosing sialadenitis, hypophysitis, and retroperitoneal fibrosis, but lacking pancreatic involvement," *Internal Medicine*, vol. 45, no. 21, pp. 1243–1247, 2006.

[8] J. Mikulicz, "Über eine eigenartige symmetrische Erkrankung der Tränen und Mundspeicheldrüsen," in *Beiträge zur Chirurgie : Festschrift gewidmet Theodor Billroth*, pp. 610–630, 1892.

[9] M. Blanco, T. Mesko, M. Cura, and B. Cabello-Inchausti, "Chronic sclerosing sialadenitis (Kuttner's tumor): unusual presentation with bilateral involvement of major and minor salivary glands," *Annals of Diagnostic Pathology*, vol. 7, no. 1, pp. 25–30, 2003.

[10] T. Tabata, T. Kamisawa, K. Takuma et al., "Serum IgG4 concentrations and IgG4-related sclerosing disease," *Clinica Chimica Acta*, vol. 408, no. 1-2, pp. 25–28, 2009.

[11] M. Yamamoto, S. Harada, M. Ohara et al., "Beneficial effects of steroid therapy for Mikulicz's disease," *Rheumatology*, vol. 44, no. 10, pp. 1322–1323, 2005.

32

Autoimmune Lymphoproliferative Syndrome and Epstein-Barr Virus-Associated Lymphoma: An Adjunctive Diagnostic Role for Monitoring EBV Viremia?

Romina Pace[1] and Donald C. Vinh[2]

[1] Department of Medicine, McGill University Health Centre, Montreal, QC, Canada H3G 1A4
[2] Division of Infectious Diseases, Division of Allergy & Clinical Immunology (Department of Medicine),
   Department of Medical Microbiology, Department of Human Genetics, McGill University Health Centre, Montreal General Hospital,
   1650 Cedar Avenue, Rm A5-156, Montreal, QC, Canada H3G 1A4

Correspondence should be addressed to Donald C. Vinh; donald.vinh@mcgill.ca

Academic Editors: N. Martinez-Quiles, A. E. Tebo, M. Trendelenburg, and A. Vojdani

Background. Autoimmune lymphoproliferative syndrome (ALPS) is a genetic disorder of lymphocyte homeostasis due to defects in FAS-mediated apoptosis. ALPS is characterized by childhood onset of chronic lymphadenopathy and splenomegaly, autoimmunity, an expanded population of double-negative T cells (DNTCs), and an increased risk of lymphoma. This propensity for lymphoma in ALPS is not well understood. It is possible that lymphomagenesis in some of these patients may result from Epstein-Barr virus (EBV) infection exploiting the defective T-cell surveillance resulting from impaired FAS-mediated apoptosis. *Case Presentation.* We report the first case, to our knowledge, of lymphoma in a patient with ALPS that was clinically heralded by progressively increasing EBV viremia. We discuss its practical implications and the possible immune pathways involved in the increased risk for EBV-associated lymphoproliferative disorders in ALPS patients. *Conclusion.* In patients with ALPS, distinguishing chronic lymphadenopathy from emerging lymphoma is difficult, with few practical recommendations available. This case illustrates that, at least for some patients, monitoring for progressively increasing EBV viremia may be useful.

1. Background

Autoimmune lymphoproliferative syndrome (ALPS) is a Mendelian disorder of lymphocyte homeostasis caused by defects in FAS-mediated apoptosis [1]. The majority of cases to date are due to heterozygous germline mutations in the *APT1* (*TNFRSF6*) gene, which encodes the cell surface-expressed transmembrane receptor, FAS (CD95) [2]. Ligation of FAS by its cognate ligand (FAS ligand; FAS-L) triggers B- and T-lymphocyte apoptosis. Mutations in FAS, FAS-L, or in the downstream molecules that constitute the apoptosis-inducing complex (i.e., Caspase-10) impair programmed cell death of lymphocytes. Consequently, ALPS is characterized by childhood onset of chronic (>6 months) noninfectious, nonmalignant lymphadenopathy and splenomegaly, associated with an increased circulating number of a unique T-cell population that is CD3+ and expresses the α/β receptor but is CD4− and CD8−, the so-called double-negative T cells (DNTCs). DNTCs are considered elevated when they are >1.5% of total lymphocytes or >2.5% of CD3+ lymphocytes in the setting of normal or elevated lymphocyte counts [2]. Additional diagnostic criteria for ALPS include polyclonal hypergammaglobulinemia, elevated vitamin B12 levels, and elevated immune biomarkers in plasma (e.g., soluble FAS-L, IL 10, and IL-18) [2]. The clinical course of ALPS is marked by increased rates of autoimmunity and of malignancy. In particular, individuals with germline FAS mutations have risks for Hodgkin's lymphoma (HL) and non-HL of 51- and

14-fold, respectively, above the general population [3]. This predisposition to lymphoma in ALPS is not fully understood. Failure of the FAS apoptotic pathway is apparently necessary, likely by providing an expanded lymphoid pool at risk for clonal transformation. However, the temporal delay between the onset of ALPS manifestations and that of lymphoma suggests a requirement for additional oncogenic events. Epstein-Barr virus (EBV) is a ubiquitous lymphotropic γ-herpesvirus. With its ability to establish lifelong latency in B cells and its growth transformation capacity, EBV is associated with various lymphoproliferative disorders (LPD). Diagnoses of some EBV-related LPD are facilitated by quantitative monitoring of EBV viral load (VL) in blood. We report the first case, to our knowledge, of lymphoma in a patient with ALPS that was heralded by progressively increasing EBV viremia and discuss its clinical implications.

2. Case Presentation

A 33-year-old French-Canadian male was referred for reevaluation of chronic lymphadenopathy and splenomegaly since the age of 4, when he had been diagnosed with "chronic EBV illness" based on serology. He had no history of unexplained fever, liver dysfunction, cytopenia, mosquito bite reactions, or hydroa vacciniforme, features that would suggest the nosologic entity "chronic active EBV." Based on elevated serum vitamin B12 level, polyclonal hypergammaglobulinemia and 15% DNTC, the diagnosis of ALPS was confirmed by identification of a heterozygous c.784A>T mutation in *TNFRSF6*, resulting in p.I262F mutation in the intracellular death domain of FAS (GeneDx). Initial whole blood EBV VL was 0 copies/mL. Baseline positron-emission tomography (PET-CT) demonstrated diffuse hypermetabolic lymphadenopathy with enlarged but not hypermetabolic spleen. Right axillary lymph node biopsy revealed paracortical expansion with DNTCs and increased number of EBV$^+$ B cells (by EBV-encoded small RNA (EBER)) but no lymphoma. At 1-year followup, he was noted to have asymptomatic EBV viremia (Figure 1). Serial monitoring of the viral load demonstrated an initial decline and then progressive increase in EBV viremia followed by worsening lymphadenopathy, without constitutional symptoms. PET-CT demonstrated nodal foci with significantly increased metabolic activity. Lymph node excision *in toto* was required because of a nondiagnostic percutaneous biopsy; histopathological analysis and molecular rearrangement studies demonstrated a composite lymphoma (i.e., follicular lymphoma, diffuse large B-cell lymphoma (DLBCL), and classical HL). Chemotherapy with Rituximab, to target the EBV$^+$ B cells, cyclophosphamide, doxorubicin, vincristine and, prednisone (R-CHOP) has led, to a dramatic improvement in his lymphomas and concomitant EBV viral load.

3. Discussion

Propensity for lymphoma in ALPS is not well understood. The role of EBV, if any, is undefined. In the general population, EBV has been implicated as the causative agent in a number of lymphomas, including HL and certain DLBCL, albeit in only a proportion of cases [4]. Certain primary (e.g., Wiskott-Aldrich syndrome) [5] or secondary immunodeficiencies (e.g. transplant; HIV) are known to be at increased risk for EBV-LPD; again, only an unexplained select subgroup of patients is affected. In the original ALPS-associated lymphoma cohort at the National Institutes of Health, 10 of 130 subjects heterozygous for germline FAS mutation developed lymphoma: three (two of B cell origin, one of T cell) were EBV-positive on pathology by *in situ* hybridization (Table 1) [3]. Although the clinical penetrance of ALPS in subjects with germline FAS mutation is variable, lymphoma appeared to principally occur in only those who manifest some or all features of ALPS, an observation echoed by Neven et al. [6]. More recently, 20 subjects constituted the ALPS/lymphoma NIH cohort [2], of which 4 had EBV-associated disease [7], while Neven et al. [6] reported one EBV-positive case among their cohort of 7 subjects. Thus, ~15–30% of lymphomas in patients with ALPS appear to be EBV-related.

Surveillance for lymphoma in ALPS patients is challenging for several reasons: the waxing/waning course of lymphadenopathy; the difficulty in distinguishing nonmalignant lymphadenopathy from malignancy on metabolic imaging [9]; and limitations associated with repeat biopsies of multiple lymph nodes (e.g., feasibility; sampling error) during a potentially insidious course of illness that may span decades. While B-type symptoms (i.e., fever, night sweats, weight loss, and itching) may be suggestive, it may not always be present (as in this case) or may manifest only later in the lymphomagenesis process. Thus, there is a need for complementary tumor-specific biomarkers. Given that some lymphoma cases in ALPS patients appear to be EBV associated, monitoring EBV VL in blood may be a useful adjunctive tool to guide the need for more aggressive diagnostic investigations. Routine monitoring of EBV VL in blood is well established as a predictor and assessment of treatment response of PTLD, as well as other EBV-related malignancies [10]. In our case, initial lymph node biopsy demonstrated cells latently infected with EBV by EBER *in situ* hybridization but without evidence of lymphoma; there was no concomitant detectable EBV viremia. EBV VL was then monitored because of the historical diagnosis of "chronic EBV illness," serendipitously illustrating a progressively increasing EBV VL in blood metachronous to lymphomatous transformation. Although no causality is implied, this case suggests that monitoring EBV VL in at least some ALPS patients may be a useful proxy test for certain types of lymphoproliferative malignancies. Nomura et al. recently reported the detection of EBV viremia in 3 patients initially diagnosed with CAEBV but subsequently found to be heterozygous for FAS mutations, suggesting that they, in fact, had ALPS [8]. However, in these patients, only a single EBV VL was reported and none had malignancy (although lymph node histopathology was not reported). Thus, if EBV VL proves clinically useful in diagnosing or predicting lymphoma in some patients with ALPS, it may be through dynamic increases on serial measurements, rather than from single values, as is seen in PTLD.

TABLE 1: Clinical and laboratory profiles of ALPS patients with EBV lymphoma and/or EBV viremia.

Patient (reference; pedigree if available)	Country	Sex	Age of ALPS manifestations	Adeno-pathy	Spleno-megaly	Anemia	Thrombo-cytopenia	% DNTC*	EBV+ Lymphoma	Lymphoma onset (years after ALPS onset)	EBV viremia	FAS mutation	Outcome
1†	Canada	M	4 years	+	+	+	−	15	Composite lymphoma (follicular lymphoma, diffuse large B-cell lymphoma, and classic Hodgkin's lymphoma)	30	+ (progressively increasing)	784A → T	Treated with chemotherapy. Alive.
2 [3] (26-II-4)	USA	M	2 years	+	+	+	+	0.7	Omental Burkitt's lymphoma	48	NR	973A → T	Treated with chemotherapy. Survived.
3 [3] (26-IV-5)	USA	M	10 months	+	+	+	NR	2.1	Classic Hodgkin's lymphoma (mixed cellularity)	7	NR	973A → T	Treated with chemotherapy; survived. Diagnosed with histiocytic sarcoma (at age 13); died from pulmonary hemorrhage after bone marrow transplant
4 [3] (45-III-2)	USA	M	5 years	+	+	+	+	11.7	Hodgkin's lymphoma	6	NR	779del11	Treated with chemotherapy. Outcome NR.
5 [3] (G3-III-4)	Germany	F	NR	+	+	−	+	75	T-cell lymphoma	2	NR	1009A → G	Treated with chemotherapy. Survived
6 [8]	Japan	M	3 months	+	+	−	+	10.4	NR	NR	+	IVS8 + 5G → T	Alive at 15 years old.
7 [8]	Japan	M	1	+	+	+	−	20.3	NR	NR	+	1020C → T	Alive at 14 years old.
8 [8]	Japan	M	2	+	+	−	+	12.5	NR	NR	+	1020C → T	NR

"+": presence. "−": absence. NR: not reported. *DNTC: double negative T cells = TCR α/β CD4- CD8-T cells.
†Current case; [3] Straus et al. Blood, 2001. [8] Nomura et al. Int J Hematol, 2011.

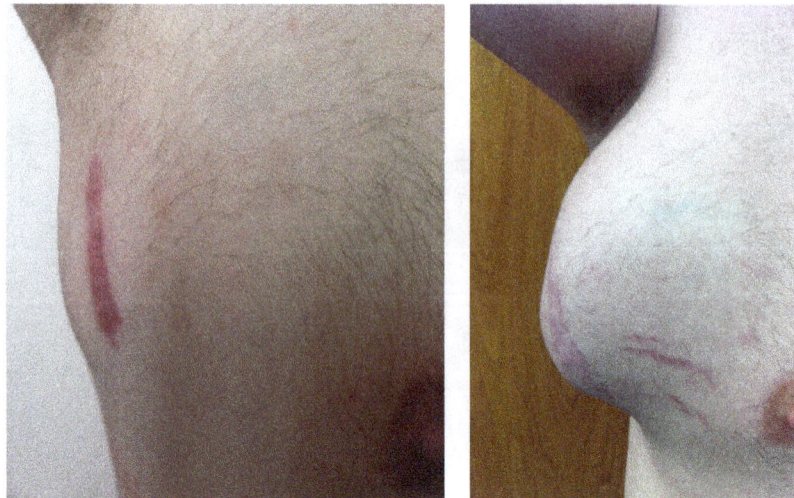

(a)

(b)

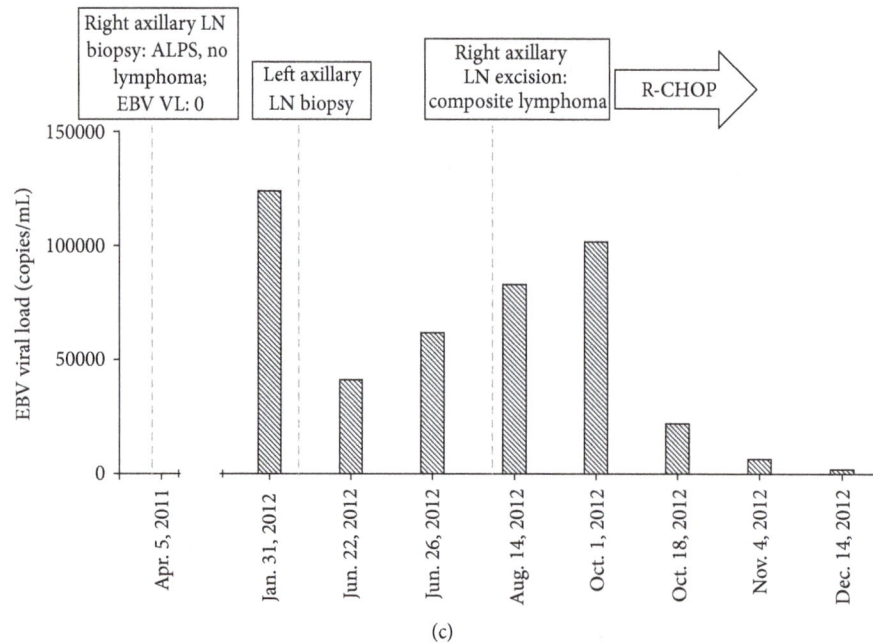

(c)

FIGURE 1: EBV viremia and EBV$^+$ lymphoma in ALPS. A 33-year-old male with ALPS-Ia developed asymptomatic worsening lymphadenopathy (Right axillary lymph node in July 2011 (a) and June 2012 (b)), with progressively increasing EBV viral load (VL). He was found to have a composite EBV$^+$ lymphoma. (c) Monitoring of whole blood EBV VL demonstrates an increasing viremia with concomitant identification of lymphoma and improvement in viremia with (rituximab, cyclophosphamide, doxorubicin, vincristine, and prednisone; R-CHOP) chemotherapy.

4. Conclusion

This case and the literature review suggest that patients with ALPS may have increased susceptibility to EBV-associated lymphomas. Further, this case fortuitously illustrates that at least in some patients with ALPS, serial monitoring of EBV VL may be a useful noninvasive biomarker to monitor for lymphomatous transformation. Further studies are needed to confirm these findings.

List of Abbreviations

ALPS: Autoimmune Lymphoproliferative Syndrome
DNTCs: Double-negative T cells
EBV: Epstein-Barr virus
LPD: Lymphoproliferative disorder
HL: Hodgkin's lymphoma
VL: Viral load
PET-CT: Baseline positron emission tomography

EBER: EBV-encoded small RNA
DLBCL: Diffuse large B-cell lymphoma
R-CHOP: Rituximab, cyclophosphamide, doxorubicin, vincristine, and prednisone
PTLD: Posttransplant lymphoproliferative disorder
CAEBV: Chronic active Epstein-Barr virus.

Conflict of Interests

The authors do not have a direct financial relation with any commercial identity mentioned in this paper that might lead to a conflict of interests for any of the authors. D. C. Vinh has received an unrestricted educational grant and speaking fees from CSL Behring Canada.

Authors' Contribution

D. C. Vinh was involved in the medical care of this patient. D. C. Vinh and R. Pace drafted the paper. All authors read and approved the final paper.

Acknowledgment

The authors are grateful for the patient and his family for participation in this study.

References

[1] W. Al-Herz, A. Bousfiha, J. L. Casanova et al. et al., "Primary immunodeficiency diseases: an update on the classification from the international union of immunological societies expert committee for primary immunodeficiency," *Frontiers in Immunology*, vol. 2, p. 54, 2011.

[2] V. K. Rao and J. B. Oliveira, "How I treat autoimmune lymphoproliferative syndrome," *Blood*, vol. 118, no. 22, pp. 5741–5751, 2011.

[3] S. E. Straus, E. S. Jaffe, J. M. Puck et al., "The development of lymphomas in families with autoimmune lymphoproliferative syndrome with germline Fas mutations and defective lymphocyte apoptosis," *Blood*, vol. 98, no. 1, pp. 194–200, 2001.

[4] M. K. Gandhi, E. Lambley, J. Burrows et al., "Plasma Epstein-Barr virus (EBV) DNA is a biomarker for EBV-positive Hodgkin's lymphoma," *Clinical Cancer Research*, vol. 12, no. 2, pp. 460–464, 2006.

[5] R. Amnueilaph, P. Boongird, M. Leechawengwongs, and A. Vejjajiva, "Heroin neuropathy," *The Lancet*, vol. 1, no. 7818, pp. 1517–1518, 1973.

[6] B. Neven, A. Magerus-Chatinet, B. Florkin et al., "Asurvey of 90 patients with autoimmune lymphoproliferative syndrome related to TNFRSF6 mutation," *Blood*, vol. 118, no. 18, pp. 4798–4807, 2011.

[7] G. Venkataraman, K. L. McClain, S. Pittaluga, V. K. Rao, and E. S. Jaffe, "Development of disseminated histiocytic sarcoma in a patient with autoimmune lymphoproliferative syndrome and associated rosai-dorfman disease," *American Journal of Surgical Pathology*, vol. 34, no. 4, pp. 589–594, 2010.

[8] K. Nomura, H. Kanegane, K. Otsubo et al., "Autoimmune lymphoproliferative syndrome mimicking chronic active Epstein-Barr virus infection," *International Journal of Hematology*, vol. 93, no. 6, pp. 760–764, 2011.

[9] V. K. Rao, J. A. Carrasquillo, J. K. Dale et al., "Fluorodeoxyglucose positron emission tomography (FDG-PET) for monitoring lymphadenopathy in the autoimmune lymphoproliferative syndrome (ALPS)," *American Journal of Hematology*, vol. 81, no. 2, pp. 81–85, 2006.

[10] H. Kimura, Y. Ito, R. Suzuki, and Y. Nishiyama, "Measuring Epstein-Barr virus (EBV) load: the significance and application for each EBV-associated disease," *Reviews in Medical Virology*, vol. 18, no. 5, pp. 305–319, 2008.

33

Successful Management of Insulin Allergy and Autoimmune Polyendocrine Syndrome Type 4 with Desensitization Therapy and Glucocorticoid Treatment: A Case Report and Review of the Literature

Joselyn Rojas,[1,2] **Marjorie Villalobos,**[1,2] **María Sofía Martínez,**[1] **Mervin Chávez-Castillo,**[1] **Wheeler Torres,**[1] **José Carlos Mejías,**[1] **Edgar Miquilena,**[1] and **Valmore Bermúdez**[1]

[1] *Endocrine and Metabolic Diseases Research Center, School of Medicine The University of Zulia, Maracaibo 4004, Venezuela*
[2] *Endocrinology Department, Maracaibo University Hospital (SAHUM), Maracaibo 4004, Venezuela*

Correspondence should be addressed to Joselyn Rojas; rojas.joselyn@gmail.com

Academic Editor: Rajni Rani

Introduction. Insulin allergy is a rare complication of insulin therapy, especially in type 1 diabetes mellitus (T1DM). Key manifestations are hypersensitivity-related symptoms and poor metabolic control. T1DM, as well as insulin allergy, may develop in the context of autoimmune polyendocrine syndrome (APS), further complicating management. *Case Report.* A 17-year-old male patient, diagnosed with T1DM, was treated with various insulin therapy schemes over several months, which resulted in recurrent anaphylactoid reactions and poor glycemic control, after which he was referred to our Endocrinology and Immunology Department. A prick test was carried out for all commercially available insulin presentations and another insulin scheme was designed but proved unsuccessful. A desensitization protocol was started with Glargine alongside administration of Prednisone, which successfully induced tolerance. Observation of skin lesions typical of vitiligo prompted laboratory workup for other autoimmune disorders, which returned positive for autoimmune gastritis/pernicious anemia. These findings are compatible with APS type 4. *Discussion.* To our knowledge, this is the first documented case of insulin allergy in type 4 APS, as well as this particular combination in APS. Etiopathogenic components shared by insulin allergy and APS beg for further research in immunogenetics to further comprehend pathophysiologic aspects of these diseases.

1. Introduction

Type 1 diabetes mellitus (T1DM) is an autoimmune disease where adaptive immunity-mediated destruction of pancreatic β cells leads to an absolute absence of insulin [1]. Infiltration of Langerhans islets by mononuclear cells, as well as antipancreatic islet antibodies and circulating islet-reactive T cells, is prominent features of this pathology [2]. Notwithstanding the key role played by genetic susceptibility for the development of T1DM, environmental and nongenetic factors are an equally relevant component in the pathophysiology of this disease [3]. Due to the irreversibility of the damage to pancreatic β cells, patients with T1DM require lifetime insulin therapy to preserve adequate metabolic control [4]. In these subjects, hypersensitivity to insulin is a rare condition, yet it represents a substantial challenge for attending physicians, since in these cases, the predominant immune component attacks not only the pancreatic islet, but also insulin itself, the main therapeutic measure for the disease.

In early documented cases of insulin allergy, hypersensitivity was developed in response to administration of animal-origin insulins, which possess a great antigenic potential due to alterations in their structure, presence of contaminants, and highly immunogenic components such as C-peptide and proinsulin [5–7]. Moreover, IgG anti-insulin antibodies can induce a primary form of insulin resistance, progressive dysglycemia, and lipoatrophy [5]. However, the introduction of human recombinant insulins in the early 1980s has led to a drastic decrease in incidence of these cases, currently

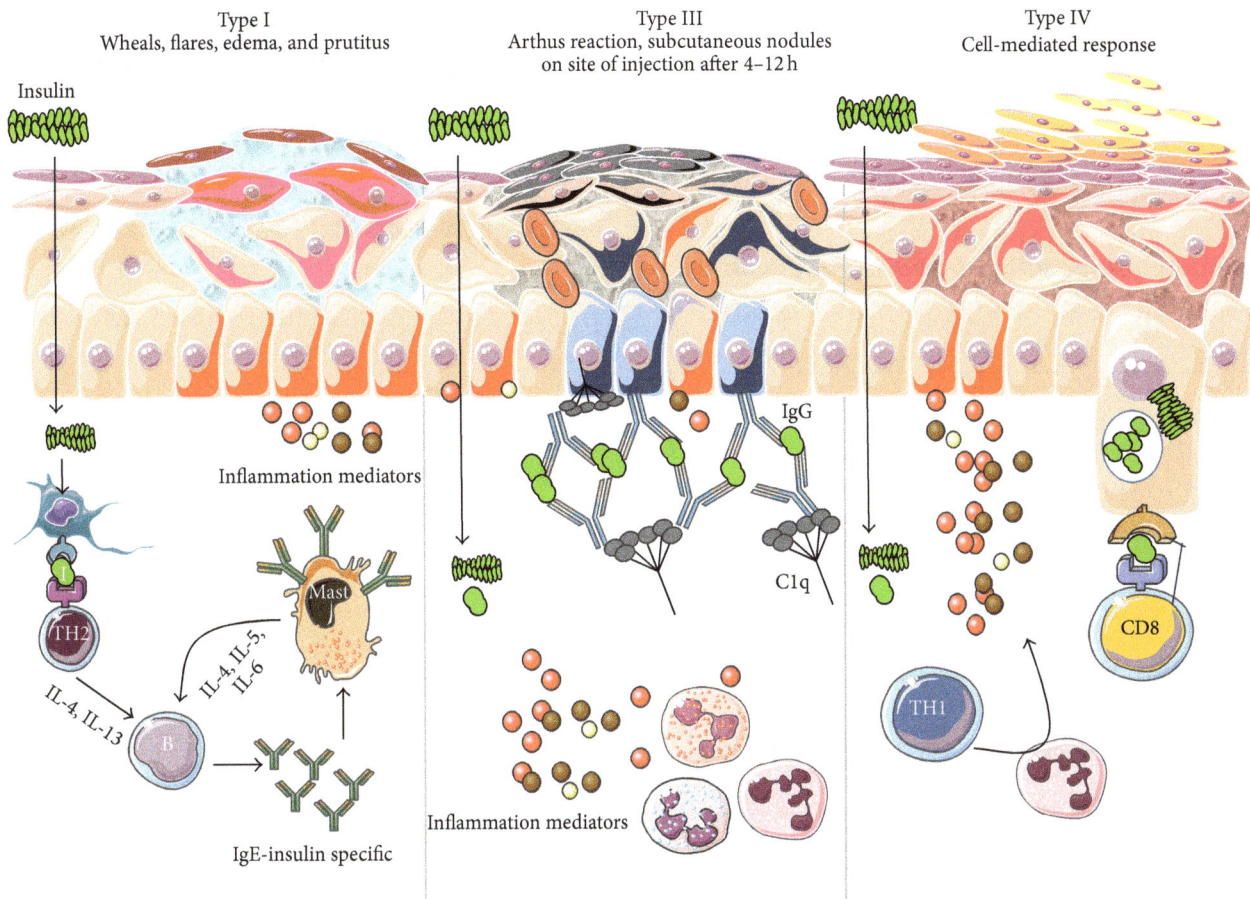

FIGURE 1: Types of hypersensitivity associated with insulin-related allergy reactions. Type I hypersensitivity reaction is characterized to be a TH2-controlled IgE-insulin specific mediated process, with local edema, itching, wheals, and flares, which could also be associated with angioedema. Type III hypersensitivity is mediated by antigen-antibody complex and recruitment of complement C1q, with subsequent edema, necrosis, and nodule formation. Finally, Type IV reactions are CD8-cytotoxic specific with subcutaneous edema, itching, and hyperkeratosis.

estimated at <1% to 2.4% [8]. Clinically, manifestations range from local reactions at the site of injection to severe cases of potentially life-threatening generalized anaphylaxis, and the disease has been described as type I hypersensitivity (IgE-mediated) [9], type III (immune complex-mediated) [10], and type IV delayed hypersensitivity to components added to insulin preparations such as cresol, protamine, and epoxy resin [7, 8, 10–25]; see Figure 1. Tendency to developing hypersensitivity towards insulin relies on its structural modifications in comparison to endogenous insulin, which would modify central tolerance for T lymphocytes [10–25] (Table 1). Management of such cases involves a change of insulin presentation, but, ultimately, most individuals are set through a desensitization protocol [7, 26].

It has been observed that T1DM can coexist with other autoimmune diseases, including vitiligo. The latter is an autoimmune skin disorder characterized by loss of pigmentation due to melanocyte destruction [27]. Several genetic factors have been involved in its pathogenesis, including polymorphisms in HLA-DRB1*07:01, HLA-B*44:03, HLA-A*02:01 y HLA-A*33:01 [27], and other intrinsic defects in melanocytes, which affect its ability to sustain UV stress [28].

Cellular immunity has been proved to participate in this scenario, along with autoreactive CD8+ T cells which are the effector cells in this disease [29]. The combination of T1DM and vitiligo can be seen as part of the autoimmune polyendocrine syndromes (APS), alongside various other glandular autoimmune dysfunctions [30], with a prevalence of 2–10% [16]. Classification of entities in the APS spectrum is complex and is based on the distinct combinations of autoimmunity-targeted organs [31]; see Table 2. In this broad spectrum of autoimmune diseases, T1DM patients can also be diagnosed with autoimmune thyroid disease (~30%), celiac disease (4–9%), autoimmune gastritis/pernicious anemia (5–10%), and Addison's disease (~0.5%) [30, 31].

The following case concerns a teenage boy with T1DM, vitiligo, and autoimmune gastritis, presenting with a severe case of allergy to multiple insulins, managed with a desensitization protocol.

2. Case Presentation

A 17-year-old teenager patient, from Los Puertos de Altagracia community (Miranda municipality, Zulia state), who was

TABLE 1: Insulin analogues and recombinant variations, structure, and related immunogenic reactions.

Immunogenic molecules	Reaction type	References
Regular human insulin		
Insulin	I	[8, 10–15]
	III	[15]
Crystalline insulin		
Insulin	I	[8, 16, 17]
Porcine insulin		
Insulin	I	[8, 16]
Bovine insulin		
Insulin	I	[8, 16]
Neutral Protamine Hagedorn (NPH) insulin		
Insulin	I	[8, 10, 11, 17]
	IV	[18]
Protamine	I	[8, 10, 19]
Lispro insulin (Humalog)		
Insulin	I	[8, 12, 15]
	III	[15]
Aspart insulin (NovoLog)		
Insulin	I	[8, 16, 20]

TABLE 1: Continued.

Immunogenic molecules	Reaction type	References
Glargine insulin (Lantus)		
Insulin	I	[11, 12, 21]
	III	[14]
Detemir insulin (Levemir)		
		$C_{14}H_{28}O_2$
Insulin	I	[12, 22]
	III	[14, 23]
	IV	[22]
Metacresol	I	[24]

diagnosed with T1DM on October 2012 after a hyperglycemic crisis complicated with diabetic ketoacidosis, treated only with fast-acting insulin (Crystalline) due to type I hypersensitivity to intermediate-lasting insulin NPH (Neutral Protamine Hagedorn), and long-lasting insulin Glargine (Lantus). He was referred to the Endocrinology and Immunology outpatient unit at our institute due to persistent bilious emesis, abdominal pain, weight loss, muscular wasting, and daily sprouts of wheals in arms, legs, and torso, usually 30 minutes after the injection of insulin. The following findings were described after written consent was obtained from his mother—his current legal guardian.

This child was the result of an uneventful pregnancy. At birth, imperforate anus was diagnosed and corrected before 3 months of life. During his infancy, he achieved all stages of neurological development satisfactorily. His height—1.83 m—is a noteworthy trait since parents do not exceed 1.70 m in this regard. Earliest manifestations of vitiligo were observed at 12 years of age, with symmetrical patches of hypopigmented skin in ankles, knees, and hands (Figure 2). His family history includes a younger brother who was born with transient hypoglycemia, low birth weight, and multiform erythema and uncle from his mother side with vitiligo.

His diabetic debut was further investigated and the mother was reinterrogated. During his first hyperglycemic crisis—October 2012—he was brought to the ER with intense tiredness, weight loss, polyuria, polydipsia, abdominal pain, emesis, and glucose levels >400 mg/mL. He was treated with fluids and one Crystalline insulin 10 U IV bolus per hour until normalization of glucose levels; afterwards, he was switched to a bimodal schedule of SC insulin therapy: 5 U of Crystalline preprandially and 14 U of NPH at bedtime. The first dose

TABLE 2: Classification of autoimmune polyglandular syndromes (APS).

Category	Subtypes	Criteria
APS-1	—	Two or more from the following (i) Addison's disease (ii) Chronic candidiasis (iii) Hypoparathyroidism Associated conditions (i) Alopecia (ii) Autoimmune gastritis/pernicious anemia (iii) Type 1 diabetes (iv) Vitiligo (v) Autoimmune thyroid disease (vi) Chronic hepatitis (vii) Autoimmune-related gonadal failure
APS-2	—	Addison's disease plus any of the following (i) Type 1 diabetes (ii) Autoimmune thyroid disease
APS-3	APS-3A APS-3B APS-3C APS-3D	Autoimmune thyroid disease plus: type 1 diabetes with/without any other endocrine organ involvement Autoimmune thyroid disease plus: autoimmune gastrohepatic disease (inflammatory bowel syndrome, pernicious anemia, autoimmune gastritis, and primary biliary cirrhosis) Autoimmune thyroid disease plus: skin autoimmune disease (vitiligo with/without alopecia areata) with/without nervous system autoimmune disease (miastenia gravis, multiple sclerosis) Autoimmune thyroid disease plus: rheumatological autoimmune disease (systemic and discoid lupus, rheumatoid arthritis, Sjögren syndrome, systemic sclerosis, vasculitis, and antiphospholipid syndrome) with/without hematological disease
APS-4	—	Any other combination of specific organ and nonorgan specific autoimmune diseases

of NPH caused immediate hypersensitivity, with urticaria lesions, pruritus, and low fever. Thus, this presentation was omitted, and IV chlorpheniramine was used twice per day for treatment of the allergic reaction; he was discharged 3 days later with SC Crystalline as sole treatment, at a dosage of 15 U 30 minutes prior to each meal.

Two weeks later, in November 2012, the patient returns to the local ER with moderate dehydration, multiple emesis, abdominal pain, and polyuria. He was started on fluids, empirical antibiotic therapy, and IV Crystalline boluses, and after normalization of glucose levels, he was administered 32 U of Glargine SC which induced an immediate anaphylactoid reaction with angioedema, wheezing, shortness of breath, and pruritic rash. He was treated with IV hydrocortisone (1 g) and chlorpheniramine (10 mg), and the allergic symptoms remitted after 36 hours. He was discharged again 1 week later with SC Lispro (Humalog, 18 U 15 minutes prior to every meal) insulin as treatment. During the first weeks of December 2012, the mother started to notice small urticaria lesions on her son's legs and torso 2 hours after insulin injection, which disappeared with the use of common oral antihistamines such as Loratadine. However, she became aware that the dosage for insulin appeared insufficient and had to be increased progressively in order to try and achieve glycemic control, but skin lesions were spreading further around his body.

During the final week of December 2012, the patient was referred to the University Hospital in the city of Maracaibo due to hyperglycemia, ketoacidosis, profound weight loss (20 kilograms since October 2012), muscular wasting, and general malaise. During physical examination the following was observed: profuse diaphoresis, pale skin, abdominal distention and flatulence, no signs of neurological focalization, or disorientation; respiratory rate: 22 bpm, heart rate: 121 bpm, blood pressure: 100/60 mmHg, and temperature: 36.8°C; regarding anthropometric measurements, height: 183 cm, weight: 47 kg, arm span: 185 cm, and BMI: 14.07 kg/m^2. He was admitted with a diagnosis of diabetic ketoacidosis and treated with both 100 U of Crystalline insulin diluted in 500 cc of 0.9% saline solution at a rate of 5 UI/kg/h and chlorpheniramine (10 mg) STAT intravenously. After 4 hours, glucose levels normalized and no signs of allergy were observed. However, the following day the patient develops symptomatic hypoglycemia and insulin treatment is modified. A bimodal scheme is installed with 5 U SC of Crystalline insulin preprandially, maintaining the dose of IV chlorpheniramine every 12 hours. Forty-eight hours later, no skin lesions resembling hypersensitivity were observed, but glycemic control was suboptimal, with reports of preprandial glycemia between 250–480 mg/dL at noon. Insulin therapy was then further modified to include a 15 U prebreakfast bolus of Crystalline insulin, 5 U before lunch and before

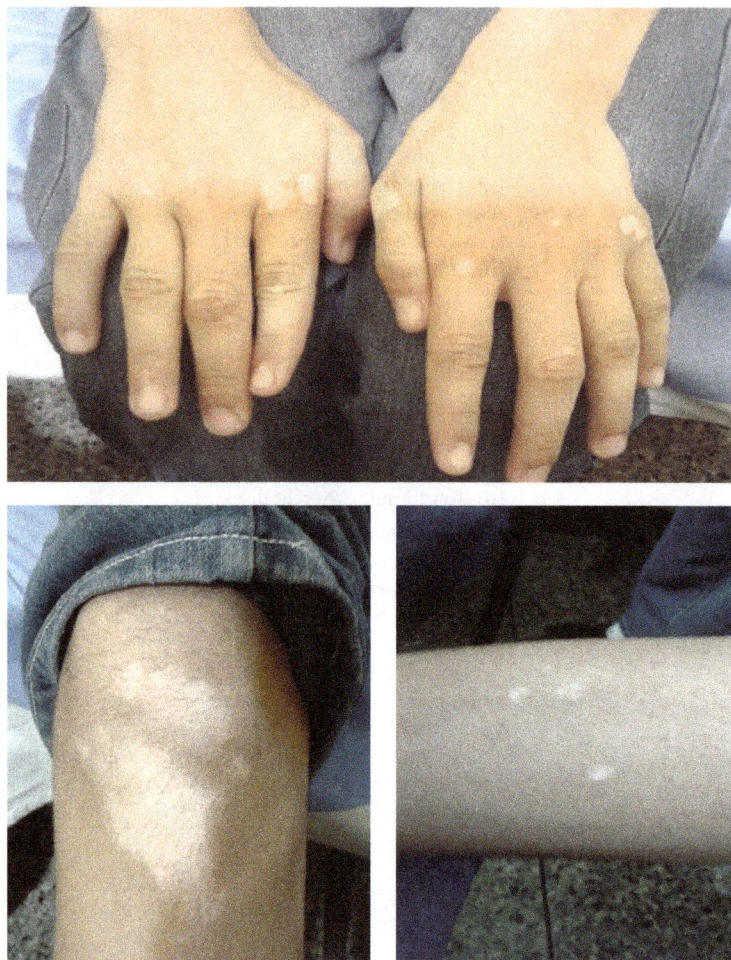

FIGURE 2: Hypochromic skin lesions associated with vitiligo.

dinner, and a final 10 U bedtime bolus of NPH insulin, both SC. However, this schedule was omitted immediately because the patient developed angioedema with the first dose of NPH.

It is after this last hypersensitivity episode that our Endocrinology and Immunology Departments were asked to evaluate the case. A Prick Test with different types of insulin was performed in order to determine which preparation would be most appropriate for the patient. All commercially available presentations were used with the exception of Aspart (NovoRapid) insulin (which was not available in the city at the time). The test was positive for NPH and Lispro, while it was negative for Glargine, Detemir (Levemir), and glulisine (Apidra). Insulin therapy was then started with a basal-bolus scheme: glulisine 10 U SC preprandially and Detemir 20 U SC at bedtime, accompanied with 10 mg of Ebastine p.o. every 8 hours, and 10 mg of Prednisone p.o. once per day. Normalization of glycemic values was obtained with this scheme with no allergic skin lesions, so the patient was discharged. During hospitalization, several laboratory panels were undertaken to further investigate insulin allergy and to exclude involvement of autoimmunity in other glands, which would suggest diagnosis of APS (Table 3); these explorations returned positive

for autoimmune gastritis/pernicious anemia. Additionally, he was evaluated for Marfan's syndrome due to his height and arm span measurements; however ophthalmologic, radiologic, and cardiologic testing ruled out this diagnosis. One week after discharge, the patient attends emergency services again due to pruriginous papules in the neck, thorax, and limbs that appeared approximately 45 minutes after the Detemir injections (Figure 3), and one event during dinnertime injection associated with intense pruritus with glulisine dosage. In light of these findings, a desensitization protocol was conceived and applied.

The desensitization protocol is described in Table 4. The purpose of this therapy is to induce skin anergy by multiple and increasing dosages of insulin until a given dosage of the medication is tolerated by cutaneous immunocytes. Since the patient tolerated Crystalline via SC, we decided to use Glargine insulin because of local availability and economic factors. The protocol included premedication with 10 mg of Ebastine and 60 mg of Prednisone 30 minutes before the first dose. Glargine was administered intradermally in the abdominal region every 20 minutes for 5 days; see Table 3 for dosages. The goal of the procedure was to induce tolerance to dosages of 12 U Glargine, given twice almost simultaneously

TABLE 3: Complementary laboratory workup.

	Results	Reference values
Immunoglobulin E (IgE)	140.60 IU/mL	0–150 IU/mL
Immunoglobulin A (IgA)	1 g/L	0.60–3.09 g/liter
Immunoglobulin M (IgM)	245 mg/dL	40–250 mg/dL
Immunoglobulin G (IgG)	1529 mg/dL	710–1520 mg/dL
Fasting C peptide	0.14 ng/mL	0.9–7.1 ng/mL
Cortisol (AM)	42.5	30–150 ng/mL
Free triiodothyronine (FT3)	1.9 pg/mL	1.4–4.2 pg/mL
Free thyroxine (FT4)	1.1	0.89–1.76 ng/mL
Thyroid stimulating hormone (TSH)	0.945 μIU/mL	0.3–4.00 mUI/mL
Anti-thyroglobulin antibody	7.0 IU/mL	<10 IU/mL
Anti-thyroperoxidase antibody	10.1 IU/mL	<30 IU/mL
Parietal cell autoantibody	Positive	
Intrinsic factor autoantibody	Positive	
Anti-gliadin antibodies	Negative	
Anti-transglutaminase antibodies	Negative	
Anti-*Saccharomyces* antibodies	Negative	

to achieve a total of 24 U of this insulin per day in two different body regions. The dose of Prednisone was then lowered to 30 mg during days 2 and 3 and suspended on day 4; glucocorticoid therapy lasted a total of 4 days. The patient was discharged seven days after admission. One year later, he is stable and without any flaring event, studying second semester at community college. Currently assisting to the outpatient consults every 4 months.

3. Discussion

Insulin allergy is a rare and complex complication of insulin therapy in diabetic patients, with a current estimated prevalence of approximately 2.4% [8], depending on case reports in type 1 and type 2 diabetes mellitus patients. The importance of insulin allergy relies on its fundamental role as a lifelong treatment. Several cases have been documented on diabetic patients, allergic to Glargine [32, 33], Detemir [34, 35], Crystalline [14, 36], NPH [14, 37], Aspart [14], Lispro [33], all available insulins [8, 12, 15, 38], and even components of such medications such as metacresol [24] and protamine [10, 19, 33], with or without presence of beta-lactam antibiotic allergy [12]. Clinical presentation varies, from local cutaneous lesions to anaphylactic shock, either IgE- or IgG-mediated [39]; see Figure 1. Type I allergy reactions are IgE-dependent, induced by the insulin molecule or other components, activating the allergy-related pathway. Nevertheless, IgG-mediated insulin allergy has also been reported [15, 40].

Heinzerling et al. [39] proposed a diagnostic flowchart, suggesting manifestations related to the acute presentation (urticaria, rash, angioedema, dyspnea, nausea, diarrhea, and cardiovascular manifestations) are likely to be IgE-mediated and suggest the need for skin prick testing and assessment of IgE-insulin-specific titers. On the other hand, type IV late signs such as induration and erythema at injection site suggest IgG-mediated allergy, relating to specific antiinsulin

TABLE 4: Desensitization protocol using Glargine insulin.

Day	Number of dosages*	Accumulated dose (IU)	Total dosage per day (IU)	Local reaction (cm) ¶
1	1	0,001	0,001	1
1	2	0,01	0,011	0
1	3	0,1	0,111	1,5
1	4	1	1,111	0
1	5	2	3,111	0
2	6	0,1	0,1	1
2	7	1	1,1	0
2	8	2	3,1	0
2	9	3	6,1	0
3	10	2	2	0
3	11	3	5	0
3	12	4	9	0
4	13	12	12	0
5	14	12	12	0
5	15°	12	24	0

*Time between injections: 20 minutes.
°Administrated almost simultaneously with dosage number 14, in a different corporal region.
¶Diameter of the flare.

and anticomponent IgG titers. In the present case, we assessed a young man who had acute presentation symptoms when treated with Glargine, NPH, Lispro, Detemir, and Glulisine, which evolved over a period of approximately 3 months. When insulin allergy is diagnosed, the general recommendation is to change to another insulin preparation and observe tolerance, which in this case failed in each attempt, demonstrated by cutaneous manifestations and severe inadequate glycemic control. An important limitation in this case, was the lack of quantification of insulin-specific IgE/IgG

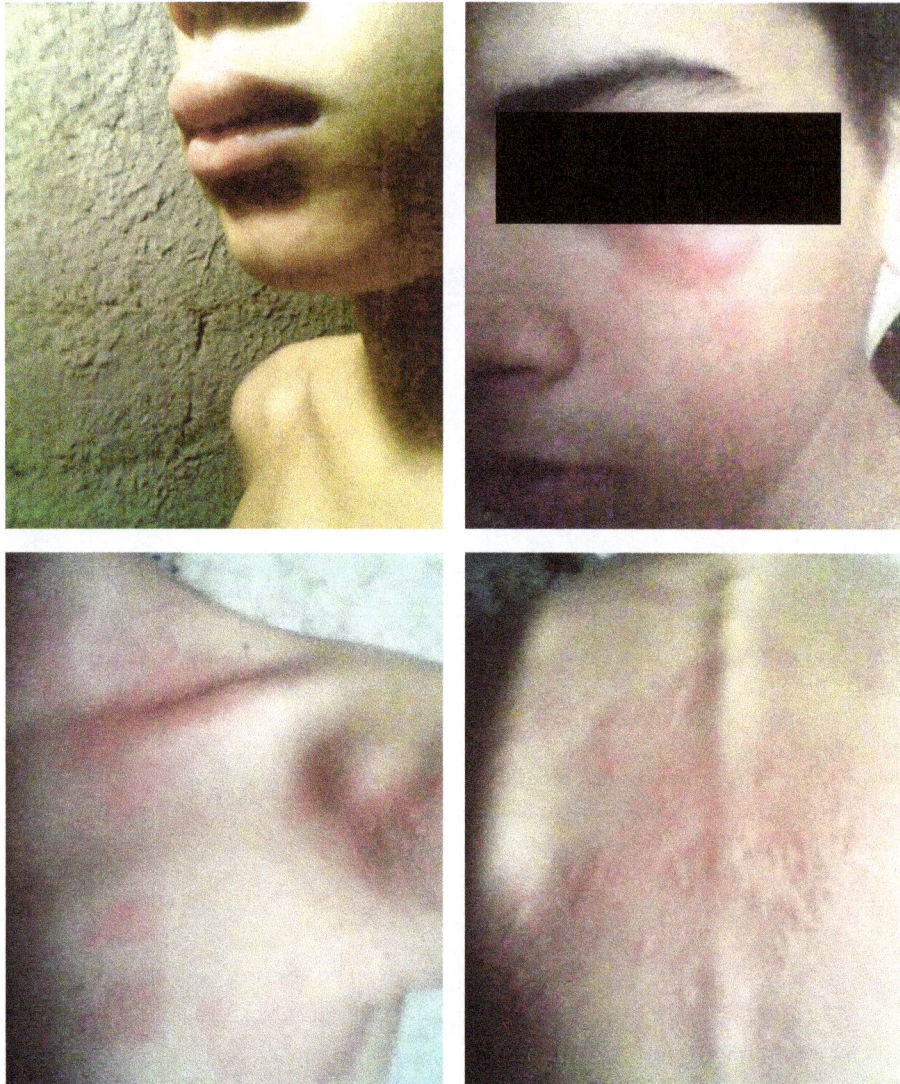

FIGURE 3: Allergic reaction to Detemir. Note distribution of wheals and flares, as well as angioedema of lips and eyelids.

antibodies, as these assay kits are not available in our country. It is noteworthy to comment about the results of the prick test. Glargine was negative in this test, even though he had experienced hypersensitivity to this type of insulin when injected with 32 U. We propose that negativity for this insulin might be due to (a) very high dosage used in this primary treatment which might have caused an adverse drug reaction, or (b) Glargine allergy-induction needs higher doses than the one used in the prick test. Previous case reports have suggested that insulin-related allergy depends on dosage, route of administration, and type of insulin and these account for discrepancies observed between allergenic crisis and skin testing [14, 39, 41].

Given the escalating insulin allergy events observed, a desensitization protocol was planned with Glargine, a long-lasting insulin formulation that is easily available in the country. The purpose of this protocol is to control local forms of insulin allergy, inducing anergy in skin immunocytes [26]. Other protocols have used Glargine [33, 39, 41] and other

insulin analogs, such as Aspart [8, 24] for their desensitization therapy, either using continuous infusion [24, 40, 41] or intradermal injections, all of them achieving immunological control and metabolic improvement.

To our knowledge, this is the first documented case of insulin allergy in type 4 APS. Both clinical entities share similar immunogenetics: insulin immunogenicity is intimately related to T1DM pathogenesis [42] and might share HLA haplotypes with APS. Although HLA-B15-DR4 boasts an important association with hyperimmune manifestations [43], insulin-allergic subjects exhibit a greater prevalence of HLA-Bw44, HLA-DR7, and HLA-A2 and their combinations, with a RR of 20.6 for developing an allergy/immune reaction to insulin [44] and the presence of a specific immune response gene for insulin [43]. On the other hand, APS encompasses a constellation of immunogenic diseases (Table 2) whose presentation and severity rely on the convergence of predisposing and protective HLA haplotypes. In regards to the present case (APS-4: vitiligo + T1DM + autoimmune gastritis/pernicious anemia), vitiligo has been associated with cytotoxic T lymphocyte-mediated melanocyte destruction in patients positive for HLA-A2 [45], HLA-DRB1*07-DQB1*02 [46], and HLA-B*44:03/DRB1*07:01 [47]. As for T1DM, several alleles have been proposed, and although they appear to be highly ethnicity-specific, HLA-A2 [48], HLA-DR4-DQ8, and DR3-DQ2 [49] are the most prevalent worldwide. Lastly, autoimmune gastritis has been described to be mainly associated with DRB1*1101/DQA1*0505 [50] and HLA-DRB1*04/DQB1*03 [51], whereas pernicious anemia is associated with higher prevalence of HLA-D/DR3 and HLA-DR5 [52].

Cases of APS type 4 have been published previously, although with different combinations when compared to ours. Krysiak et al. [53] published a case concerning primary hypoparathyroidism and T1DM, associated with positive anti-transglutaminase and anti-parietal cell antibodies, while Hsu et al. [54] reported a peculiar case of T1DM, anti-GAD-related dystonia, vitiligo, *alopecia areata,* and *myasthenia gravis.* The present case is characterized by the primary development of vitiligo, followed by T1DM, and the detection of autoimmune gastritis/pernicious anemia while investigating insulin allergy, making this case one of a kind.

4. Conclusions

Insulin allergy is considered a rare complication during insulin therapy, yet it should always be suspected in patients with nonspecific cutaneous and systemic symptoms after insulin injections, where appropriate insulin-specific IgE assays should be carried out. The presence of two or more autoimmune-related diseases must prompt further evaluation for other affected organs and classification of the patient. Ultimately, this scenario begs the question: is insulin allergy a sign of an underlying major autoimmune disease, such as APS and nonconventional organ-specific autoimmunity? Further immunogenetic and pathophysiologic studies may help clarify this enigma, especially in the case of this pair of disorders, which seem to be more prevalent in current medical practice.

Conflict of Interests

The authors declare that there is no conflict of interests regarding the publication of this paper.

References

[1] American Diabetes Association, "Executive summary: standards of medical care in diabetes—2014," *Diabetes Care*, vol. 37, supplement 1, pp. S5–S13, 2014.

[2] J.-W. Yoon and H.-S. Jun, "Autoimmune destruction of pancreatic β cells," *American Journal of Therapeutics*, vol. 12, no. 6, pp. 580–591, 2005.

[3] M. Aguirre, J. Rojas, R. Cano, M. Villalobos, and L. Berrueta, "Diabetes mellitus tipo 1 y factores ambientales: la gran emboscada," *Revista Venezolana de Endocrinología y Metabolismo*, vol. 10, pp. 122–134, 2012.

[4] T. L. van Belle, K. T. Coppieters, and M. G. von Herrath, "Type 1 diabetes: etiology, immunology, and therapeutic strategies," *Physiological Reviews*, vol. 91, no. 1, pp. 79–118, 2011.

[5] G. Schernthaner, "Immunogenicity and allergenic potential of animal and human insulins," *Diabetes Care*, vol. 16, no. 3, pp. 155–165, 1993.

[6] R. Patterson, M. RobertsI, and L. C. Grammer, "Insulin allergy: re-evaluation after two decades," *Annals of Allergy*, vol. 64, no. 5, pp. 459–462, 1990.

[7] M. K. Ghazavi and G. A. Johnston, "Insulin allergy," *Clinics in Dermatology*, vol. 29, no. 3, pp. 300–305, 2011.

[8] V. Matheu, E. Perez, M. Hernández et al., "Insulin allergy and resistance successfully treated by desensitisation with Aspart insulin," *Clinical and Molecular Allergy*, vol. 3, article 16, 2005.

[9] A.-Y. Lee, W.-Y. Chey, J. Choi, and J.-S. Jeon, "Insulin-induced drug eruptions and reliability of skin tests," *Acta Dermato-Venereologica*, vol. 82, no. 2, pp. 114–117, 2002.

[10] M. E. Bollinger, R. G. Hamilton, and R. A. Wood, "Protamine allergy as a complication of insulin hypersensitivity: a case report," *Journal of Allergy and Clinical Immunology*, vol. 104, no. 2, pp. 462–465, 1999.

[11] A. Teixeira Rodrigues, L. F. Chiaverini Ensina, L. Sabino Garro, L. Kase Tanno, P. Giavina-Bianchi, and A. Abilio Motta, "Human insulin allergy: four case reports," *European Annals of Allergy and Clinical Immunology*, vol. 42, no. 6, pp. 221–223, 2010.

[12] P. Andrade, L. Barros, and M. Gonçalo, "Type 1 Ig-E mediated allergy to human insulin, insulin analogues and beta-lactam antibiotics," *Anais Brasileiros de Dermatologia*, vol. 87, no. 6, pp. 917–919, 2012.

[13] J. H. Hong, J. H. Lee, J. H. Shin et al., "Maintenance of insulin therapy by desensitization in insulin allergy patient," *Korean Diabetes Journal*, vol. 32, pp. 529–531, 2008.

[14] H. Yokoyama, S. Fukumoto, H. Koyama, M. Emoto, Y. Kitagawa, and Y. Nishizawa, "Insulin allergy; desensitization with crystalline zinc-insulin and steroid tapering," *Diabetes Research and Clinical Practice*, vol. 61, no. 3, pp. 161–166, 2003.

[15] C. Pföhler, C. S. L. Müller, D. O. Hasselmann, and W. Tilgen, "Successful desensitization with human insulin in a patient with an insulin allergy and hypersensitivity to protamine: a case report," *Journal of Medical Case Reports*, vol. 2, article 283, 2008.

[16] P. J. Raubenheimer and N. S. Levitt, "Insulin allergy," *South African Medical Journal*, vol. 94, no. 6, pp. 428–429, 2004.

[17] K.-N. Durand-Gonzalez, N. Guillausseau, C. Pecquet, and J.-P. Gayno, "Glargine insulin is not an alternative in insulin allergy," *Diabetes Care*, vol. 26, no. 7, article 2216, 2003.

[18] M. Maheshwari, D. Goyal, P. Desouza, and R. K. Goyal, "Spotted dermopathy in a diabetic patient due to insulin allergy," *Journal of Association of Physicians of India*, vol. 52, pp. 926–927, 2004.

[19] Y. Q. Chu, L. J. Cai, D. C. Jiang, D. Jia, S. Y. Yan, and Y. Q. Wang, "Allergic shock and death associated with protamine administration in a diabetic patient," *Clinical Therapeutics*, vol. 32, no. 10, pp. 1729–1732, 2010.

[20] "Insulin detemir/insulin glargine/insulin protamine aspart," *Reactions Weekly*, no. 1412, p. 26, 2012.

[21] E. Alfadhli, "Allergy to insulin glargine: a case report," *Journal of Medical Cases*, vol. 2, pp. 4–6, 2011.

[22] A. Sola-Gazagnes, C. Pecquet, J. M'Bemba, E. Larger, and G. Slama, "Type I and type IV allergy to the insulin analogue detemir," *The Lancet*, vol. 369, no. 9562, pp. 637–638, 2007.

[23] P. Darmon, V. Castera, M.-C. Koeppel, C. Petitjean, and A. Dutour, "Type III allergy to insulin detemir," *Diabetes Care*, vol. 28, no. 12, article 2980, 2005.

[24] B. J. Wheeler and B. J. Taylor, "Successful management of allergy to the insulin excipient metacresol in a child with type 1 diabetes: a case report," *Journal of Medical Case Reports*, vol. 6, article 263, 2012.

[25] M. E. R. Silva, M. J. M. Mendes, M. J. M. Ursich et al., "Human insulin allergy-immediate and late type III reactions in a long-standing IDDM patient," *Diabetes Research and Clinical Practice*, vol. 36, no. 2, pp. 67–70, 1997.

[26] I. Eguíluz-Gracia, M. Rodríguez-Álvarez, M. Cimarra-Álvarez, M. C. Sanabria-Pérez, and C. Martínez-Cócera, "Desensitization for Insulin allergy: a useful treatment also for local forms," *Journal of Investigational Allergology and Clinical Immunology*, vol. 22, no. 3, pp. 215–235, 2012.

[27] R. Begum, Y. S. Marfatia, N. C. Laddha, M. Dwivedi, M. S. Mansuri, and M. Singh, "Vitiligo: a complex disease and a complex approach," *Molecular Cytogenetics*, vol. 7, article 157, 2014.

[28] N. Karsli, C. Akcali, O. Ozgoztasi, N. Kirtak, and S. Inaloz, "Role of oxidative stress in the pathogenesis of vitiligo with special emphasis on the antioxidant action of narrowband ultraviolet B phototherapy," *Journal of International Medical Research*, vol. 42, pp. 799–805, 2014.

[29] B. X. Zhang, M. Lin, X. Y. Qi et al., "Characterization of circulating CD8+T cells expressing skin homing and cytotoxic molecules in active non-segmental vitiligo," *European Journal of Dermatology*, vol. 23, no. 3, pp. 331–338, 2013.

[30] A. van den Driessche, V. Eenkhoorn, L. van Gaal, and C. de Block, "Type 1 diabetes and autoimmune polyglandular syndrome: a clinical review," *Netherlands Journal of Medicine*, vol. 67, no. 11, pp. 376–387, 2009.

[31] G. J. Kahaly, "Polyendocrine autoimmune syndromes," *European Journal of Endocrinology*, vol. 61, pp. 11–20, 2009.

[32] G. Petrovski, M. Zivkovic, T. Milenkovic, I. Ahmeti, and I. Bitovska, "Successful desensitization in patient with type 2 diabetes with an insulin allergy using insulin pump and glargine," *Acta Diabetologica*, 2014.

[33] C. Hasselmann, C. Pecquet, E. Bismuth et al., "Continuous subcutaneous insulin infusion allows tolerance induction and diabetes treatment in a type 1 diabetic child with insulin allergy," *Diabetes & Metabolism*, vol. 39, no. 2, pp. 174–177, 2013.

[34] M. P. Aujero, S. Brooks, N. Li, and S. Venna, "Severe serum sickness-like type III reaction to insulin detemir," *Journal of the American Academy of Dermatology*, vol. 64, no. 6, pp. e127–e128, 2011.

[35] S. Ghosh, V. McCann, L. Bartle, A. Collier, and I. Malik, "Allergy to insulin detemir," *Diabetic Medicine*, vol. 24, no. 11, p. 1307, 2007.

[36] H. Takatsuki, H. Ishii, T. Yamauchi et al., "A case of insulin allergy: the crystalline human insulin may mask its antigenicity," *Diabetes Research and Clinical Practice*, vol. 12, no. 2, pp. 137–139, 1991.

[37] C. Blanco, R. Castillo, J. Quiralte et al., "Anaphylaxis to subcutaneous neutral protamine Hagedorn insulin with simultaneous sensitization to protamine and insulin," *Allergy: European Journal of Allergy and Clinical Immunology*, vol. 51, no. 6, pp. 421–424, 1996.

[38] M. A. Mollar-Puchades and I. L. Villanueva, "Insulin glulisine in the treatment of allergy to rapid acting insulin and its rapid

acting analogs," *Diabetes Research and Clinical Practice*, vol. 83, no. 1, pp. e21–e22, 2009.

[39] L. Heinzerling, K. Raile, H. Rochlitz, T. Zuberbier, and M. Worm, "Insulin allergy: clinical manifestations and management strategies," *Allergy*, vol. 63, no. 2, pp. 148–155, 2008.

[40] M. F. Madero, J. Sastre, J. Carnés, S. Quirce, and J. L. Herrera-Pombo, "IgG4-mediated allergic reaction to glargine insulin," *Allergy*, vol. 61, no. 8, pp. 1022–1023, 2006.

[41] M. Asai, M. Yoshida, and Y. Miura, "Immunologic tolerance to intravenously injected insulin," *The New England Journal of Medicine*, vol. 354, no. 3, pp. 307–309, 2006.

[42] V. M. Cambuli, M. Incani, E. Cossu et al., "Prevalence of type 1 diabetes autoantibodies (GADA, IA2, and IAA) in overweight and obese children," *Diabetes Care*, vol. 33, no. 4, pp. 820–822, 2010.

[43] B. Bruni, P. Barolo, G. Gadaleta et al., "HLA typing and insulin antibody production in insulin-dependent diabetics," *Annali dell'Ospedale Maria Vittoria di Torino*, vol. 27, no. 7–12, pp. 185–213, 1984.

[44] C. R. Kahn, D. Mann, A. S. Rosenthal, J. A. Galloway, A. H. Johnson, and N. Mendell, "The immune response to insulin in man. Interaction of HLA alloantigens and the development of the immune response," *Diabetes*, vol. 31, no. 8, pp. 716–723, 1982.

[45] R. L. Mandelcorn-Monson, N. H. Shear, E. Yau et al., "Cytotoxic T lymphocyte reactivity to gp100, MelanA/MART-1, and tyrosinase, in HLA-A2-positive vitiligo patients," *Journal of Investigative Dermatology*, vol. 121, no. 3, pp. 550–556, 2003.

[46] A. Bouayad, L. Benzekri, S. Hamada, C. Brick, B. Hassam, and M. Essakalli, "Association of HLA alleles and haplotypes with vitiligo in Moroccan patients: a case-control study," *Archives of Dermatological Research*, vol. 305, no. 10, pp. 925–932, 2013.

[47] A. Singh, P. Sharma, H. K. Kar et al., "HLA alleles and amino-acid signatures of the peptide-binding pockets of HLA molecules in vitiligo," *The Journal of Investigative Dermatology*, vol. 132, no. 1, pp. 124–134, 2012.

[48] P. van Endert, Y. Hassainya, V. Lindo et al., "HLA class I epitope discovery in type 1 diabetes," *Annals of the New York Academy of Sciences*, vol. 1079, pp. 190–197, 2006.

[49] A. Huber, F. Menconi, S. Corathers, E. M. Jacobson, and Y. Tomer, "Joint genetic susceptibility to type 1 diabetes and autoimmune thyroiditis: from epidemiology to mechanisms," *Endocrine Reviews*, vol. 29, no. 6, pp. 697–725, 2008.

[50] H.-W. Lee, K.-B. Hahm, J. S. Lee, Y.-S. Ju, K. M. Lee, and K. W. Lee, "Association of the human leukocyte antigen class II alleles with chronic atrophic gastritis and gastric carcinoma in Koreans," *Journal of Digestive Diseases*, vol. 10, no. 4, pp. 265–271, 2009.

[51] A. M. Oksanen, K. E. Haimila, H. I. K. Rautelin, and J. A. Partanen, "Immunogenetic characteristics of patients with autoimmune gastritis," *World Journal of Gastroenterology*, vol. 16, no. 3, pp. 354–358, 2010.

[52] M. Thomsen, F. Jørgensen, M. Brandsborg et al., "Association of pernicious anemia and intrinsic factor antibody with HLA-D," *Tissue Antigens*, vol. 17, no. 1, pp. 97–103, 1981.

[53] R. Krysiak, I. Kobielusz-Gembala, and B. Okopień, "Atypical clinical presentation of autoimmune polyglandular syndrome type 4," *Przegląd Lekarski*, vol. 68, no. 6, pp. 339–341, 2011.

[54] Y.-T. Hsu, J.-R. Duann, M.-K. Lu, M.-C. Sun, and C.-H. Tsai, "Polyglandular autoimmune syndrome type 4 with GAD antibody and dystonia," *Clinical Neurology and Neurosurgery*, vol. 114, no. 7, pp. 1024–1026, 2012.

34

Differentiation between Celiac Disease, Nonceliac Gluten Sensitivity, and Their Overlapping with Crohn's Disease: A Case Series

Aristo Vojdani[1,2] and David Perlmutter[3]

[1] Deptartment of Immunology, Immunosciences Lab., Inc., Los Angeles, CA 90035, USA
[2] Cyrex Laboratories, Phoenix, AZ 85015, USA
[3] Perlmutter Health Center, Naples, FL 34102, USA

Correspondence should be addressed to Aristo Vojdani; drari@msn.com

Academic Editors: N. Martinez-Quiles, M. T. Perez-Gracia, and H. L. Trivedi

Celiac disease (CD) and nonceliac gluten sensitivity (NCGS) are two distinct conditions triggered by the ingestion of gliadin. Although symptoms of nonceliac gluten sensitivity may resemble those of celiac disease, due to the lack of objective diagnostic tests, NCGS is associated with overlapping symptomatologies of autoimmunities and Crohn's disease. Furthermore, a gluten-free diet is only recommended for those who meet the criteria for a diagnosis of CD. Unfortunately, that leaves many nonceliac gluten-sensitive people suffering unnecessarily from very serious symptoms that put them at risk for complications of autoimmune disorders that might be resolved with a gluten-free diet. Thus, a new paradigm is needed for aid in diagnosing and distinguishing among various gut-related diseases, including CD, NCGS (also known as silent celiac disease), and gut-related autoimmunities. Herein, we report three different cases: the first, an elderly patient with celiac disease which was diagnosed based on signs and symptoms of malabsorption and by a proper lab test; second, a case of NCGS which was initially misdiagnosed as lupus but was detected as NCGS by a proper lab test with its associated autoimmunities, including gluten ataxia and neuromyelitis optica; third, a patient with NCGS overlapping with Crohn's disease. The symptomatologies of all three patients improved significantly after 12 months of gluten-free diet plus other modalities.

1. Introduction

Wheat allergy, celiac disease (CD), and nonceliac gluten sensitivity (NCGS) are three distinct conditions that are triggered by the ingestion of wheat gliadin [1–3]. In these conditions, the reaction to gluten is mediated by both cellular and humoral immune responses, resulting in the presentation of different symptomatologies. For example, in wheat allergy a specific sequence of gliadin peptides cross-links two IgE molecules on the surface of mast cells and basophils that trigger the release of mediators such as histamines and leukotrienes [4].

Celiac disease (CD) is an autoimmune condition with known genetic makeup and environmental triggers, such as gliadin peptides. CD affects between 1-2% of the general population.

Markers for confirming a diagnosis of this disorder are IgA against native, deamidated gliadin peptides, and IgA antitissue transglutaminase (tTg) autoantibody. In comparison with CD, nonceliac gluten sensitivity (NCGS) may affect from 6 to 7% of the population, [5–7]. According to two articles published in 2010 and 2011 by Sapone et al. [5, 6], symptoms in GS may resemble some of the gastrointestinal symptoms that are associated with CD or wheat allergy, but it is emphasized that objective diagnostic tests for nonceliac gluten sensitivity are currently missing [5, 6]. While studying the innate and immune responses in CD compared to those in NCGS, the researchers found that TLR1, TLR2, and TLR4, which are associated with innate immunity, were elevated in mucosal NCGS but not in CD, while biomarkers of adaptive immunity such as IFN-γ, IL-21, and IL-17A were expressed in mucosal tissue in CD but not NCGS. They believed that measurements of toll-like receptors and IFN-γ, IL-21, and IL-17A would enable them to differentiate between CD and NCGS [5, 6] with a method that is highly invasive and would require a biopsy. Immediate type 1 hypersensitivity to gluten is IgE mediated, while delayed type hypersensitivity to gluten is an antibody- (IgG, IgA) and T-cell-mediated reaction, which is called celiac disease or nonceliac gluten sensitivity with enteropathy [8]. In the absence of IgG and IgA against tTg, elevated IgG and IgA against various wheat antigens and peptides indicate the loss of mucosal immune tolerance against wheat peptides and the development of nonceliac gluten sensitivity [8]. Due to antigenic similarities between wheat antigens and human tissue, both CD and NCGS can result in many autoimmune conditions, including type 1 diabetes, arthritis, thyroiditis, and even neuroautoimmune conditions such as gluten ataxia and multiple sclerosis [9–11].

While NCGS patients, similar to CD patients, are unable to tolerate gluten and can develop the same or similar sets of gastrointestinal symptoms, in NCGS this immune reaction does not lead to small intestine damage [5, 6]. This lack of induction of intestinal damage in NCGS and the association of CD with genetic markers HLA DQ2/DQ8 plus small intestinal damage make the diagnosis of CD much easier than NCGS. The less severe clinical picture in NCGS, the absence of tTg autoantibodies, and the dismissal of the significance of elevated IgG and IgA autoantibodies against various wheat proteins and peptides by many clinicians make NCGS an extremely dangerous disorder. This is because the persistence of IgG and/or IgA antibodies in the blood for long periods of time along with inducers of inflammatory cascades can result in full-blown autoimmunity. If this were to be the case, due to the severity of the resulting tissue damage, even implementation of a gluten-free diet (GFD) might not be able to help reverse the course of the autoimmune reaction induced by IgG and IgA antibodies against different wheat antigens and peptides.

Several studies have evaluated the possible neurological complications of CD, with emphasis on both the central nervous system and peripheral nervous system, particularly the involvement of small fiber neuropathy that seems to play a more important role in the pathogenesis of neurological complications of CD [9–16]. In some of these studies, the important finding was made that some patients who adopted a GFD and had CD in good remission still had an increased risk of clinical or subclinical neuropathy despite good adherence to the GFD [14]. These data reinforce the previous report of Volta et al., in which peripheral nervous disorders persisted in a 46-year-old female but improved significantly in a 38-year-old female despite a GFD [15]. This means that the duration of exposure to wheat antigens and antibody reactivity against the central and peripheral nervous systems, in particular cerebellar and ganglioside antibodies, plays a significant role in the recovery of patients from neurological manifestations of gluten reactivity after a GFD [10].

Similar results have been described for the association between CD and antineuronal antibodies. Their prevalence ranges from 22.22 to 61% in adults [10, 14], whereas in children the prevalence is about 5% [16]. The interesting finding of these reports is that in most cases these antibodies did not disappear after adoption of a GFD, except in a child reported by Briani et al. [16]. However, in their already mentioned study, Volta et al. [15] described the disappearance of antibodies within 1 year in most patients, as well as the regression of these antibodies in pediatric CD patients. Contrarily, in a more recent report [12], antineuronal antibodies did not disappear in any of the adult CD patients and in fact correlated with the persistence of neurological picture.

This raises the question: why does the GFD seem to work in some cases and not in others? Why do antineuronal antibodies disappear a year after implementation of a GFD in some patients and not in others? The first hypothesis is that 12 months may be sufficient for mucosal recovery but not for gluten-associated pathological conditions. But it is also possible that persistence of antibodies, as well as persistence of neurological symptoms, may be related to the duration of gluten exposure. There may be a first stage of neurological disease in CD when it is still gluten sensitive. During this stage a GFD may still result in both regression of neurological symptoms and the disappearance of antineuronal antibodies. The succeeding more advanced stage may, however, be considered gluten insensitive; in this phase both neurological symptoms and antineuronal antibodies persist despite a GFD, perhaps due to autoimmunity resulting from gluten. Thus, the key to explaining this apparent inconsistency in the efficacy of a GFD may be the duration of gluten ingestion [12].

Since, then, as in many autoimmune disorders the key seems to be the duration of exposure to the environmental triggers, in this case gluten exposure, our recommendation is to use the most sensitive biomarkers to diagnose CD or NCGS as early as possible, because in many adult patients delays in the diagnosis may cause severe and irreversible damage to various tissues, including the central and peripheral nervous systems [12, 17].

A comparison between celiac disease and gluten immune reactivity/sensitivity is shown in Figure 1. According to this model, if two children, one with a negative genetic makeup (HLA DQ2/DQ8$^-$), and the other with positive (HLA DQ2/DQ8$^+$), are exposed to environmental factors, such as Rota virus, bacterial endotoxins, and some medications or their synergistic effects, the result can be a breakdown of mucosal immune tolerance in both children. The induction of mucosal immune tolerance against gliadin results in the production of IgA and/or IgG against native wheat proteins and peptides.

However, in the individual with the positive genetic makeup, the IgG and IgA antibodies against gliadin along with biomarkers of inflammation can activate tTg, induce damage to the villi, and result in villous atrophy. Deamidation of a specific gliadin peptide leads to the formation of a complex between it and the tTg; the presentation of this complex by antigen-presenting cells to T cells and B cells results in IgA or IgG production against tTg, deamidated gliadin, and the gliadin-tTg complex. The formation of these antibodies and their detection in blood is the hallmark of CD, which is an inherited condition detected in 1-2% of the population. If CD is left untreated, the outcome could be autoimmunities and cancer.

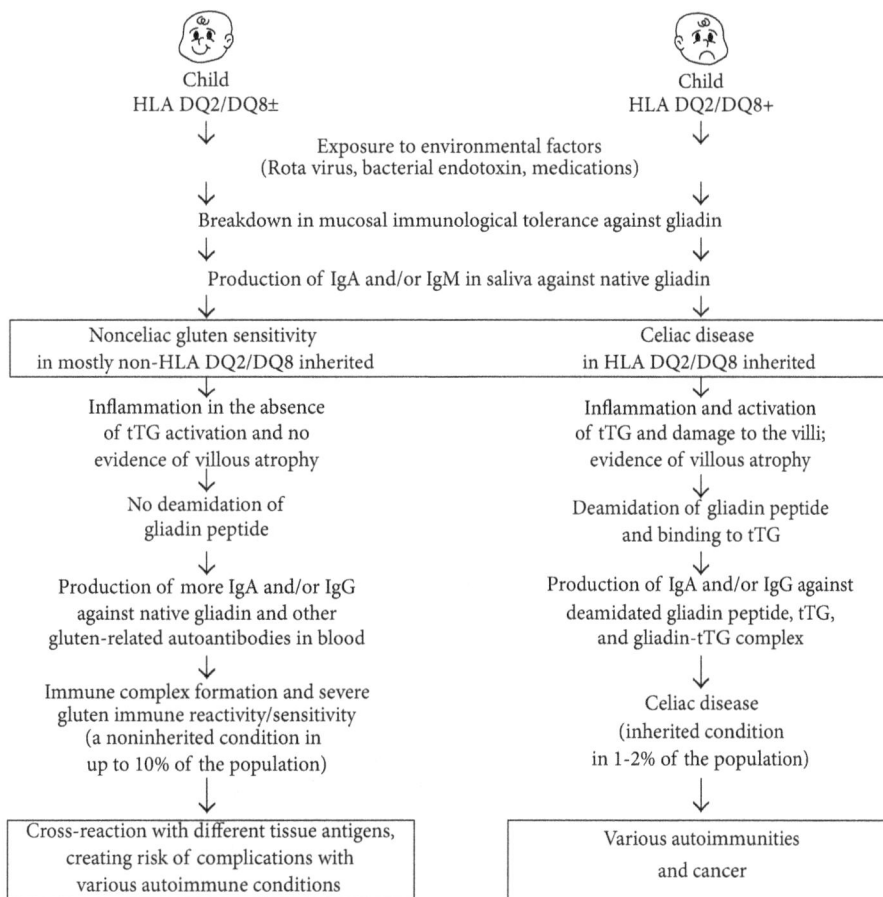

FIGURE 1: Differentiation between nonceliac gluten sensitivity and celiac disease.

In comparison, in an individual negative for HLA DQ2/DQ8, this breakdown in immunological tolerance and the concomitant production of IgA and or IgG against native wheat proteins and peptides may activate an inflammatory cascade. In the absence of tTg activation, however, villous atrophy does not occur. Furthermore, gliadin peptides do not go through deamidation, and consequently IgG and IgA antibodies are produced only against native wheat and gliadin peptides.

With continuous exposure to wheat antigens and continuous mucosal immune tolerance, the wheat antigens and reacting antibodies form an unholy alliance of immune complexes, resulting in severe NCGS. This immune reactivity and sensitivity are a noninherited condition detected in up to 10% of the population. If this disorder is left unchecked, prolonged exposure to IgG and IgA antibodies against wheat antigens and peptides and their cross-reaction with different tissue antigens can result in various autoimmune disorders.

2. Materials and Methods

The ELISA methodology for measuring antibodies against various wheat proteomes and tissue antigens has been described previously [17]. Briefly, the microwell plates were prepared and coated with the desired number of wheat-associated antigens and/or peptides. Calibrator and positive controls and diluted patient samples were added to the wells and autoantibodies recognizing different wheat antigens bound during the first incubation. After washing the wells to remove all unbound proteins, purified alkaline phosphatase-labeled rabbit anti-human IgG/IgA was added; unbound conjugate was then removed by a further wash step.

Bound conjugate was visualized with paranitrophenyl phosphate (PNPP) substrate, which gives a yellow reaction product; the intensity of which is proportional to the concentration of autoantibody in the sample. Sodium hydroxide was added to each well to stop the reaction. The intensity of color was read at 405 nm.

3. Case Study Examples

Three different case reports, the first on a patient with celiac disease, the second with nonceliac gluten sensitivity and autoimmunity, and the third with nonceliac gluten sensitivity overlapping with Crohn's disease are shown next.

3.1. Case Report No. 1: Diagnosis of Celiac Disease in the Elderly by the Use of IgA against Gliadin and Tissue Transglutaminase with Improvement on a Gluten-Free Diet. A 76-year-old man with longstanding dyspepsia, indigestion, tiredness, and rapid weight loss was referred for gastrointestinal evaluation. Blood tests showed macrocytic anemia with low concentrations of folate and vitamin B-12. The patient's hemoglobin concentration was 7.9 g/dL, albumin 32 g/L, and transglutaminase 212 mg/mL (normal range = 0–10 mg/mL). An urgent colonoscopy and duodenal biopsy were performed, which yielded macroscopically normal results. At this level his IgG and IgA concentrations against gliadin and transglutaminase were checked using FDA-approved kits. Both IgG and IgA against α-gliadin were very high; against transglutaminase, IgA but not IgG was 3.8-fold higher than the reference range. In view of the IgA positivity against gliadin and transglutaminase and diagnosis of celiac disease he was transfused with 2 units of packed cells and started on both a gluten-free diet and 20 mg of prednisone daily. Six months later he had gained about 12 pounds and showed few GI symptoms. Because of this improvement the patient became committed to the GFD. One year after the first performance of IgG and IgA antibody testing against gliadin and transglutaminase the repeat tests for these antibodies were negative, which is a further indication that disease management plus a GFD was instrumental in the treatment of this elderly patient with silent celiac disease.

3.1.1. Discussion.

According to Catassi et al. [1, 18], celiac disease (CD) is one of the most common lifelong disorders in western countries. However, most cases of CD remain undiagnosed mostly due to the poor awareness of the primary care physician regarding this important affliction. Celiac disease is perceived as presenting GI symptoms accompanied by malabsorption. But many patients with celiac disease do not present GI symptoms. These individuals may have silent or atypical celiac disease, and the condition may present with iron deficiency, anemia, increased liver enzymes, osteoporosis, or neurological symptoms [19]. As used herein, the term "atypical celiac disease" refers to celiac disease in patients who have only subtle symptoms, and the term "silent celiac disease" refers to celiac disease in patients who are asymptomatic.

The increasing recognition of celiac disease is attributed to the use of new serological assays with higher sensitivity and specificity. Until recently celiac disease was incorrectly perceived as being uncommon and detected mainly during infancy or childhood. However, it is now recognized that most cases of CD occur in adults 40–60 years old. Patients in this age group may present their symptoms, lab test results, and other examination signs in atypical fashion. In fact, according to a very recent publication, less than one in seven patients is correctly diagnosed with CD [20].

Consequently, as this case shows, if an adult patient presents with symptoms and signs suggesting malabsorption, testing for IgA antibody against gliadin and transglutaminase should be considered. If the test results are positive, celiac diseases should then be made a part of the differential diagnosis, based on which a gluten-free diet should be recommended. If the gluten-free diet should produce an improvement in symptoms, the patient should commit to the diet regardless of age.

3.2. Case Report No. 2: A Patient with Nonceliac Gluten Sensitivity and Autoimmunity.

Here, a case report is described in which the original presentation led to an erroneous diagnosis of irritable bowel syndrome, resulting in incorrect medical intervention. The correct diagnosis of nonceliac gluten sensitivity (NCGS) was made after years of mistreatment. A 49-year-old woman with abdominal pain, constipation, acid reflux, and headache was examined by an internist. Investigation revealed normal CBC with hemoglobin of 10.8 g/dL and normal chemistry profile including liver enzyme. Over several visits detailed biochemical and immunological profiles including ANA, rheumatoid factor, T3, T4, and TSH levels were performed, all testing within the normal range. After repeated complaints about GI discomfort, the patient was referred for GI evaluation. Both endoscopy and *H. pylori* test results were normal. The patient was diagnosed with irritable bowel syndrome and put on β-blockers and esomeprazole magnesium, which moderately improved her symptomatologies. Four years later, however, in addition to the old GI symptoms and headache, she presented symptoms of malaise, blurred vision, and facial rash. She was intermittently sleepy and irritable and experienced breathing problems. Further lab tests revealed that her hemoglobin was 9.7 g/dL with MCV of 72 fL, a raised erythrocyte sedimentation rate at 46 mm/1st hour (normal range 0–20 mm/1st hour), ANA of 1 : 80 (normal range < 40), mild elevation in IgA smooth muscle antibody, double-stranded DNA, and extractable nuclear antibodies were negative. Based on the available evidence, a diagnosis of systemic lupus erythematosus (SLE) was made by a rheumatologist, and treatment with steroids was commenced. There was some improvement in her overall state but her hemoglobin level continued to be low, while her ESR fluctuated. Two years later she developed difficulty in passing urine accompanied by tingling and sensory disturbance in her trunk and legs, which led to her being referred to a neurologist. The patient reported a band-like sensation in the trunk and reduced visual acuity (8/46 in the right eye, 8/23 in the left eye) with minimal eye pain but normal eye movement. Lab investigation revealed low hemoglobin, abnormal MCV, and low serum ferritin at 14 mg/L (normal range 10–150 mg/L), which confirmed iron deficiency. MRI scan of the brain showed extensive white matter abnormalities not typical of multiple sclerosis, and no abnormalities were detected in CSF examination. Blood and CSF examination showed no evidence of bacterial and viral infection including syphilis, mycobacteria, borrelia, EBV, CMV, HTLV, and herpes type-6. Visual evoked potentials showed delay in both optic nerves. In view of these abnormalities, and since tests for nonceliac gluten sensitivity had not been performed during the earlier investigations, the possibility of nonceliac gluten sensitivity was considered. A comprehensive IgG and IgA panel was ordered against a repertoire of wheat proteins and peptides, as well as against tTg and various tissue antigens. This comprehensive nonceliac gluten sensitivity and immune reactivity screen revealed IgG against wheat

TABLE 1: IgG and IgA antibody patterns of a patient with gluten immune reactivity/sensitivity/autoimmunity reacting against various wheat antigens, peptides, and tissue antigens expressed as optical density with calculation of indices.

	Wheat antigens	Alpha gliadin 33 mer	Alpha gliadin 17 mer	Gamma Gliadin 15 mer	Omega Gliadin 17 mer	Glutenin 21 mer	Gluteomorphin	Prodynorphin	Gliadin-tTg complex	*tTg	Wheat germ agglutinin	**GAD-65
						IgG						
Cal 1	0.33	0.42	0.34	0.33	0.38	0.38	0.36	0.35	0.33	0.35	0.35	0.36
Cal 2	0.36	0.48	0.36	0.38	0.42	0.44	0.39	0.40	0.45	0.38	0.38	0.43
(OD)	3.85	2.44	2.38	3.86	2.41	2.50	3.86	2.49	1.49	1.00	3.86	3.88
	3.85	2.36	2.33	3.86	2.40	2.40	3.86	2.40	1.58	0.96	3.86	3.87
Index	**11.10**	**5.33**	**6.81**	**10.79**	**6.05**	**5.99**	**10.23**	**6.60**	**3.91**	**2.69**	**10.59**	**9.79**
Ref. range	1.3	1.4	1.5	1.5	1.6	1.5	1.5	1.7	1.6	1.4	1.5	1.3
						IgA						
Cal 1	0.392	0.462	0.401	0.368	0.400	0.449	0.467	0.445	0.400	0.430	0.485	0.397
Cal 2	0.421	0.462	0.414	0.379	0.418	0.453	0.479	0.481	0.392	0.402	0.455	0.404
(OD)	3.862	0.429	0.350	0.208	0.364	0.269	0.401	0.336	0.335	0.438	3.868	0.359
	3.828	0.426	0.397	0.245	0.325	0.290	0.546	0.372	0.360	0.473	3.833	0.438
Index	**9.459**	**0.925**	**0.917**	**0.606**	**0.842**	**0.620**	**1.001**	**0.765**	**0.878**	**1.095**	**8.193**	**0.995**
Ref. range	2.4	1.8	2.0	1.9	1.8	1.7	1.8	1.8	1.6	1.5	1.9	1.5

*Transglutaminase.
**Glutamic acid decarboxylase.
Index = mean OD of patients/mean OD of calibrators.

TABLE 2: IgG and IgA antibody patterns of a Patient with crohn's disease reacting against various wheat antigens, peptides, and tissue antigens expressed as optical density with calculation of indices.

	Wheat antigens	Alpha gliadin 33 mer	Alpha gliadin 17 mer	Gamma gliadin 15 mer	Omega gliadin 17 mer	Glutenin 21 mer	Gluteomorphin	Prodynorphin	Gliadin-tTg complex	*tTg	Wheat germ agglutinin	**GAD-65
IgG												
Cal 1	0.45	0.41	0.38	0.39	0.36	0.39	0.55	0.47	0.71	0.49	0.41	0.55
Cal 2	0.38	0.33	0.44	0.44	0.37	0.40	0.54	0.56	0.60	0.49	0.48	0.46
(OD)	3.86	3.79	3.86	3.67	3.85	3.24	3.84	3.86	1.71	3.80	3.82	3.84
(OD)	3.84	3.79	3.84	3.59	3.85	3.25	3.83	3.83	1.73	3.74	3.80	3.59
Index	9.31	10.23	9.33	8.67	10.51	8.22	7.03	7.43	2.62	7.71	8.60	7.34
Ref. range	1.3	1.4	1.5	1.5	1.6	1.5	1.5	1.7	1.6	1.4	1.5	1.3
IgA												
Cal 1	0.37	0.39	0.40	0.39	0.43	0.43	0.46	0.47	0.41	0.42	0.48	0.42
Cal 2	0.45	0.44	0.46	0.42	0.47	0.51	0.54	0.50	0.48	0.48	0.49	0.47
(OD)	3.89	3.56	0.99	0.99	2.25	1.05	1.12	3.85	1.00	1.18	3.73	3.87
(OD)	3.89	3.48	0.99	0.99	2.25	1.03	1.10	3.82	0.99	1.20	3.83	3.85
Index	9.48	8.43	2.27	2.45	4.98	2.20	2.23	7.90	2.25	2.65	7.79	8.69
Ref. range	2.4	1.8	2.0	1.9	1.8	1.7	1.8	1.8	1.6	1.5	1.9	1.5

*Transglutaminase.
**Glutamic acid decarboxylase.
Index = mean OD of patients÷mean OD of calibrators.

antigens, α-gliadin 33 and 17 mer, γ- and ω-gliadin, glutenin, gluteomorphin, prodynorphin, gliadin-tTg complex, wheat germ agglutinin, and glutamic acid decarboxylase 65 (GAD-65). IgA antibodies were detected against wheat antigens and wheat germ agglutinin (see Table 1). Interestingly, both IgG and in particular IgA tested against tTg were within the normal range.

Furthermore, antibodies against ganglioside, cerebellar, synapsin, myelin basic protein, collagen, thyroglobulin, thyroid peroxidase, and aquaporin-4 were tested, and all were 2–4 fold above the reference range. Upper GI endoscopy and biopsy revealed normal histology and intraepithelial lymphocytes. Overall the patient was diagnosed as having nonceliac gluten sensitivity with its associated autoimmunities, including gluten ataxia, headache, white matter abnormalities, and neuromyelitis optica. A five-day course of intravenous methylprednisolone was implemented, and gradually the sensory, motor, and visual symptoms improved. In addition, based on the very high levels of IgG and some IgA antibodies against a repertoire of wheat antigens and peptides, a gluten-free diet was introduced, and 12 weeks later marked improvement was observed in the patient's clinical symptomatology. She continued the 100% gluten-free diet under the observation of a dietitian, and the steroid treatment was stopped. Six months after introduction of the diet antibody tests against wheat antigens, peptides, and human tissue were repeated; more than 60% reduction in some antibody levels was observed, and the patient became almost asymptomatic.

3.2.1. Discussion. From this data we concluded that a patient may suffer from NCGS without having abnormal tissue histology or flat erosive gastritis and antibody against tTg based on which a diagnosis of celiac disease is normally made. If patients with NCGS are not detected in time based on the proper lab tests, in particular IgG and IgA antibodies against a repertoire of wheat proteins and peptides, patients' symptomatologies may mislead many clinicians into treating their patients for lupus, MS-like syndrome, neuromyelitis optica, and many other autoimmune disorders. Therefore, measurement of IgG and IgA antibodies against a repertoire of wheat antigens, peptides, and neuronal antigens is recommended for patients with signs and symptoms of autoimmunities so that intervention with a gluten-free diet will be instrumental in reversing the autoimmune conditions associated with NCGS. Otherwise, untreated and/or mistreated, the patient may develop multiple autoimmune disorders.

3.3. Case Report No. 3: A Patient with Nonceliac Gluten Sensitivity Overlapping with Crohn's Disease. Crohn's disease is an inflammatory disorder that often emerges during the second or third decade of life, affecting the terminal ileum in more than two-thirds of patients [21]. A combination of genetic and environmental factors, including a shift in gut microbiota and dysfunctional responses against them, is believed to lead to dysregulated immunity, altered intestinal barrier function, and possibly autoimmunity [22].

A 32-year-old man presented with gastrointestinal discomfort and diarrhea 2-3 times per month. Laboratory results including chemistry panel, CBC, iron, ferritin, transferrin, vitamin B-12, thyroid function, and urine analysis were within the median level of the normal range. Upon the second visit and continuation of GI symptoms he was referred to a GI specialist who ordered additional lab examinations, including microbiological evaluation of the stool and blood tests for antibodies against *H. pylori, Saccharomyces,* and gliadin. Stool testing for *Salmonella, Shigella, Yersinia, Campylobacter,* enteropathogenic and enterohemorrhagic *E. coli,* or *Clostridium difficile* came out negative. Regarding antibody examinations in the blood, IgG against *H. pylori* and IgA against Saccharomyces and gliadin were negative, but IgG against gliadin was moderately elevated at 59 U/mL (normal value $\leq$ 20 U/mL). The IgG antibody elevations were considered nonspecific or protective, and the patient was put on painkillers and sent home with no diagnosis of any specific disorder.

Three years later after seeing the frequency of the watery diarrhea increase to 3–5 times daily and losing 12 pounds of his body weight in the last two months, the patient went to another GI specialist for a second opinion. Gastric and duodenal biopsies were performed. While the endoscopy of the upper GI tract revealed gastritis of the antrum, histologically, gastric and duodenal biopsy turned out to be negative. D-xylose absorption test was performed; the resulting value of 1.89 g/5 h in urine was suggestive of malabsorption. Immunoserologically ANA titers were below 1 : 40, p-ANCA and c-ANCA were negative, but the IgA anti-*Saccharomyces* antigen (ASCA) was positive at 85 U/mL (normal $\leq$ 10 U/mL). Based on the increased frequency of watery diarrhea, abnormal D-xylose absorption, and positive IgA anti-ASCA, the diagnosis of Crohn's disease was made. A therapeutical trial using cholestyramine was initiated, but the frequency of the diarrhea remained unchanged. In addition the patient was treated with 230 mg of methylprednisolone and 2 × 1000 mg of mesalazine. Two years after this treatment the patient developed enteroenteric fistulae in the terminal ileum with sigmoid affection. After admission to the hospital, ileocolectomy was performed, and 22 cm of the ileum was resected. Upon his release remission maintenance with 3 × 500 mg of mesalazine was implemented.

For eight years following this treatment the patient continued to suffer from increasing frequency of watery diarrhea and lost an additional 14 pounds. During this period several additional treatment attempts were made using aspirin, loperamide, and budesonide, unfortunately without significant clinical improvement. Furthermore, the patient was losing more weight on a monthly basis. A complete review of the medical history revealed the fact that almost thirteen years earlier, gliadin IgG antibody had been found to be elevated, which was considered normal at the time. Since all classical treatments for Crohn's disease had failed to improve the clinical picture over all the years, a comprehensive test for the assessment of gluten immune reactivity and sensitivity was ordered. This included IgG and IgA against wheat, native, and deamidated α-gliadin peptides, γ-gliadin, ω-gliadin, glutenin, gluteomorphin, prodynorphin, gliadin-tTg complex, transglutaminase, wheat germ agglutinin, and GAD-65.

Results depicted in Table 2 show that the patient had a significant elevation of IgG antibodies against 11 out of 12 tested antigens, and IgA antibodies against wheat, α-gliadin 33 mer, ω-gliadin, prodynorphin, wheat germ agglutinin, and GAD-65 were detected at 2–5 fold above the normal range. Based on these results, in addition to Crohn's disease a diagnosis of nonceliac gluten sensitivity was also made. A diet consisting of rice, potato, and other gluten-free/yeast-free foods was commenced immediately, which led after six weeks to a complete cessation of diarrhea. Upon continuation of the gluten-free diet, not only did stool consistency become normal, but the patient also started gaining weight. On followup one year later the patient was back to a normal state and had regained more than 80% of his lost weight.

3.3.1. Discussion. This case demonstrates the association of Crohn's disease with nonceliac gluten sensitivity but not with celiac disease. Based on the impressive clinical response to the gluten-free diet plus the detection of IgG and IgA antibodies against various wheat antigens, and upon re-evaluation of the IgG antibody level detected 14 years earlier, the diagnosis of Crohn's disease with secondary malabsorption and NCGS was finally established. Since IgG antibodies against gliadin but not transglutaminase were detected, it can be argued that in this patient the disease was initiated with nonceliac gluten sensitivity and not Crohn's disease.

It is contemplated herein that continuous exposure to environmental factors, such as wheat antigen-induced inflammation for a prolonged period of time, may result in inflammatory bowel disease or Crohn's disease.

4. Conclusions Regarding Case Reports

The case studies presented demonstrate the importance of expanding the understanding of the etiology and pathophysiology of the autoimmune disorders described and highlight the utility of novel laboratory evaluations described herein.

Disclosure

Dr. A. Vojdani is the CEO and coowner of Immunosciences Lab., Inc. in Los Angeles, CA, USA. Dr. D. Permutter is a board-certified neurologist and is the medical director of the Perlmutter Health Center in Naples, FL, USA.

References

[1] C. Catassi and A. Fasano, "Celiac disease," *Current Opinion in Gastroenterology*, vol. 24, no. 6, pp. 687–691, 2008.

[2] L. A. Anderson, S. A. McMillan, R. G. P. Watson et al., "Malignancy and mortality in a population-based cohort of patients with coeliac disease or 'gluten sensitivity'," *World Journal of Gastroenterology*, vol. 13, no. 1, pp. 146–151, 2007.

[3] J. F. Ludvigsson, D. A. Leffler, and J. C. Bai, "The Oslo definitions for coeliac disease and related terms," *Gut*, vol. 62, pp. 43–45, 2013.

[4] S. Tanabe, "Analysis of food allergen structures and development of foods for allergic patients," *Bioscience, Biotechnology and Biochemistry*, vol. 72, no. 3, pp. 649–659, 2008.

[5] A. Sapone, K. M. Lammers, G. Mazzarella et al., "Differential mucosal IL-17 expression in two gliadin-induced disorders: gluten sensitivity and the autoimmune enteropathy celiac disease," *International Archives of Allergy and Immunology*, vol. 152, no. 1, pp. 75–80, 2010.

[6] A. Sapone, K. M. Lammers, V. Casolaro et al., "Divergence of gut permeability and mucosal immune gene expression in two gluten-associated conditions: celiac disease and gluten sensitivity," *BMC Medicine*, vol. 9, article 23, 2011.

[7] R. L. Chin, N. Latov, P. H. R. Green et al., "Neurological complications of celiac disease," *Journal of Clinical Neuromuscular Disease*, vol. 5, pp. 129–137, 2004.

[8] A. Vojdani, T. O'Bryan, and G. H. Kellermann, "The immunology of immediate and delayed hypersensitivity reaction to gluten," *European Journal of Inflammation*, vol. 6, no. 1, pp. 1–10, 2008.

[9] D. B. A. Shor, O. Barzilai, M. Ram et al., "Non-celiac gluten sensitivity in multiple sclerosis: experimental myth or clinical truth?" *Annals of the New York Academy of Sciences*, vol. 1173, pp. 343–349, 2009.

[10] A. Vojdani, T. O'Bryan, J. A. Green et al., "Immune response to dietary proteins, gliadin and cerebellar peptides in children with autism," *Nutritional Neuroscience*, vol. 7, no. 3, pp. 151–161, 2004.

[11] M. Hadjivassiliou, R. A. Grünewald, M. Lawden, G. A. B. Davies-Jones, T. Powell, and C. M. L. Smith, "Headache and CNS white matter abnormalities associated with gluten sensitivity," *Neurology*, vol. 56, no. 3, pp. 385–388, 2001.

[12] A. Tursi, G. M. Giorgetti, C. Iani et al., "Peripheral neurological disturbances, autonomic dysfunction, and antineuronal antibodies in adult celiac disease before and after a gluten-free diet," *Digestive Diseases and Sciences*, vol. 51, no. 10, pp. 1869–1874, 2006.

[13] G. Holmes, "Neurological and psychiatric complications in celiac disease," in *Epilepsy and Other Neurological Disorders in Celiac Disease*, pp. 251–264, John Libbey, London, UK, 1997.

[14] L. Luostarinen, S. L. Himanen, M. Luostarinen, P. Collin, and T. Pirttilä, "Neuromuscular and sensory disturbances in patients with well treated coeliac disease," *Journal of Neurology Neurosurgery and Psychiatry*, vol. 74, no. 4, pp. 490–494, 2003.

[15] U. Volta, R. De Giorgio, N. Petrolini et al., "Clinical findings and antineuronal antibodies in celiac disease with neurological disorders," *Scandinavian Journal of Gastroenterology*, vol. 37, pp. 1276–1281, 2002.

[16] C. Briani, S. Riggero, G. Zara et al., "Anti-ganglioside antibodies in children with celiac disease: correlation with gluten-free diet and neurological complications," *Alimentary Pharmacology and Therapeutics*, vol. 20, pp. 231–235, 2004.

[17] A. Vojdani, "The characterization of the repertoire of wheat antigens and peptides involved in the humoral immune responses in patients with non-celiac gluten sensitivity and Crohn's disease," *ISRN Allergy*, vol. 2011, Article ID 950104, 12 pages, 2011.

[18] C. Catassi, D. Kryszak, O. Louis-Jacques et al., "Detection of Celiac disease in primary care: a multicenter case20 finding

study in North America," *American Journal of Gastroenterology*, vol. 102, pp. 1454–1460, 2007.

[19] D. S. Sanders, D. P. Hurlstone, M. E. McAlindon et al., "Antibody negative coeliac disease presenting in elderly people-an easily missed diagnosis," *British Medical Journal*, vol. 330, pp. 775–776, 2005.

[20] T. Matthias, S. Neidhofer, S. Pfeiffer et al., "Novel trends in celiac disease," *Cellular and Molecular Immunology*, vol. 8, pp. 121–125, 2011.

[21] C. E. Egan, K. J. Maurer, S. B. Cohen et al., "Synergy between intraepithelial lymphocytes and lamina propria T cells drives intestinal inflammation during infection," *Mucosal Immunology*, vol. 4, pp. 658–670, 2011.

[22] A. Kaser, S. Zeissig, and R. S. Blumberg, "Inflammatory bowel disease," *Annual Review of Immunology*, vol. 28, pp. 573–621, 2010.

35

Increased IL-17, a Pathogenic Link between Hepatosplenic Schistosomiasis and Amyotrophic Lateral Sclerosis: A Hypothesis

Oswald Moling,[1] **Alfonsina Di Summa,**[2] **Loredana Capone,**[2] **Josef Stuefer,**[3] **Andrea Piccin,**[4] **Alessandra Porzia,**[5] **Antonella Capozzi,**[5] **Maurizio Sorice,**[5] **Raffaella Binazzi,**[1] **Lathá Gandini,**[1] **Giovanni Rimenti,**[1] **and Peter Mian**[1]

[1] *Division of Infectious Diseases, Ospedale Generale, 39100 Bolzano, Italy*
[2] *Division of Neurology, Ospedale Generale, 39100 Bolzano, Italy*
[3] *Radiology, Ospedale Generale, 39100 Bolzano, Italy*
[4] *Division of Hematology, Ospedale Generale, 39100 Bolzano, Italy*
[5] *Department of Experimental Medicine, Sapienza University, 00161 Rome, Italy*

Correspondence should be addressed to Oswald Moling; molosw@hotmail.com

Academic Editor: Takahisa Gono

The immune system protects the organism from foreign invaders and foreign substances and is involved in physiological functions that range from tissue repair to neurocognition. However, an excessive or dysregulated immune response can cause immunopathology and disease. A 39-year-old man was affected by severe hepatosplenic schistosomiasis *mansoni* and by amyotrophic lateral sclerosis. One question that arose was, whether there was a relation between the parasitic and the neurodegenerative disease. IL-17, a proinflammatory cytokine, is produced mainly by T helper-17 CD4 cells, a recently discovered new lineage of effector CD4 T cells. Experimental mouse models of schistosomiasis have shown that IL-17 is a key player in the immunopathology of schistosomiasis. There are also reports that suggest that IL-17 might have an important role in the pathogenesis of amyotrophic lateral sclerosis. It is hypothesized that the factors that might have led to increased IL-17 in the hepatosplenic schistosomiasis *mansoni* might also have contributed to the development of amyotrophic lateral sclerosis in the described patient. A multitude of environmental factors, including infections, xenobiotic substances, intestinal microbiota, and vitamin D deficiency, that are able to induce a proinflammatory immune response polarization, might favor the development of amyotrophic lateral sclerosis in predisposed individuals.

1. Introduction

Schistosomiasis is a major tropical parasitic disease caused by blood-dwelling fluke worms of the genus *Schistosoma*. It is contracted by humans when wading in bodies of water contaminated with the free-swimming cercariae, the larval and infective form of the schistosomes, released from aquatic vector snails. Cercariae penetrate the skin, reach the blood circulation, and mature into adult worms and in the case of *Schistosoma mansoni* home to the mesenteric venous vasculature, where male and female mate and lay 100–300 eggs per day [1, 2]. The lifespan of an adult schistosome averages 3–5 years but can be as long as 30 years [3]. The eggs then exit the vasculature to enter the intestinal lumen and are set free in search of appropriate vector snails. However, many eggs embolize and are trapped mostly in the liver (hepatosplenic schistosomiasis), less frequently in the central nervous system (neuroschistosomiasis), where they precipitate an immune reaction of varying degree. Most individuals develop a relative mild "intestinal" schistosomiasis, whereas 5–10% suffer the severe hepatosplenic form of disease, in which there is progressive liver fibrosis, portal hypertension, splenomegaly, esophageal varicose veins, gastrointestinal hemorrhage, and death [4, 5].

Amyotrophic lateral sclerosis (ALS) is a fatal neurodegenerative disease characterized by progressive and selected loss of both upper and lower motor neurons. Patients experience signs and symptoms of progressive muscle atrophy and weakness and increased fatigue, which typically lead to respiratory failure and death. Median survival is 2–4 years from onset; only 1–10% of patients survive beyond 10 years. Less than 10% of ALS cases are familial with 20% of these cases linked to various mutations in the Cu/Zn superoxide dismutase 1 (SOD1) gene [6, 7]. The etiology of ALS is unknown. A wide range of contributing factors including genetic mutations and polymorphisms, oxidative stress, and neuroinflammation have been identified; however the initiating or most relevant ones are unknown [6–12]. There were more than 2000 publications on ALS only in 2013. This growing knowledge will hopefully move towards the discovery of an effective treatment and prevention of this tragic disease. We report on a 39-year-old man who presented with progressive hemiparesis of unknown origin, lupus-like autoimmune phenomena, and a suspected reactivation of *M. tuberculosis* infection. He was subsequently diagnosed as suffering from severe hepatosplenic schistosomiasis *mansoni* and amyotrophic lateral sclerosis. In an attempt to understand the diseases recent advances in immunology were reviewed and it may be that common pathogenic mechanisms might underlie the different diseases.

2. Case Report

A 39-year-old man from Ghana, who had been resident in Italy for five years, was admitted to hospital in April 2013 because of slowly progressive gait disturbances and right hemiparesis which had developed within the last two months. His past medical history was unremarkable. No cerebral vascular lesions were seen neither on magnetic resonance angiography or Doppler sonography. Instead, liver cirrhosis with portal hypertension, esophageal varicose veins, and splenomegaly was detected. He was a mild occasional alcohol drinker and viral hepatitis screening was negative (for laboratory values see Table 1). Hematologic malignancy and leishmaniasis were excluded by bone marrow examination. The presence of antinuclear antibodies, anticardiolipin antibodies detected by TLC immunostaining [13], and lupus anticoagulant, the decrease of the complement factors C3 and C4 were reminiscent of systemic lupus erythematosus (Table 1). Findings of apical scars and calcification of hilar lymph nodes of the right lung detected by computer tomography (CT) and a 15 mm cutaneous tuberculin reaction indicated a *Mycobacterium tuberculosis* infection. Therefore standard antituberculous therapy was initiated, considered also as chemoprophylaxis in the perspective of future corticosteroid treatment. 25-hydroxy-vitamin D 10,000 IU (250 μg) weekly was added to treatment. Sufficient criteria for the diagnosis of systemic lupus erythematosus (SLE) would had been fulfilled [14]; however, such extreme liver and spleen changes as in this patient are not usually seen in SLE.

Indeed, a high titer of anti-*Schistosoma* antibodies was demonstrated. Retrospectively, the ultrasound-, CT-, and

MR-imaging that showed the extensive periportal fibrosis of the liver and the huge spleen with a diameter of 24 cm and unusual spots (Figure 1) turned out to be characteristic for hepatosplenic schistosomiasis *mansoni*. Seven years earlier in the district of Dunkwa in Offin, Ghana, the patient had to wade through water for about 10 minutes daily for more than one year while going to work to cut large trees and requiring physical exertion. Praziquantel 60 mg/kg daily for three days, methyl-prednisolone 1 g daily for five days, and then prednisone 1 mg/kg, tapered in the next three months, were given [15]. Subsequently an improvement in the strength of the right arm was observed for only a few weeks, followed by a worsening of the movement disorder.

Physical examination four months following his first hospitalization revealed muscle weakness also on the left side. There was increased muscle rigidity, hypotrophic thenar muscles of the right hand, hyperreflexia, and spontaneous and triggered muscle fasciculations. Spirometry showed evidenced deficits of the inspiratory and exspiratory musculature. The patient did not report neither sphincter dysfunction nor pain or sensitivity alterations. This pattern was indicative of motor neuron disease and of amyotrophic lateral sclerosis, as were the electromyographic findings. Repeated MRI showed mild diffuse signal hyperintensities of the white matter in the centrum semiovale regions by FLAIR imaging. The gadolinium enhancement of the meninges at the vertebral level D4-D6 was compatible with a reaction to embolized ova of schistosome, but these alterations did not explain the neurological symptoms. Because praziquantel had been given without considering the interaction with rifampin [16], rifampin was stopped. One month later praziquantel was repeated at a dose of 80 mg/kg daily for three days considering the interaction with prednisone [17] at that time given at a dose of 25 mg daily. The movement disorder did not improve despite daily physiotherapy exercises. In the absence of any effective treatment for amyotrophic lateral sclerosis being available to the patient, he returned to Ghana in November 2013.

Thereafter IL-17 has been determined in four serum samples previously stored, which were taken at monthly intervals. IL-17 cytokine was assayed by human-specific ELISA kit (R&D Systems) at the Department of Experimental Medicine, Sapienza University, Rome. The first sample was taken before initiating treatment with praziquantel and high dose corticosteroids. The results were IL-17 672.2 pg/mL, 36.5 pg/mL, <10 pg/mL, and 32.9 pg/mL, respectively, (normal value <31.2 pg/mL).

3. Discussion

3.1. Diagnostic Considerations. According to the new SLICC classification criteria for systemic lupus erythematosus (SLE) at least 4 out of 17 criteria are necessary for the diagnosis of SLE [14]. Of these 17 classification criteria the described patient satisfied the following 7 criteria: neurologic symptoms, leukopenia, lymphopenia, thrombocytopenia, antinuclear antibodies, antiphospholipid antibodies (anticardiolipin antibodies, lupus anticoagulant), and reduced complement

TABLE 1: Laboratory data.

Analyte	Reference range	Month 1	Month 4	Month 8
Leukocyte count ($\times 10^3/\mu$L)	4.3–11.0	**1.30**	**1.50**	**1.70**
Lymphocytes ($\times 10^3/\mu$L)	1.0–3.7	**0.50**	**0.70**	**0.70**
CD4 T cells %	31–60	50		53
CD4 T cells (/μL)	410–1590	**311**		**315**
Hemoglobin (g/dL)	12–16	12.9	13.4	13.8
Platelet count ($\times 10^3/\mu$L)	140–450	**36**	**33**	**51**
PT INR	<1.20	**1.49**	**1.44**	**1.22**
PTT RATIO	<1.20	**1.21**	1.15	1.05
CRP (mg/dL)	<0.50	**1.4**	0.01	0.03
γ-GT (U/L)	<60	**157**	**246**	**100**
AST (IU/liter)	<40	**56**	33	19
ALT (IU/liter)	<40	**59**	**87**	17
Gamma-globulin (%)	8–16.7	**19.6**	14.6	12.1
IgE (IU/mL)	<120	81	**175**	63
Vitamin B12 (pg/mL)	191–663		1.057	
Folic acid (ng/mL)	4.6–18.7		3.89	
25-OH-vitamin D (ng/mL)	31–100	**14**		
CPK (IU/liter)	40–230	**1,277**	**253**	84
ANA titer	<1:80	**1:320**	**1:160**	**1:320**
C3 (mg/dL)	79–152	**68**	**73**	**78**
C4 (mg/dL)	16–38	**12**	**11**	**12**
Lupus anticoagulant panel				
aPTT-low phospholipid	<1.15	0.85		0.66
DRVVT ratio	<1.10	**1.20**		**1.14**
Anticardiolipin-Ab		**positive**		
Schistosoma-Ab			**positive**	

HIV-Ab, HTLV-I/II-Ab, HAV-IgM, HBs-Ag, HCV-Ab, HEV-Ab, CMV-IgM, TPPA, *Toxoplasma*-Ab, EBV-DNA, *Plasmodium falciparum*-Ag, and emoscopy for plasmodia: all negative.
Values out of the reference range are in bold.
ALT: alanine transaminase; AST: aspartate transaminase; ANA: antinuclear antibodies; CPK: creatine phosphokinase; CRP: C-reactive protein; DRVVT: dilute viper venome time; γ-GT: γ-glutamyltransferase; PT: prothrombine time; HTLV-I/II: human T lymphotropic virus I/II; PTT: partial thromboplastine time; and TPPA: Treponema pallidum particle agglutination.

C3, C4. But such extreme hepatosplenomegaly (Figure 1) is usually not seen in SLE. Indeed, the extensive periportal fibrosis, the marked hypertrophy of the left hepatic and caudate lobe, the marked hypotrophy of the right hepatic lobe, and the huge spleen with spots (siderotic nodules, Gamna-Gandy bodies), which was a pattern of abnormalities that had never been seen at the General Hospital of Bolzano, turned out to be characteristic for hepatosplenic schistosomiasis and allowed the distinction of hepatosplenic schistosomiasis from viral or alcohol induced liver cirrhosis [18–20]. Splenic Gamna-Gandy bodies can also be observed in sickle cell anemia [21]. In endemic areas these sonographic findings are used as a noninvasive diagnostic test, replacing invasive liver biopsy [18]. Because of the thrombocytopenia and the altered coagulation tests (Table 1), liver biopsy and lumbar puncture were not carried out in the patient.

The nonspecific mild diffuse white matter hyperintensities seen in the MR-FLAIR-imaging of the patient, can be seen in SLE [22], in neurologically asymptomatic hepatosplenic schistosomiasis *mansoni* [23], and in other cerebral small vessel disease [24], and are not indicative of motor neuron disease. The antiphospholipid antibodies might have caused cerebral microangiopathy and favored blood brain barrier disruption and neuroimflammation [25]. Schistosome eggs can reach the CNS trough retrograde venous flow in the valveless Batson vertebral venous plexus, which connects the portal venous system and the venae cavae to the spinal cord and cerebral veins [2]. The gadolinium enhancement of the meninges at the vertebral level D4-D6 of the patient might have reflected an immunoreaction to schistosome eggs but do not explain the selective motor neuron disease. Spinal neuroschistosomiasis of *Schistosoma mansoni* usually manifests with lumbar pain, lower limb radicular pain, muscle weakness, sensory loss, and bladder dysfunction [2, 14]. The question was whether there was a link between hepatosplenic schistosomiasis and ALS.

3.2. Hepatosplenic Schistosomiasis mansoni and IL-17.

In schistosomiasis the host mounts a pathogenic immune response

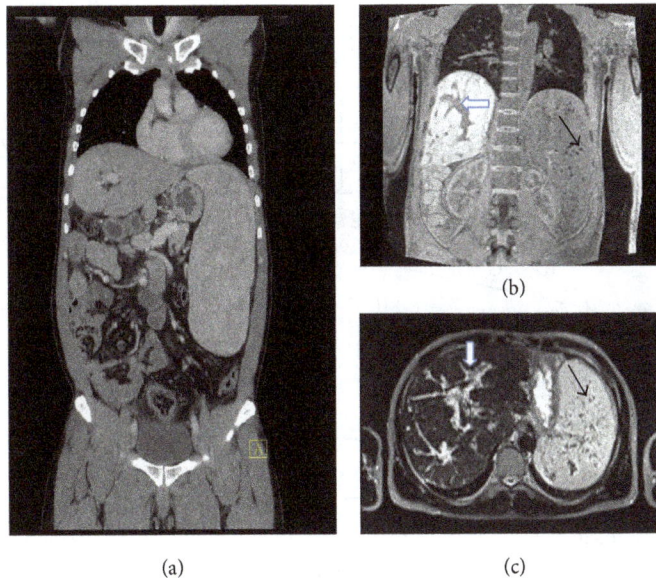

FIGURE 1: (a) Computerized tomography (CT) imaging showing the enlarged spleen (b) and (c) magnetic resonance imaging (MRI) demonstrating the periportal fibrosis (white arrows) and the Gamna-Gandy bodies (siderotic nodules) in the spleen (black arrows).

against tissue-trapped parasite eggs. The CD4 T cell mediated granulomatous inflammation varies greatly in magnitude in humans and among mouse strains in experimental models [5]. Mouse strains which develop severe immunopathology show substantial Th17 as well as Th1 and Th2 cell responses; a solely Th2-polarized response is only observed in low-pathology strains such as the C57BL/6 mice [26]. The ability to mount pathogenic Th17 cell responses depends on the production of IL-23 and IL-1β by antigen presenting cells following recognition of egg antigens by pathogen associated molecular patterns (PAMPs) recognition receptors (PRRs) [27]. IL-1β contributes to the induction of Th17 cells and IL-23 is necessary for their maintenance and proliferation. Low-pathology C57BL/6 mice immunized subcutaneously with a soluble schistosome egg antigen preparation in complete Freund's adjuvant (CFA), that contains mainly heat killed *M. tuberculosis,* prior to and during infection with schistosomes, were shown to develop severe immunopathology. If in these mice the genes for p40 or p19, the two peptide components of IL-23 were knocked out, they became resistant to the induction of the severe immunopathology. Knocking out IL-12p35, a component of IL-12, did not prevent the severe schistosomiasis induced immunopathology. This indicates that an IL-17 producing T cell population, likely driven by IL-23, significantly contributes to the severe immunopatology in schistosomiasis [28]. T-helper 17 cells have been associated with pathology in *Schistosoma haematobium*-infected children [29].

In other experiments it was demonstrated that schistosome-specific IL-17 induction by dendritic cells from low-pathology C57BL/6 mice is normally inhibited by their induction of IL-10. In vitro, simultaneous stimulation of schistosome-exposed C57BL/6 dendritic cells with a heat-killed bacterium enables these cells to overcome IL-10 inhibition and to induce IL-17. This schistosome specific

IL-17 was dependent on IL-6 production by the copulsed dendritic cells [30]. In vivo, coimmunisation of C57BL/6 animals with bacterial and schistosome antigens also resulted in schistosome-specific IL-17 production and this response was enhanced in the absence of IL-10 mediated immune regulation [30]. These experiments suggest that the balance of pro- and anti-inflammatory cytokines that determines the severity of pathology during schistosome infection can be influenced not only by the host and parasite, but also by concurrent bacterial or mycobacterial stimulation. On the other side, coinfection with intestinal nematodes was shown to reduce hepatic egg-induced immunopathology due to damping pathogenic Th17 cell responses by promoting regulatory mechanisms such as those afforded by alternatively activated macrophages and T regulatory cells [31]. It can be concluded that the pathological immune response to schistosome infection, represented by increased IL-17, is affected by multiple factors including intestinal parasite exposure, host variability, bacterial or mycobacterial infection, and commensal microbiota.

3.3. Amyotrophic Lateral Sclerosis and IL-17. There is compelling evidence that neuroinflammation is involved in the pathogenesis of ALS [32–34]. But neuroinflammation can exert both neuroprotective and neurodestructive effects, depending on the balance and timing of the different immune responses [32–34]. IL-17 was discovered to be a key player in the pathogenesis of multiple sclerosis (MS). P40 or p19 gene knockout mice are resistant to induction of experimental autoimmune encephalomyelitis, the experimental model of multiple sclerosis [35]. As mentioned above, p40 and p19 are the two peptide components of IL-23, the cytokine necessary for maintenance and proliferation of Th17 cells [35].

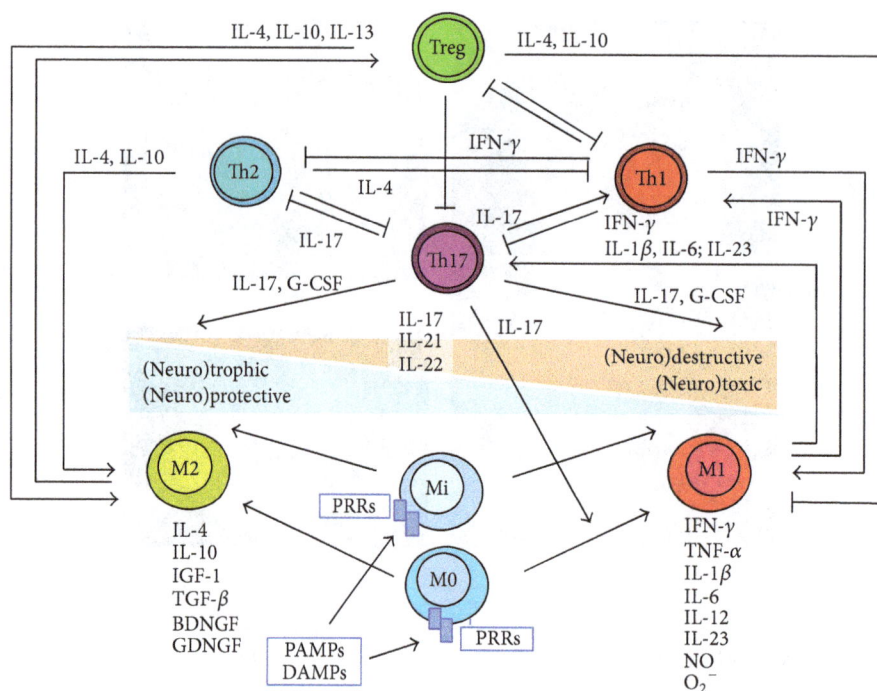

FIGURE 2: Simplified hypothetical model of immune cell interaction. ↑ = activation, induction; T = inhibition, reduction; BDNF = brain derived neurotrophic factor; DAMP = danger associated molecular pattern; G-CSF = granulocyte-colony stimutating factor; GDGF = glial-cell-derived neurotrophic factor; IGF-1 = insulin-like growth factor; IL = interleukin; Mi = microglia; M0 = nonactivated macrophages; M1 = classically activated macrophages; M2 = alternatively activated macrophages; PAMP = pathogen associated molecular pattern; PRRs = PAMP recognition receptors; and TGF-β = transforming growth factor-β.

Recently, increased levels of IL-17 have been found in the blood and in the CSF of the majority of patients affected by ALS [35–37]. But there are only few reports on IL-17 in ALS. Fiala and colleagues reported that the IL-17 serum level was increased above the highest observed level in control subjects of 40 pg/mL in 65% of 32 patients with ALS and in 4 of 4 patients with autoimmune disease [37]. In the described patient the IL-17 serum level was 672.2 pg/mL in the first blood sample, which was taken before treatment with praziquantel, and high dose corticosteroids were initiated. The normalization of the IL-17 values observed in the following three samples may be a consequence of treatment with high dose corticosteroids, with praziquantel, or a consequence of other unknown reasons. In vitro, mononuclear cells treated with superoxide dismutase 1 (SOD1) aggregates, misfolded SOD1, oxidized SOD1, or with mutant SOD1 produced IL-1β, IL-6, and IL-23, the cytokines that induce IL-17 [37, 38]. Stimulation of peripheral blood mononuclear cells by mutant SOD1 induced higher transcripts of IL-1α and IL-6, but lower transcripts of IL-10 in mononuclear cells of ALS patients as compared to controls [37]. This suggests that the vulnerability to ALS may be linked to the mode of the immune response. In the transgenic mouse model CNS-targeted production of IL-17 induces activation of astrocytes and microglia, microvascular pathology and enhances the neuroinflammatory response to systemic endotoxemia [39].

3.4. IL-17. IL-17, produced also by non-Th17 cells, functions as a first line of defense and represents a bridge between innate and adaptive immune response (for immune cell interaction see Figure 2) [40–43]. IL-17 protects the host from bacterial and fungal infections, particularly at the mucosal surfaces. IL-17 has also potent inflammatory potential and was shown to be the "superstar" in chronic inflammatory conditions [40–44]. Multiple pathogen associated molecular pattern (PAMP) recognition receptors (PRRs), for example, Toll-like receptors, NOD-like receptors, C-type lectins, on macrophages and other innate immune cells sense pathogen associated molecular patterns (PAMPs), xenobiotic substances, and endogenous "danger" associated molecular patterns (DAMPs) (e.g. aggregated, misfolded, oxidized, or mutant SOD1), and activate the immune response. Disease susceptibility or disease outcome may result from exposure to one or multiple infectious pathogens, xenobiotic substances (e.g. heavy metals), and/or endogenous "danger" associated molecular patterns (DAMPs) [44]. Polarization towards a proinflammatory immune response may lead to immunopathology, to infectious, allergic, or autoimmune disease (Figure 2). An already infection-arouse immune system may be more reactive to subsequent exogenous and endogenous immune stimulation [44].

Therefore it is possible that in the described patient the *M. tuberculosis* infection due to stimulation of PRRs contributed to the severe pathology of hepatosplenic schistosomiasis *mansoni* and that both *M. tuberculosis* and schistosome infection might have contributed to the development of ALS. Interestingly, the increased levels of IL-17 observed in individuals with latent *M. tuberculosis* infection compared to patients with tuberculosis were suggested to have a protective effect against tuberculosis [45]. The complete Freund's adjuvant, that consists of heat killed *M. tuberculosis,* has for long time been known to enhance the immune response. Other potential environmental triggers like vitamin D deficiency [46–48], a hypothetical loss of intestinal helminths after his transfer from Ghana to Italy [31], a hypothetical decreased induction of oral immune tolerance due to a reduced amount oral antigens [49], a possible induction of IL-17 due to changes of the intestinal flora [50–52], might have promoted a proinflammatory immune response polarization, thus contributing to ALS development in the described patient. Increased IL-17 levels have been detected in the circulation and tissues of human and murine lupus [53]. It was demonstrated that IL-17 promotes B cell survival and differentiation into antibody producing cells. Therefore IL-17 is suspected to promote humoral immunity against self-antigens [53]. It is possible that increased IL-17 has contributed to the development of autoantibodies detected in the described patient.

4. Conclusion

Because ALS is not a disease of infancy, it is probable that contributing factors have to accumulate over time and/or have to combine with each other in order to overcome the various physiologic compensation-, and repair-mechanisms, and cause disease. Besides the genetic background, environmental factors such as infections, xenobiotic substances, changes in the gut microbiota and vitamin D deficiency, may contribute to shift the balance of the immune response from a protective to a more destructive one [54]. Autoimmune disease associations with ALS raise the possibility of shared genetic or environmental risk factors [55]. Recent progress in immunology suggests that in the described patient an increased IL-17 level may have been a common pathogenic feature of the different diseases. If we consider ALS as a common outcome of a multitude of different risk factors, so in the future we have to learn to recognize and differentiate the various combinations of the contributing factors or subcategories of the disease. This will be a precondition for a combined therapeutic approach from different fronts and for interventions of immune modulation without abrogation of the protective part of the immune response. The reported clinical case suggests that the analytic methods of immunology, for example, measuring of cytokines and chemokines, will have to be introduced into daily clinical practice in order to progress towards better understanding and towards an effective treatment and prevention of amyotrophic lateral sclerosis.

Conflict of Interests

The authors declare that there is no conflict of interests regarding the publication of this paper.

References

[1] J. E. H. Pittella, "Neuroschistosomiasis," *Brain Pathology*, vol. 7, no. 1, pp. 649–662, 1997.

[2] A. G. Ross, D. P. McManus, J. Farrar, R. J. Hunstman, D. J. Gray, and Y. Li, "Neuroschistosomiasis," *Journal of Neurology*, vol. 259, no. 1, pp. 22–32, 2012.

[3] B. Gryseels, K. Polman, J. Clerinx, and L. Kestens, "Human schistosomiasis," *The Lancet*, vol. 368, no. 9541, pp. 1106–1118, 2006.

[4] I. Bica, D. H. Hamer, and M. J. Stadecker, "Hepatic schistosomiasis," *Infectious Disease Clinics of North America*, vol. 14, no. 3, pp. 583–604, 2000.

[5] B. M. Larkin, P. M. Smith, H. E. Ponichtera, M. G. Shainheit, L. I. Rutitzky, and M. J. Stadecker, "Induction and regulation of pathogenic Th17 cell responses in schistosomiasis," *Seminars in Immunopathology*, vol. 34, no. 6, pp. 873–888, 2012.

[6] P. H. Gordon, "Amyotrophic lateral sclerosis: an update for 2013 clinical features, pathophysiology, management and therapeutic trials," *Aging and Disease*, vol. 4, no. 5, pp. 295–310, 2013.

[7] J. Ravits, S. Appel, R. H. Baloh et al., "Deciphering amyotrophic lateral sclerosis: what phenotype, neuropathology and genetics are telling us about pathogenesis," *Amyotrophic Lateral Sclerosis and Frontotemporal Degeneration*, vol. 14, supplement 1, pp. 5–18, 2013.

[8] M. R. Turner, O. Hardiman, M. Benatar et al., "Controversies and priorities in amyotrophic lateral sclerosis," *The Lancet Neurology*, vol. 12, no. 3, pp. 310–322, 2013.

[9] S. D. Rao and J. H. Weiss, "Excitotoxic and oxidative cross-talk between motor neurons and glia in ALS pathogenesis," *Trends in Neurosciences*, vol. 27, no. 1, pp. 17–23, 2004.

[10] Y. R. Li, O. D. King, J. Shorter, and A. D. Gitler, "Stress granules as crucibles of ALS pathogenesis," *The Journal of Cell Biology*, vol. 201, no. 3, pp. 361–372, 2013.

[11] S. M. Kim, H. Kim, J. S. Lee et al., "Intermittent hypoxia can aggravate motor neuronal loss and cognitive dysfunction in ALS mice," *PLoS ONE*, vol. 8, no. 11, Article ID e81808, 2013.

[12] K. V. Luong and L. T. Nguyễn, "Roles of vitamin D in amyotrophic lateral sclerosis: possible genetic and cellular signaling mechanisms," *Molecular Brain*, vol. 6, article 16, 2013.

[13] F. Conti, C. Alessandri, M. Sorice et al., "Thin-layer chromatography immunostaining in detecting anti-phospholipid antibodies in seronegative anti-phospholipid syndrome," *Clinical and Experimental Immunology*, vol. 167, no. 3, pp. 429–437, 2012.

[14] M. Petri, A. M. Orbai, G. S. Alarcón et al., "Derivation and validation of the systemic lupus international collaborating clinics classification criteria for systemic lupus erythematosus," *Arthritis and Rheumatism*, vol. 64, no. 8, pp. 2677–2686, 2012.

[15] T. C. A. Ferrari, P. R. R. Moreira, and A. S. Cunha, "Clinical characterization of neuroschistosomiasis due to *Schistosoma mansoni* and its treatment," *Acta Tropica*, vol. 108, no. 2-3, pp. 89–97, 2008.

[16] W. Ridtitid, M. Wongnawa, W. Mahatthanatrakul, J. Punyo, and M. Sunbhanich, "Rifampin markedly decreases plasma concentrations of praziquantel in healthy volunteers," *Clinical Pharmacology and Therapeutics*, vol. 72, no. 5, pp. 505–513, 2002.

[17] M. L. Vazquez, H. Jung, and J. Sotelo, "Plasma levels of praziquantel decrease when dexamethasone is given simultaneously," *Neurology*, vol. 37, no. 9, pp. 1561–1562, 1987.

[18] A. Manzella, K. Ohtomo, S. Monzawa, and J. H. Lim, "Schistosomiasis of the liver," *Abdominal Imaging*, vol. 33, no. 2, pp. 144–150, 2008.

[19] J. R. Lambertucci, L. C. D. S. Silva, L. M. Andrade et al., "Imaging techniques in the evaluation of morbidity in schistosomiasis mansoni," *Acta Tropica*, vol. 108, no. 2-3, pp. 209–217, 2008.

[20] A. S. D. A. Bezerra, G. D'Ippolito, R. P. Caldana et al., "Differentiating cirrhosis and chronic hepatosplenic schistosomiasis using MRI.," *The American journal of roentgenology*, vol. 190, no. 3, pp. W201–207, 2008.

[21] A. Piccin, H. Rizkalla, O. Smith et al., "Composition and significance of splenic γ-Gandy bodies in sickle cell anemia," *Human Pathology*, vol. 43, no. 7, pp. 1028–1036, 2012.

[22] S. Appenzeller, A. V. Faria, M. L. Li, L. T. L. Costallat, and F. Cendes, "Quantitative magnetic resonance imaging analyses and clinical significance of hyperintense white matter lesions in systemic lupus erythematosus patients," *Annals of Neurology*, vol. 64, no. 6, pp. 635–643, 2008.

[23] A. Manzella, P. Borba-Filho, C. T. Brandt, and K. Oliveira, "Brain magnetic resonance imaging findings in young patients with hepatosplenic schistosomiasis mansoni without overt symptoms," *The American Journal of Tropical Medicine and Hygiene*, vol. 86, no. 6, pp. 982–987, 2012.

[24] S. Debette and H. S. Markus, "The clinical importance of white matter hyperintensities on brain magnetic resonance imaging: systematic review and meta-analysis," *British Medical Journal*, vol. 341, no. 7767, Article ID c3666, 2010.

[25] L. L. Horstman, W. Jy, C. J. Bidot et al., "Antiphospholipid antibodies: paradigm in transition," *Journal of Neuroinflammation*, vol. 6, article 3, 2009.

[26] L. I. Rutitzky and M. J. Stadecker, "Exacerbated egg-induced immunopathology in murine Schistosoma mansoni infection is primarily mediated by IL-17 and restrained by IFN-γ," *European Journal of Immunology*, vol. 41, no. 9, pp. 2677–2687, 2011.

[27] M. G. Shainheit, K. W. Lasocki, E. Finger et al., "The pathogenic Th17 cell response to major schistosome egg antigen is sequentially dependent on IL-23 and IL-1β," *Journal of Immunology*, vol. 187, no. 10, pp. 5328–5335, 2011.

[28] L. I. Rutitzky, L. Bazzone, M. G. Shainheit, B. Joyce-Shaikh, D. J. Cua, and M. J. Stadecker, "IL-23 is required for the development of severe egg-induced immunopathology in schistosomiasis and for lesional expression of IL-17," *The Journal of Immunology*, vol. 180, no. 4, pp. 2486–2495, 2008.

[29] M. Mbow, B. M. Larkin, L. Meurs et al., "T-helper 17 cells are associated with pathology in human schistosomiasis," *Journal of Infectious Diseases*, vol. 207, no. 1, pp. 186–195, 2013.

[30] G. Perona-Wright, R. J. Lundie, S. J. Jenkins, L. M. Webb, R. K. Grencis, and A. S. MacDonald, "Concurrent bacterial stimulation alters the function of helminth-activated dendritic cells, resulting in IL-17 induction," *Journal of Immunology*, vol. 188, no. 5, pp. 2350–2358, 2012.

[31] L. E. Bazzone, P. M. Smith, L. I. Rutitzky et al., "Coinfection with the intestinal nematode Heligmosomoides polygyrus markedly reduces hepatic egg-induced immunopathology and proinflammatory cytokines in mouse models of severe schistosomiasis," *Infection and Immunity*, vol. 76, no. 11, pp. 5164–5172, 2008.

[32] S. H. Appel, D. R. Beers, and J. S. Henkel, "T cell-microglial dialogue in Parkinson's disease and amyotrophic lateral sclerosis:

are we listening?" *Trends in Immunology*, vol. 31, no. 1, pp. 7–17, 2010.

[33] T. Philips and W. Robberecht, "Neuroinflammation in amyotrophic lateral sclerosis: Role of glial activation in motor neuron disease," *The Lancet Neurology*, vol. 10, no. 3, pp. 253–263, 2011.

[34] S. H. Appel, W. Zhao, D. R. Beers, and J. S. Henkel, "The microglial-motoneuron dialogue in ALS," *Acta Myologica*, vol. 30, no. 1, pp. 4–8, 2011.

[35] S. Zhu and Y. Qian, "IL-17/IL-17 receptor system in autoimmune disease: mechanisms and therapeutic potential," *Clinical Science*, vol. 122, no. 11, pp. 487–511, 2012.

[36] M. Rentzos, A. Rombos, C. Nikolaou et al., "Interleukin-17 and interleukin-23 are elevated in serum and cerebrospinal fluid of patients with ALS: a reflection of Th17 cells activation?" *Acta Neurologica Scandinavica*, vol. 122, no. 6, pp. 425–429, 2010.

[37] M. Fiala, M. Chattopadhay, A. La Cava et al., "IL-17A is increased in the serum and in spinal cord CD8 and mast cells of ALS patients," *Journal of Neuroinflammation*, vol. 7, article 76, 2010.

[38] G. Liu, M. Fiala, M. T. Mizwicki et al., "Neuronal phagocytosis by inflammatory macrophages in ALS spinal cord: inhibition of inflammation by resolvin D1," *American Journal of Neurodegenerative Disease*, vol. 1, no. 1, pp. 60–74, 2010.

[39] J. Zimmermann, M. Krauthausen, M. J. Hofer, M. T. Heneka, I. L. Campbell, and M. Müller, "CNS-targeted production of IL-17A induces glial activation, microvascular pathology and enhances the neuroinflammatory response to systemic endotoxemia," *PLoS ONE*, vol. 8, no. 2, Article ID e57307, 2013.

[40] P. Miossec, T. Korn, and V. K. Kuchroo, "Interleukin-17 and type 17 helper T cells," *The New England Journal of Medicine*, vol. 361, no. 9, pp. 888–898, 2009.

[41] S. A. Khader, S. L. Gaffen, and J. K. Kolls, "Th17 cells at the crossroads of innate and adaptive immunity against infectious diseases at the mucosa," *Mucosal Immunology*, vol. 2, no. 5, pp. 403–411, 2009.

[42] K. Hirota, H. Ahlfors, J. H. Duarte, and B. Stockinger, "Regulation and function of innate and adaptive interleukin-17-producing cells," *EMBO Reports*, vol. 13, no. 2, pp. 113–120, 2012.

[43] S. K. Bedoya, B. Lam, K. Lau, and J. Larkin III, "Th17 cells in immunity and autoimmunity," *Clinical and Developmental Immunology*, vol. 2013, Article ID 986789, 16 pages, 2013.

[44] N. Y. Hemdan, A. M. Abu El-Saad, and U. Sack, "The role of T helper (T_H)17 cells as a double-edged sword in the interplay of infection and autoimmunity with a focus on xenobiotic-induced immunomodulation," *Clinical and Developmental Immunology*, vol. 2013, Article ID 374769, 13 pages, 2013.

[45] A. Bandaru, K. P. Devalraju, P. Paidipally et al., "Phosphorylated STAT3 and PD-1 regulate IL-17 production and IL-23 receptor expression in *Mycobacterium tuberculosis* infection," *European Journal of Immunology*, vol. 44, no. 7, pp. 2013–2024, 2014.

[46] D. L. Kamen and V. Tangpricha, "Vitamin D and molecular actions on the immune system: modulation of innate and autoimmunity," *Journal of Molecular Medicine*, vol. 88, no. 5, pp. 441–450, 2010.

[47] D. Bruce, S. Yu, J. H. Ooi, and M. T. Cantorna, "Converging pathways lead to overproduction of IL-17 in the absence of vitamin D signaling," *International Immunology*, vol. 23, no. 8, pp. 519–528, 2011.

[48] J. H. Ooi, J. Chen, and M. T. Cantorna, "Vitamin D regulation of immune function in the gut: why do T cells have vitamin D receptors?" *Molecular Aspects of Medicine*, vol. 33, no. 1, pp. 77–82, 2012.

[49] O. Moling and P. Mian, "Induction of oral tolerance as treatment or prevention of chronic diseases associatet with Chlamydia pneumoniae infection: hypothesis," *Medical Science Monitor*, vol. 9, no. 5, pp. HY15–HY18, 2003.

[50] I. I. Ivanov, K. Atarashi, N. Manel et al., "Induction of intestinal Th17 cells by segmented filamentous bacteria," *Cell*, vol. 139, no. 3, pp. 485–498, 2009.

[51] A. Sczesnak, N. Segata, X. Qin et al., "The genome of Th17 cell-inducing segmented filamentous bacteria reveals extensive auxotrophy and adaptations to the intestinal environment," *Cell Host and Microbe*, vol. 10, no. 3, pp. 260–272, 2011.

[52] J. U. Scher, A. Sczesnak, R. S. Longman et al., "Expansion of intestinal *Prevotella copri* correlates with enhanced susceptibility to arthritis," *eLife*, vol. 2, Article ID e01202, 2013.

[53] M. S. Shin, N. Lee, and I. Kang, "Effector T-cell subsets in systemic lupus erythematosus: update focusing on Th17 cells," *Current Opinion in Rheumatology*, vol. 23, no. 5, pp. 444–448, 2011.

[54] A. Vojdani, "A potential link between environmental triggers and autoimmunity," *Autoimmune Diseases*, vol. 2014, Article ID 437231, 18 pages, 2014.

[55] M. R. Turner, R. Goldacre, S. Ramagopalan, K. Talbot, and M. J. Goldacre, "Autoimmune disease preceding amyotrophic lateral sclerosis: an epidemiologic study," *Neurology*, vol. 81, no. 14, pp. 1222–1225, 2013.

36

A Rare Case of Prototheca Algaemia in a Patient with Systemic Lupus Erythematosus and Recent Belimumab Infusion

Carolina Mejia-Otero,[1] **Shelley Singh,**[1] **Luis Arias Urdaneta,**[2] **Carlos Sesin,**[2] **Anindita Chakrabarti,**[3] **Nanci Mae Miller,**[4] **and Claudio Tuda**[5]

[1] *Internal Medicine Department, Mount Sinai Medical Center, Miami, FL 33140, USA*
[2] *Division of Rheumatology, Internal Medicine Department, Mount Sinai Medical Center, Miami, FL, USA*
[3] *Department of Infectious Disease, University of Miami Miller School of Medicine, Miami, FL 33136, USA*
[4] *Department of Pathology, Mount Sinai Medical Center, Miami, FL, USA*
[5] *Division of Infectious Disease, Internal Medicine Department, Mount Sinai Medical Center, Miami, FL, USA*

Correspondence should be addressed to Carolina Mejia-Otero, caroliname85@gmail.com

Academic Editors: A. M. Mansour, A. E. Tebo, and M. Trendelenburg

Novel agents for the treatment of immune-mediated diseases such as systemic lupus erythematosus (SLE) have been increasingly used as an alternative to or in combination with conventional therapies. Belimumab, a human monoclonal antibody that inhibits B-cell activating factor (BAFF), has demonstrated efficacy in moderate-to-severe SLE with similar adverse effects when compared to other biologic agents and conventional SLE therapies. Here, we describe a woman with SLE and diabetes mellitus (DM) on immunosuppressive therapy for five years who was admitted to the hospital for pneumonia but had a complicated hospital course with multiple infections and, most notably, a nosocomial algaemia due to *Prototheca wickerhamii*, which was treated successfully with amphotericin B. She had recently received three belimumab infusions as an outpatient prior to admission to the hospital. To the best of our knowledge no cases of human protothecosis in patients receiving belimumab have been described in the English literature; however, unusual infections have to be considered in all patients undergoing immunosuppressive therapies who persist with fever despite conventional antimicrobials.

1. Introduction

SLE is a heterogeneous disease caused by an aberrant autoimmune response that spares no organ and affects people of African, Hispanic, and Asian ancestry more than other racial or ethnic groups [1, 2]. Genetic, environmental, hormonal, and immunoregulatory factors contribute to the expression of tissue injury and clinical manifestations. Both T and B cell antigen receptor-mediated activation are altered and early signaling events are amplified [1, 3]. All B-cell subgroups contribute to the production of autoantibodies. These play an important role in the presentation of antigens and autoantigens to T cells, thus mediating tissue damage and contributing to disease expression [1].

A better understanding of the pathogenesis of immune-mediated diseases has led to the development of a new therapeutic approach to SLE, B-cell-targeted therapy. This acts through two principal mechanisms: direct killing by monoclonal antibodies specific for B-cell surface molecules CD19, CD20 (rituximab, ocrelizumab), and CD22 (epratuzumab) and attrition due to the inhibition of B-cell survival factors BLyS (belimumab) and APRIL (atacicept) [4]. Belimumab is the first targeted biological treatment that is FDA approved specifically for the treatment of SLE [5]. Previous randomized controlled trials have shown reductions in disease activity and prevention of flares [6, 7], with an acceptable safety profile [8]; however, malignancies, serious or severe infections, and infusion reactions have been described [4, 5].

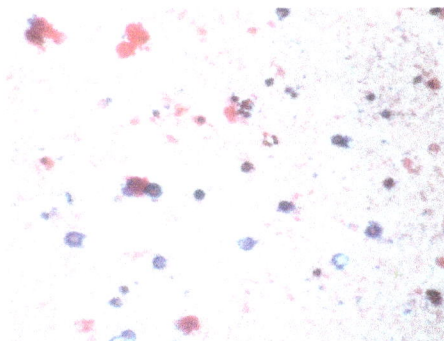

FIGURE 1: Gram stain of yeast-like colonies from blood and chocolate agar showing large gram-positive spherical cells of varied sizes from 8 uM to 24 uM in diameter. *Courtesy of the Department of Pathology-Microbiology at Mount Sinai Medical Center of Florida.*

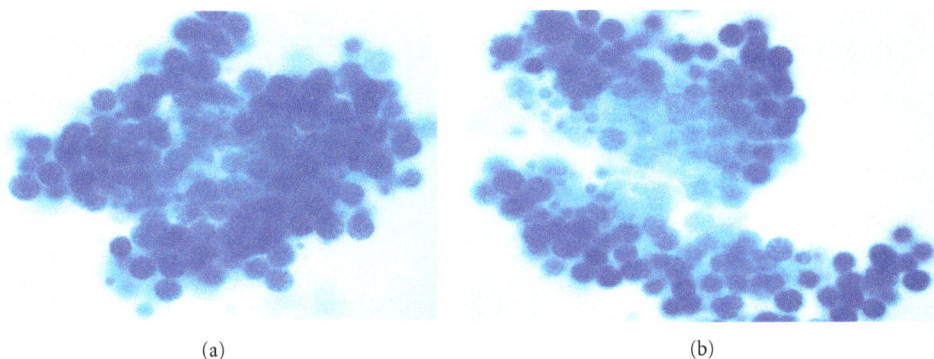

(a)   (b)

FIGURE 2: Yeast-like cells of variable sizes resembling endospores contained in a sporangiospore seen on a wet mount prepared using lactophenol cotton blue, reported as *Prototheca* based on the morphology of the organism. *Courtesy of the Department of Pathology-Microbiology at Mount Sinai Medical Center of Florida.*

A case of algaemia with *P. wickerhamii* after belimumab infusion is reported here.

2. Case Presentation

We describe a case of a 67-year-old female with SLE on immunosuppressive therapy for more than five years who presented to the hospital with a two-day history of cough, fever, and fatigue. One week prior to admission, she received her third belimumab infusion (10 mg/kg) without acute complications. Her first two loading doses of belimumab were four and two weeks earlier, again, without incident. The patient was diagnosed with SLE over five years ago, based upon a history of immune thrombocytopenia and autoimmune hemolytic anemia (Evan's syndrome), hypocomplementemia, polyarthralgias, and a positive ANA in a 1 : 160 speckled pattern. She had multiple flares of hemolytic anemia requiring high doses of steroids as well as several immunosuppressive therapies. Her regimen at the time of her admission consisted of azathioprine 50 mg twice daily and prednisone 60 mg daily. Her comorbidities included DM, essential hypertension, drug-induced osteoporosis, and cataracts, as well as a history of a left middle cerebral artery aneurysm status after clipping. Other medications were long-acting insulin, tramadol, lisinopril, metoprolol, and folic acid.

At admission, the patient was tachycardic with a low-grade fever and hypoxemia. Physical examination revealed coarse breath sounds bilaterally. Laboratory data and imaging showed leukocytosis and bilateral infiltrates consistent with multifocal pneumonia. IV antibiotics were initiated; however, the patient subsequently developed respiratory failure leading to multiple intubations throughout her hospital course and eventual tracheostomy. Results of bronchoalveolar lavages revealed *Pneumocystis jiroveci*, *Cytomegalovirus*, and *Herpes simplex virus*; blood cultures grew *E. faecalis* and *K. pneumoniae* (see Table 1). Multiple antimicrobials were employed to treat the numerous infections, including clindamycin, gancyclovir, linezolid, ceftaroline, ampicillin, valacyclovir, and trimethoprim-sulfa. The patient had persistent fevers despite multiple antimicrobial therapies and subsequent blood cultures yielded the growth of P. wickerhamii (Figures 1 and 2), which was treated with amphotericin B for two weeks. Repeat blood cultures remained negative after treatment.

3. Discussion

Human protothecosis is a rare infection caused by members of the genus *Prototheca*, a microscopic single-celled heterotrophic, achlorophyllic algae that belongs to the family Chlorellaceae. It reproduces by endosporulation and binary

TABLE 1: Positive microbiology cultures during hospitalization.

Date	Source of culture	Organism
5/27/12	Urine	*Escherichia coli*
5/31/12	Bronchoalveolar lavage	*Cytomegalovirus*
6/1/12	Blood	*Cytomegalovirus*
6/12/12	Bronchoalveolar lavage	*Pneumocystis jiroveci*
7/3/12	Bronchoalveolar lavage	*Herpes simplex virus*
7/9/12	Blood	*Cytomegalovirus*
7/15/12	Urine	*Yeast, Enterococcus species*
7/15/12	Blood	*Enterococcus faecalis*
7/19/12	Urine	*Yeast, Enterococcus species*
7/19/12	Blood	*Enterococcus faecalis, Klebsiella pneumonia*
7/20/12	Blood	*Prototheca wickerhamii, Klebsiella pneumonia*

fission and is ubiquitous in nature; the most common species causing infection in humans is *P. wickerhamii* [9–11]. The appearance of *Prototheca* is similar to yeast on routine media but may be distinguished from yeast on wet mounts with lactophenol cotton blue staining if typical morula forms are observed [12].

Patients at risk for developing prototheosis are those with chronic steroid use, hematological or solid tissue malignancy, or other immunocompromised states such as DM, autoimmune disease, or primary immunodeficiency; however, cases in immunocompetent patients have also been described [13]. In the immunosuppressed individual, opportunistic infection with *Prototheca* species may be associated with bacterial, viral, or fungal coinfection, complicating both diagnosis and treatment [12].

Cellular immunity and polymorphonuclear leukocytes (PMNs), along with IgG antibodies and serum opsonins, are involved in the host defense against *Prototheca spp.* Optimal phagocytosis and killing of *P. wickerhamii* by PMNs require the presence of both specific IgG antibody and heat-labile opsonins observed after ultrastructural studies [14].

To date, there are 160 reported cases of human prototheosis, six (4%) of which have documented algaemia [13]. Most *Prototheca* infections occur on the skin or bursae; blood infections are rare and are highly associated with an immunocompromised state, such as that which occurred with this patient with SLE, DM, and on immunosuppressive therapy. Nonetheless, only after receiving belimumab did she develop prototheosis. We propose that belimumab may have contributed to the development of this *Prototheca* infection, as her longstanding immunosuppressed state had not led her to this rare opportunistic infection in the past.

One case report of prototheosis in a hematopoietic stem cell transplant recipient has been described after infliximab treatment, another biologic agent that can lead to immunosuppression [9, 15]. No cases of human prototheosis in patients receiving belimumab have been described in the literature thus far, but the correlation does not necessarily mean causation in our patient since she was on corticosteroids and azathioprine prior to the first dose of belimumab. Nevertheless, this paper illustrates that unusual infections have to be considered in all patients undergoing immunosuppressive therapy who persist with fever despite conventional antibiotic, antiviral, and antifungal treatments. Further studies or observation of uncommon adverse events in patients with belimumab are needed.

Conflict of Interests

The authors declare that they have no conflict of interests.

Acknowledgments

The authors gratefully acknowledge the assistance of Francisco Yuri Bulcao de Macedo, MD, from Jackson Memorial Hospital, Miami, FL, USA, and Alicia Hirzel, MD, from the Department of Pathology at Mount Sinai Medical Center.

References

[1] G. Tsokos, "Mechanism of disease: systemic lupus erythematosus," *The New England Journal of Medicine*, vol. 365, pp. 2110–2121, 2011.

[2] C. Duarte, M. Couto, L. Ines, and M. H. Liang, "Epidemiology of systemic lupus erythematosus," in *Systemic Lupus Erythematosus*, R. G. Lahita, G. Tsokos, J. Buyon, and T. Koike, Eds., pp. 673–696, Elsevier, London, UK, 5th edition, 2011.

[3] J. C. Crispín, S. N. C. Liossis, K. Kis-Toth et al., "Pathogenesis of human systemic lupus erythematosus: recent advances," *Trends in Molecular Medicine*, vol. 16, no. 2, pp. 47–57, 2010.

[4] M. Ramos-Casals, I. Sanz, X. Bosch, J. Stone, and M. Khamashta, "B-cell-depleting therapy in systemic lupus erythematosus," *The American Journal of Medicine*, vol. 125, pp. 327–336, 2012.

[5] S. V. Navarra, R. M. Guzmán, A. E. Gallacher et al., "Efficacy and safety of belimumab in patients with active systemic lupus erythematosus: a randomised, placebo-controlled, phase 3 trial," *The Lancet*, vol. 377, no. 9767, pp. 721–731, 2011.

[6] W. Stohl, F. Hiepe, K. Latinis et al., "Belimumab reduces autoantibodies, normalizes low complement levels, and reduces select B cell populations in patients with systemic lupus erythematosus," *Arthritis & Rheumatism*, vol. 64, no. 7, pp. 2328–2337, 2012.

[7] D. 'Cruz, S. Manzi, J. Sánchez-Guerrero et al., "Belimumab reduced disease activity across multiple organ domains in patients with SLE: combined results from BLISS-52 and BLISS-76," *Annals of the Rheumatic Diseases*, vol. 71, no. 11, pp. 1833–1838, 2012.

[8] J. Merrill, E. Ginzler, D. Wallace et al., "Long-term safety profile of belimumab plus standard therapy in patients with systemic lupus erythematosus," *Arthritis & Rheumatism*, vol. 64, no. 10, pp. 3364–3373, 2012.

[9] C. Lass-Flörl and A. Mayr, "Human prototheosis," *Clinical Microbiology Reviews*, vol. 20, no. 2, pp. 230–242, 2007.

[10] S. M. Kantrow and A. S. Boyd, "Prototheosis," *Dermatologic Clinics*, vol. 21, no. 2, pp. 249–255, 2003.

[11] J. Mayorga, J. F. Barba-Gómez, A. P. Verduzco-Martínez, V. F. Muñoz-Estrada, and O. Welsh, "Prototheosis," *Clinics in Dermatology*, vol. 30, no. 4, pp. 432–436, 2012.

A Rare Case of Prototheca Algaemia in a Patient with Systemic Lupus Erythematosus...

171

[12] B. McMullan, K. Muthiah, D. Stark, L. Lee, and D. Marriott, "Prototheca wickerhamii mimicking yeast: a cautionary tale," *Journal of Clinical Microbiology*, vol. 49, no. 8, pp. 3078–3081, 2011.

[13] J. R. Todd, J. W. King, A. Oberle et al., "Protothecosis: report of a case with 20-year follow-up, and review of previously published cases," *Medical Mycology*, vol. 50, no. 7, pp. 673–689, 2012.

[14] J. P. Phair, J. E. Williams, and H. P. Bassaris, "Phagocytosis and algicidal activity of human polymorphonuclear neutrophils against Prototheca wickerhamii," *Journal of Infectious Diseases*, vol. 144, no. 1, pp. 72–76, 1981.

[15] V. Nwanguma, K. Cleveland, and V. Baselski, "Fatal case of protothecosis in a hematopoietic stem cell transplant recipient after infliximab treatment for graft-versus-host disease," *Journal of Clinical Microbiology*, vol. 49, no. 11, p. 4024, 2011.

37

Rare Cause of Seizures, Renal Failure, and Gangrene in an 83-Year-Old Diabetic Male

Stalin Viswanathan and Kandan Balamurugesan

Indira Gandhi Medical College, Kadhiramam, Pondicherry 605009, India

Correspondence should be addressed to Stalin Viswanathan; stalinviswanathan@ymail.com

Academic Editors: A. M. Mansour and H. Narimatsu

We report an 83-year-old diabetic male who presented with acute-onset renal failure, seizures, psychosis, pneumonia, and right foot gangrene. Investigations revealed thrombocytopenia, CSF lymphocytosis, ANA and dsDNA positivity, hypocomplementemia, and pneumonitis following which he was treated with pulse methylprednisolone. He was treated for *Pseudomonas*-related ventilator-associated pneumonia, candiduria, and *E. coli*-related bedsore infection prior to discharge. He was discharged at request and died 17 days later due to a respiratory infection.

1. Introduction

Onset of systemic lupus erythematosus (SLE) after the age of 50 (late-onset SLE) constitutes 6–18% of the lupus population [1]. Most cases of lupus over 65 years have been described as case reports. Renal failure is the initial presentation only in 25% patients of SLE [2]. Neuropsychiatric SLE (NSLE) in the elderly is very rare. Infections, malignancies, and atherosclerotic disease account for most deaths in SLE patients [3]. Here we describe an 83-year-old diabetic who presented with acute-onset seizures, psychosis, pneumonitis, foot gangrene, and renal failure and improved with immunosuppressive therapy for SLE but succumbed to another respiratory infection 17 days after discharge from hospital.

2. Case

This 83-year-old diabetic of 10 years' duration (on metformin 750 mg OD) was brought from another hospital by his relatives for mechanical ventilation. Fifteen days prior, he had complained of fatigue and anorexia and was admitted in a local nursing home where he was told to have early renal failure (creatinine 202 μmol/L). Four days later he had had a generalized tonic-clonic seizure for which he was taken to the referring hospital for management. Computed tomography

(CT) of brain was normal and the patient was commenced on phenytoin; he was uncooperative for magnetic resonance imaging (MRI). He had developed acute psychosis and delirium in hospital and was managed with risperidone. Three days later he was intubated for altered sensorium and respiratory distress following acute cough, breathlessness, and fever. He was mechanically ventilated and administered ceftriaxone and metronidazole; his seizures remained under control but altered sensorium persisted. During his stay in intensive care, he developed discoloration of his right foot and warfarin had been initiated. His renal parameters had continued to worsen (creatinine 350 μmol/L) and his relatives requested discharge and brought him to our hospital.

He was a cigar smoker (>40 years) and drank occasionally. He had had a left hip fracture six years ago which had been treated conservatively. On admission, his pulse was 104 bpm, BP 92/60 mm Hg, respiratory rate 42 breaths/min with SpO$_2$ 92% on FiO2 of 100, temperature 99°F, and central venous pressure (CVP) was 6 cm. Chest examination revealed left-sided coarse crackles. The Glasgow Coma Scale (GCS) of 2T/15, bilaterally 3 mm sluggishly reacting pupils, generalized hypotonia, and areflexia were observed on neurological examination. There was no papilledema. He had dry gangrene of right foot (Figure 1) with weak right popliteal pulse. Investigations are listed in Table 1. Doppler of right lower limb

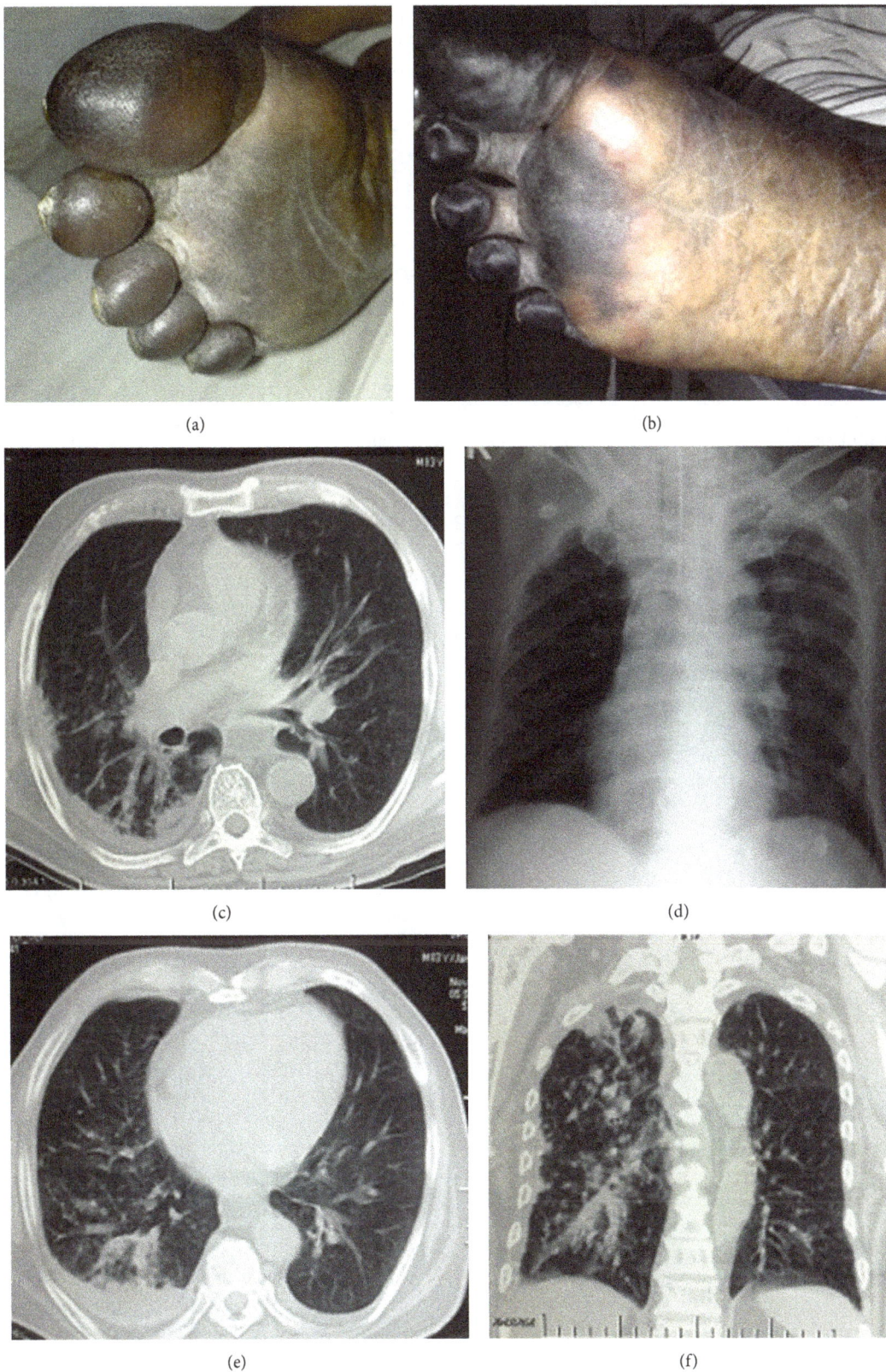

FIGURE 1: (a) Right foot discoloration at admission. (b) Right forefoot dry gangrene on day 4. (c) CT chest on day 2 showing airway dilatation (right predominant), patchy infiltrates, and ground glassing. (d) Chest radiograph on day 4 of admission shows clearing of infiltrates in the right side. (e) CT chest revealing right-sided pleural effusion, reticular infiltrates, bilateral ground glassing, and tree-in-bud appearance. (f) CT chest shows reticulonodular infiltrates in the entire right lung and ground glassing in left lung.

TABLE 1: Lab investigations of patient.

Day of admission	1	4	5	7	10	16	18
Urea (2.5–7.1 mmol/L)	67.8	61.7	47.1	38.7	33.2	26.4	21.1
Creatinine (44–80 μmol/L)	616	422	360	281	290	202	167
HbA1c (5.7–6.5%)	7.9						
Bil total (1.7–6.8 μmol/L)	1.53						
Bil dir (3.4–15.2 μmol/L)	8.5						
SGOT (0.20–0.65 μkat/L)	1.5			1.4			
SGPT (0.12–0.70 μkat/L)	0.87			0.92			
ALP (0.56–1.63 μkat/L)	3.88			9.02			
Protein (67–86 g/L)	63						
Albumin (40–50 g/L)	18	21	22	22			
GGT (0.15–0.99 μkat/L)	4.48						
K$^+$ (3.5–5.0 mmol/L)	5.6	3.3	3.9	3.2	145	137	138
Na$^+$ (136–146 mmol/L)	155	151	150	143	5.7	3.8	3.2
Calcium (2.2–2.6 mmol/L)	2.2						
Mg (0.62–0.95 mmol/L)	0.78						
Pi (0.81–1.4 mmol/L)	1.45						
LDH (114–240 IU/L)	506			269			
CK (25–200 U/L)	363			103			

Urine

Spot K$^+$ (25–120 mEq/L)	30.5
Spot Na$^+$ (40–220 mEq/L)	116
Bence-Jones	Negative
Myoglobin	Negative
Heme	Negative
Eosinophils	Negative
Culture	3 organisms
Stool occult blood	Negative
Endotracheal asp AFB	Negative
Endotracheal asp culture	Pseudomonas
Hb (130–160 g/L)	81
TC ($3.50–9 \times 10^9$/L)	10.2
Neutrophilia (%)	81
Plat ($165–415 \times 10^9$/L)	100
MCV (79–93.3 fL)	77
MCH (26.7–31.9 pg)	27.8
MCHC (323–359 g/L)	358
Reticulocyte (%)	0.5
INR	1.3
aPTT (control 25.1 s)	40
D dimer (200 ng/mL)	3200
FDP	Positive

TABLE 1: Continued.

Day of admission	1	4	5	7	10	16	18
Blood cultures				Sterile			
dsDNA (<20)				28			
ANA (<1.0)				1.8			
cANCA				Negative			
C3 (0.83–1.77 g/L)				0.78			
C4 (0.16–0.47 g/L)				0.20			
Cortisol (5–25 μg/dL)				26.1			
Ferritin (28–397 ng/L)				1328			
Direct Coombs				Negative			

Cerebrospinal fluid

Cells	103
Sugar (mg)	115
Protein (<60 mg)	39
Lymphocytes (<5)	100%
ADA	1.0
AFB	Negative
Gram	Negative
India ink	Negative

HbA1c: glycated haemoglobin; bil: bilirubin; dir: direct; SGOT: serum glutamic oxaloacetic transaminase; SGPT: serum glutamic pyruvate transaminase; ALP: alkaline phosphatase; GGT: gamma-glutamyl transferase; K$^+$: potassium; Na$^+$: sodium; Mg: magnesium; Pi-inorganic phosphate; LDH: lactate dehydrogenase; CK: creatine kinase; Hb: haemoglobin; TC: total cells; plat: platelets; MCV: mean corpuscular volume; MCH: mean corpuscular haemoglobin; MCHC: mean corpuscular haemoglobin concentration; INR: international normalized ratio; aPTT: activated partial thromboplastin time; FDP: fibrinogen degradation products; dsDNA: double-stranded DNA; ANA: antinuclear antibody; c-ANCA: antineutrophil cytoplasmic autoantibody; C3: complement C3; C4: complement C4; ADA: adenosine deaminase; AFB: acid-fast bacilli; asp: aspirate.

and echocardiography were normal. Pending cultures, he was initiated on piperacillin-tazobactam and levofloxacin, along with subcutaneous heparin, warfarin, and pentoxifylline. CT chest (day2) showed bilateral pleural thickening, bilateral ground glassing (right ≫ left), airway dilatation, and reticulonodular infiltrates (right predominant) with minimal pleural effusion (Figure 1). In view of seizures, psychosis, thrombocytopenia, renal failure, pneumonitis, ANA, and dsDNA positivity, a diagnosis of systemic lupus was made and pulse methyl prednisolone (1 g × 3 days) was initiated on day 3, followed by oral steroids (60 mg). Tracheal aspirate grew *Pseudomonas aeruginosa* and imipenem was administered on day 5 for probable ventilator-associated pneumonia. Weaning was done on 8th day of admission. Fluconazole 300 mg/day was administered for persisting candiduria. Hypernatremia was managed with dextrose saline, while sugars were controlled with infusion of regular insulin. By day 12, his power had improved to 3/5 in all limbs; he occasionally spoke a few words to his relatives but continued to be extremely afraid of hospital personnel. MRI and nerve conduction studies could not be performed due to poor cooperation. He developed an infected gluteal bedsore (*E. coli*) that necessitated amikacin. We acceded to his son's request to be discharged to home with modified doses of intramuscular amikacin therapy, twice-daily premixed insulin, warfarin, phenytoin, risperidone, clonezepam, and oral prednisolone 40 mg/day. Seventeen days later he succumbed to another respiratory infection.

3. Discussion

The 9 : 1 female predominance in SLE decreases prior to puberty and late in life [4]. Female : male ratio in late-onset SLE is about 5 : 1 [5], while another study showed a ratio of 1 : 1.1 when the age of onset was >65 years [6]. Four to 18% of cases from reported series are male [7]. In a Hong Kong study, the mean age of late-onset SLE was 62 years and onset was generally insidious [1]. Insidious onset of disease and lower index of suspicion lead to delayed diagnosis in the elderly. A study of 39 Indian male SLE subjects showed only one patient with late-onset SLE [8].

It is generally agreed that SLE in the elderly is a mild disease [9]. Prevalence of organ involvement in males depends upon the ethnic population being studied, study setting (tertiary versus primary), selection criteria of female controls, and sample size of male subjects [10]. Fever, fatigue, and weight loss are common symptoms in elderly SLE patients [5]. Serositis, muscle pains, and arthritis are more common in this age group as are secondary Sjögren's syndrome but with a lower incidence of cutaneous manifestations and Raynaud's phenomenon [9]. Males in a Thai study tended to have a shorter duration of symptoms prior to presentation, with alopecia, arthralgia and Raynaud's phenomenon being less common [10]. Psychosis, hypocomplementemia, and diffuse proliferative glomerulonephritis (DPGN) were less common in Indians [8], while renal disease and vascular thrombosis were common among Latin American males [11]. Rheumatoid arthritis, polymyalgia rheumatic, and sicca syndromes are close differentials of SLE in the elderly [5]. Late-onset lupus may have fewer major organ involvement and fewer major relapses [12].

Among patients with SLE, 60% of adults develop kidney disease [2]. SLE prevalence in India was low at 3.2/100000 population [13]; contrastingly, renal involvement among Indian SLE patients was the highest in the world [13]. Neuropsychiatric manifestations are similar in the young and the elderly [9]. Neuropsychiatric SLE (NSLE) at presentation in the elderly population has been described only as case reports. Similar to our case, seizures, coma, and pneumonia have been reported in a 72-year-old lady who had pneumonitis, hypocomplementemia, elevated fibrinogen, and FDP but with normal renal function and negative dsDNA [14]. Presence of NSLE is generally associated with a poor prognosis [9]. NSLE can be either focal (stroke, neuropathy, and transient ischemic attack) or diffuse (confusion, dementia, and psychosis) or can present with seizures (partial or generalized) [9]. Seizures are reported in 15 to 30% of patients with SLE [9]. Cognitive impairment may be the initial manifestation of SLE in the elderly [5]. The neurological manifestations seen in Indian studies were cerebrovascular accidents, myeloradiculopathies, movement disorders, seizures, coma, and psychosis [13]. Lower numbers of Raynaud and NSLE were seen in the South Indian population [13]. Our patient's cognition did not improve completely at time of discharge.

His respiratory symptoms could have also been contributed by diabetes-related pneumonia or seizure-related aspiration pneumonia but his chest radiograph (Figure 1) cleared on the 4th day of admission (after two methyl prednisolone pulses). The cause of foot gangrene could not be pinpointed. Antiphospholipid antibody testing was unavailable in our hospital. Since warfarin had been initiated prior to admission, protein C and protein S were not done. High levels of D-dimer and FDP like in our patient may indicate vascular involvement due to emboli and/or inflammation [14]. It is possible that diabetes, old age, smoking, sepsis, and SLE predisposed him towards thrombosis.

Age did not affect serological findings in a study [5]. False positive ANA can be seen in the elderly [5]. Prevalence of dsDNA positivity and hypocomplementemia may be lower [5, 9] and complement levels are inversely proportional to the age [9]. Our patient's C3 levels were borderline low, while ANA and dsDNA were positive. Anti-Ro and anti-La antibodies can be useful adjuncts in the elderly when dsDNA levels are less frequently positive [9]. The American Rheumatological Association (ARA) criteria may be too strict in the elderly population with NSLE and hence more attention is given to serology in the elderly [15]. Also, patients may not satisfy the current ARA classification criteria at presentation and hence diagnosis may be uncertain; they would need a longer duration of followup for the diagnosis to be made [12].

CNS disease and renal involvement contributed towards mortality [3]. Nonrenal factors like younger age, male sex, and hematological complications like thrombocytopenia were prognostic factors in lupus nephritis [2]. Cardiovascular disease and infections are common causes of mortality in the elderly [5]. In a retrospective Indian study, mortality in SLE patients was due to disease activity, infection, or both [3]. Hospital-acquired Gram-negative septicaemia contributed most in this study. Our patient had disease activity along with candiduria and *Pseudomonas*-related pneumonia which improved prior to discharge, but our patient finally succumbed to an infection. Septic shock due to high-dose immunosuppressants was the major cause of morality in older-onset SLE.

In conclusion, we report an elderly male diabetic with late-onset NSLE, gangrene, and sepsis (respiratory and urinary) that improved with immunosuppressant therapy. Systemic lupus erythematosus is an autoimmune disease involving women of childbearing age with highly variable clinical presentations and with 10% of cases occurring in older patients. Arthritis, fever, serositis, Raynaud's syndrome, lung disease, neuropsychiatric symptoms, positive antinuclear antibody tests, positive rheumatoid factor, positive anti-Ro/Sjögren's syndrome (SS) A, and positive anti-La/SSB are more common in patients with elderly-onset lupus. Autoimmune diseases are very rare in elderly males and need to be considered in the differential diagnoses when confronted with multisystem disease even in the presence of diabetes and systemic sepsis. The diagnosis of elderly-onset lupus is often delayed for several months because of insidious onset and similarity to other more common disorders.

Conflict of interests

The authors declare that they have no conflict of interests.

References

[1] S. K. Mak, E. K. M. Lam, and A. K. M. Wong, "Clinical profile of patients with late-onset SLE: not a benign subgroup," *Lupus*, vol. 7, no. 1, pp. 23–28, 1998.

[2] C. Molino, F. Fabbian, and C. Longhini, "Clinical approach to lupus nephritis: recent advances," *European Journal of Internal Medicine*, vol. 20, no. 5, pp. 447–453, 2009.

[3] A. Sharma, S. B. Shamanna, S. Kumar et al., "Causes of mortality among inpatients with systemic lupus erythematosus in a tertiary care hospital in North India over a 10-year period," *Lupus*, vol. 22, no. 2, pp. 216–222, 2013.

[4] C. C. Mok, C. S. Lau, T. M. Chan, and R. W. S. Wong, "Clinical characteristics and outcome of southern Chinese males with systemic lupus erythematosus," *Lupus*, vol. 8, no. 3, pp. 188–196, 1999.

[5] D. Lazaro, "Elderly-onset systemic lupus erythematosus: prevalence, clinical course and treatment," *Drugs and Aging*, vol. 24, no. 9, pp. 701–715, 2007.

[6] S. J. Pu, S.-F. Luo, Y. J. J. Wu, H. S. Cheng, and H. H. Ho, "The clinical features and prognosis of lupus with disease onset at age 65 and older," *Lupus*, vol. 9, no. 2, pp. 96–100, 2000.

[7] G. Medina, O. Vera-Lastra, L. Barile, M. Salas, and L. J. Jara, "Clinical spectrum of males with primary antiphospholipid syndrome and systemic lupus erythematosus: a comparative study of 73 patients," *Lupus*, vol. 13, no. 1, pp. 11–16, 2004.

[8] I. Pande, A. N. Malaviya, N. G. Sekharan, S. Kailash, S. S. Uppal, and A. Kumar, "SLE in indian men: analysis of the clinical and laboratory features with a review of the literature," *Lupus*, vol. 3, no. 3, pp. 181–186, 1994.

[9] M. Dennis, "Neuropsychiatric lupus erythematosus and the elderly," *International Journal of Geriatric Psychiatry*, vol. 9, no. 2, pp. 97–106, 1994.

[10] J. Mongkoltanatus, S. Wangkaew, N. Kasitanon, and W. Louthrenoo, "Clinical features of Thai male lupus: an age-matched controlled study," *Rheumatology International*, vol. 28, no. 4, pp. 339–344, 2008.

[11] M. A. Garcia, J. C. Marcos, A. I. Marcos et al., "Male systemic lupus erythematosus in a Latin-American inception cohort of 1214 patients," *Lupus*, vol. 14, no. 12, pp. 938–946, 2005.

[12] C. T. K. Ho, C. C. Mok, C. S. Lau, and R. W. S. Wong, "Late onset systemic lupus erythematosus in southern Chinese," *Annals of the Rheumatic Diseases*, vol. 57, no. 7, pp. 437–440, 1998.

[13] A. N. Malaviya, A. N. Chandrasekaran, A. Kumar, and P. N. Shamar, "Occasional series—lupus around the world systemic lupus erythematosus in India," *Lupus*, vol. 6, no. 9, pp. 690–700, 1997.

[14] M. Yamaya, M. Yoshida, M. Yamasaki, H. Kubo, K. Furukawa, and H. Arai, "Seizure and pneumonia in an elderly patient with systemic lupus erythematosus," *Journal of the American Geriatrics Society*, vol. 57, no. 9, pp. 1709–1711, 2009.

[15] M. S. Dennis, E. J. Byrne, N. Hopkinson, and P. Bendall, "Neuropsychiatric systemic lupus erythematosus in elderly people: a case series," *Journal of Neurology Neurosurgery and Psychiatry*, vol. 55, no. 12, pp. 1157–1161, 1992.

38

Visceral Leishmaniasis or Systemic Lupus Erythematosus Flare?

Sunny Garg,[1] Mousumi Kundu,[1] Amit Nandan Dhar Dwivedi,[2] Lalit Prashant Meena,[1] Neeraj Varyani,[1] Asif Iqbal,[1] and Kamlakar Tripathi[1]

[1] *Department of General Medicine, Institute of Medical Sciences, Banaras Hindu University, Varanasi 221005, India*
[2] *Department of Radiology, Institute of Medical Sciences, Banaras Hindu University, Varanasi 221005, India*

Correspondence should be addressed to Sunny Garg, sunnygarg1987@gmail.com

Academic Editors: B. Sarov and A. Vojdani

Systemic lupus erythematosus (SLE) is a multisystem disorder characterised by B-cell hyperactivity with production of multiple autoantibodies. Fever in SLE may be caused by disease exacerbation or by infection. We report a patient of SLE that was later complicated by fever, pancytopenia, and massive splenomegaly. Corticosteroid therapy for SLE might have masked the underlying infection at earlier stage. Despite negative results of rk-39 test and bone marrow biopsy, a very high suspicion for visceral leishmaniasis (VL) led us to go for direct agglutination test (DAT) and polymerase chain reaction (PCR) for leishmanial antigen that revealed positive results. Moreover, significant improvement in clinical and biochemical parameters was noted on starting the patient on antileishmanial therapy.

1. Introduction

Systemic lupus erythematosus (SLE) is a chronic autoimmune disease of unknown aetiology, characterised by B cell hyperactivity and production of multiple autoantibodies. Haematological abnormalities of SLE include haemolytic anemia, leucopenia or lymphopenia, and thrombocytopenia, due to the production of autoantibodies [1]. Splenomegaly is not a common sign of SLE, unless there is concurrent infection.

On the other hand, visceral leishmaniasis is a chronic parasitic infection caused by *Leishmania donovani*. There is B cell hyperactivity, resulting in production of autoantibodies such as ANA and others [2]. It is characterised by fever, cytopenias, and splenomegaly. Splenomegaly and hypersplenism are mainly responsible for cytopenias. Immunocompromised patients due to acquired immunodeficiency syndrome, after kidney-transplantation or leukemia are more commonly affected [3].

We report a case of SLE complicated by visceral leishmaniasis, with sharp clinical resemblance to a flare of SLE. A high suspicion for kala azar should always be kept when a patient comes from an endemic area of the disease with fever and splenomegaly, especially when superimposed on a background of an immunocompromised state.

2. Case Report

A 30-years-old female presented with complaints of low grade fever, multiple painful small joints with periorbital puffiness and bilateral pedal swelling for one month. She had history of distal phalangeal amputation 1 year back for bilateral upper limb digital infarcts. General examination revealed pallor and bilateral pitting pedal oedema. Palpable spleen 2 cm below subcostal margin was the only significant systemic finding. Haematological investigations revealed haemoglobin 2.56 mmol/L, total leukocyte count 3.4×10^9/L, platelets 59×10^9/L and, albumin : globulin (A : G) ratio 2.0 : 5.6. Renal, liver, and thyroid function tests were normal. 24 hours urinary protein excretion was 581 mg. Antinuclear antibodies (ANA) and anti-double-stranded DNA (Anti dsDNA) antibodies were positive, titres being 7.3 and 6.8 times of upper limit of normal range. Anti-Ro, anti-La, and p-ANCA were also positive. Lupus anticoagulant (LA) and anticardiolipin antibody (ACLA) were negative. Renal biopsy was suggestive of lupus nephritis of mixed type

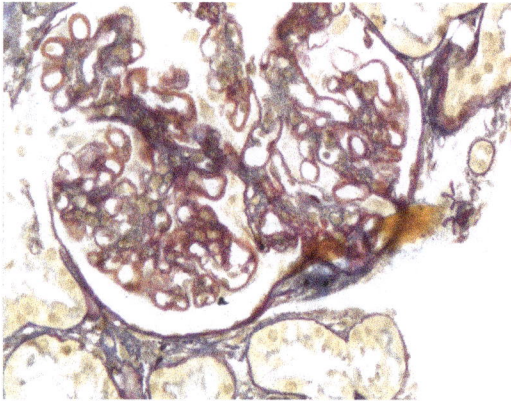

FIGURE 1: Acid fuchsin or Masson's trichome staining showing reddish coloured deposits on basement membrane.

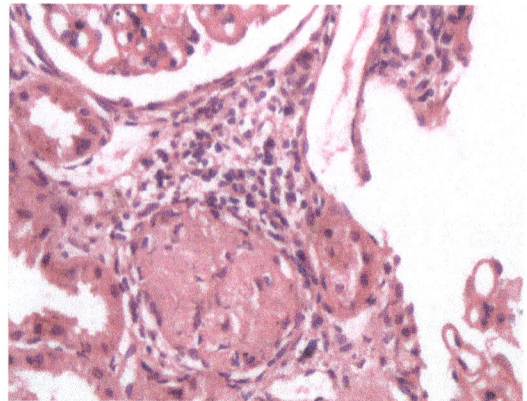

FIGURE 2: Renal biopsy showing glomerular basement membrane thickening with mesangial proliferation.

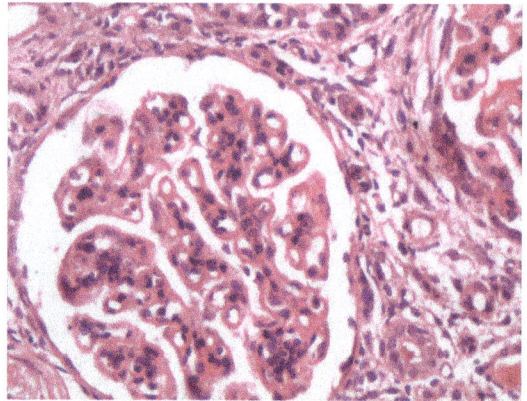

FIGURE 3: Mononuclear cell infilteration with sclerosed, hyalinised glomeruli indicating chronic disease.

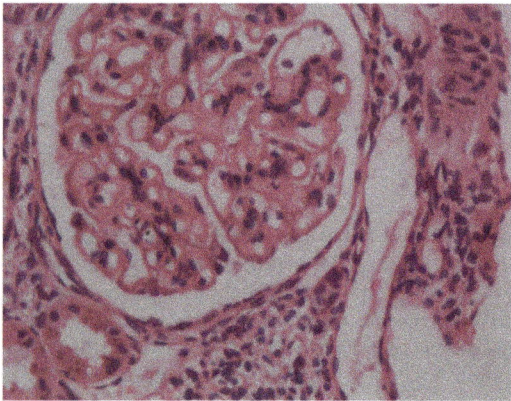

FIGURE 4: Giant mononuclear cells with pyknosis of nuclei indicating active disease process.

(grade v and ii, predominantly membranous, and mesangial cell proliferation, Figures 1, 2, 3, and 4). She was treated with methylprednisolone pulse therapy followed by oral prednisolone and hydroxychloroquine. One year later, she was again admitted in our ward with history of 1 month of high-grade fever. Low dose of steroids was given without improvement. Liver and spleen was palpable, 3 cm and 10 cm below subcostal margin, respectively, and hepatosplenomegaly was confirmed on ultrasonography. Pancytopenia, A : G reversal and slightly raised autoantibody titres still persisted. Deterioration of patient despite immunosuppressive therapy along with massive splenomegaly, normal C3 and C4, and reduced 24 hour urinary protein, almost ruled out an SLE flare. These features coupled with residence in endemic zone led to a high suspicion of kala azar. Immunochromatographic dipstick test (rK-39) and bone marrow aspiration for LD bodies was negative. Patient did not give the consent for splenic aspiration. However, Direct Agglutination Test (DAT, titre 1 : 1600) and PCR were positive for kala-azar. Patient was started on amphotericin B deoxycholate infusion following which rapid resolution of fever and hepatosplenomegaly was noticed along with improvement in haematological parameters.

3. Discussion

Visceral leishmaniasis (VL) has already been reported with SLE [4, 5]. In such cases, it mimics a lupus flare [6]. IL-10 secreted by T-cells promotes B cell survival and plasma cell differentiation. Due to polyclonal activation of B cells, there is formation of several autoantibodies like ANA, and others [2]. Presence of ANA and anti-dsDNA can mislead the diagnosis of SLE in a patient of VL and immunosuppression, as a part of therapy of SLE can be detrimental in these patients. So development of fever, pancytopenia, and splenomegaly due to VL in a patient of SLE on immunosuppressive therapy can mimic disease flare which can lead to increase in dose of immunosuppressive therapy. In our patient fever, small joint pain, facial puffiness, past history of digital infarcts, pancytopenia, positivity of ANA, anti-dsDNA, proteinuria, and biopsy proven lupus nephritis lead to primary diagnosis of SLE. Initially, patient showed slight improvement on steroid therapy but gradual deterioration followed over next few months. Moreover, the derangement in laboratory parameters persisted after 1 year of therapy, along with massive splenomegaly. The suspicion for VL was so high that we went for DAT and PCR despite negative results in rK-39 test and bone marrow studies.

This was not the case with earlier reports in which VL was diagnosed easily with the latter tests. Therefore, we conclude that a high suspicion of kala-azar should always be kept in a patient of SLE, especially when he comes from an endemic area, and immunosuppressive therapy should be started only after ruling it out diligently.

Authors' Contributions

All the authors have contributed equally in preparing this manuscript.

Conflict of Interests

There are no conflict of interests for any of the author in relation to this manuscript.

Disclosure

There is no role of any funding source in the writing of the manuscript of the decision to submit it for publication. The corresponding author had full access to all the data in the study and had final responsibility for the decision to submit for publication.

References

[1] C. Mohan, S. Adams, V. Stanik, and S. K. Datta, "Nucleosome: a major immunogen for pathogenic autoantibody-inducing T cells of lupus," *Journal of Experimental Medicine*, vol. 177, no. 5, pp. 1367–1381, 1993.

[2] E. Liberopoulos, G. Pappas, A. Kostoula, A. Drosos, E. Tsianos, and M. Elisaf, "Spectrum of autoimmunity and dysproteinemia in patients with visceral leishmaniasis," *Clinical Microbiology and Infection*, vol. 9, supplement 1, p. 417, 2003.

[3] L. J. Martinez de Letona, C. M. Vazquez, R. P. Maestu et al., "Visceral leishmaniasis as an opportunistic infection," *The Lancet*, vol. 1, no. 8489, p. 1094, 1986.

[4] B. Granel, J. Serratrice, L. Swiader et al., "Crossing of antinuclear antibodies and anti-leishmania antibodies," *Lupus*, vol. 9, no. 7, pp. 548–550, 2000.

[5] P. V. Voulgari, G. A. Pappas, E. N. Liberopoulos, M. Elisaf, F. N. Skopouli, and A. A. Drosos, "Visceral leishmaniasis resembling systemic lupus erythematosus," *Annals of the Rheumatic Diseases*, vol. 63, no. 10, pp. 1348–1349, 2004.

[6] J. Braun, J. Sieper, K. L. Schulte, E. Thiel, and K. Janitschke, "Visceral leishmaniasis mimicking a flare of systemic lupus erythematosus," *Clinical Rheumatology*, vol. 10, no. 4, pp. 445–448, 1991.

39

Multiple Thromboses in a Patient with Systemic Lupus Erythematosus after Splenectomy

Deng-Ho Yang[1,2]

[1] Division of Rheumatology/Immunology/Allergy, Department of Internal Medicine, Armed-Forces Taichung General Hospital, Number 348, Section 2, Chung Shan Road, Taiping District, Taichung City 411, Taiwan
[2] Institute of Medicine, Chung Shan Medical University, Taichung city, Taiwan

Correspondence should be addressed to Deng-Ho Yang, deng6263@ms71.hinet.net

Academic Editors: M. Hummel, N. Kutukculer, A. M. Mansour, and M. Trendelenburg

Antiphospholipid syndrome is a disorder presenting with arterial or venous thrombus and a history of fetal loss. Early diagnosis and adequate treatment is important to prevent multiple organ failures. Here, we described a woman with a two-year history of systemic lupus erythematosus with severe nephrotic syndrome, manifested multiple thrombi over the portal vein and the inferior vena cava, combined with acute renal infarction. The patient underwent splenectomy 10 months ago. Initially, she received anticoagulant treatment and low-dose glucocorticoid, but multiple organ failure progressed. After emergency plasma exchange followed by glucocorticoid pulse therapy, the patient recovered.

1. Introduction

Systemic lupus erythematosus (SLE) is an autoimmune disease with multiple organ involvement and is a common cause of secondary antiphospholipid syndrome (APS). APS is defined by arterial or venous thrombus, recurrent fetal loss, and thrombocytopenia with positive antibodies including lupus anticoagulant (LA), anticardiolipin antibodies (aCL), and antibodies to β2-glycoprotein-I (anti-β2GPI) [1, 2]. Thrombus-induced various organ infarctions such as deep vein thrombosis, stroke, pulmonary embolism, bowel, or heart ischemia, which are common in SLE patients with secondary APS. Here, we report a patient with SLE and secondary APS with coexisting renal infarction and a large thrombus over the portal vein and the inferior cava.

2. Case Report

In January 2006, a 33-year-old woman was diagnosed with SLE, based on malar rash, positive ANA (1 : 640, mixed pattern), high titer of anti-dsDNA (140 IU/mL, normal <10), and autoimmune hemolytic anemia. Since then, she received immunosuppressive medications including prednisolone, azathioprine, and hydroxychloroquine. In January 2007, splenectomy was performed on account of refractory hemolytic anemia and thrombocytopenia. In June 2007, severe nephritic syndrome with urine daily protein loss (DPL) 8 g developed. She received renal biopsy, and the biopsy revealed membranous glomerulonephritis. Monthly pulses of cyclophosphamide combined with pulse corticosteroids therapy was initiated thereafter; however, the response was poor. Persistent proteinuria (urine DPL: 5 to 10 g) was still found. In November 2007, she presented with intermittent abdominal pain in the emergency room. Physical examination revealed decreased bowel sound, positive shifting dullness, rebounding tenderness in the right lower quadrant, left costovertebral-angle tenderness, and peripheral bilateral leg edema. Laboratory data revealed the following results: WBC, 4,700/mm^3 (normal 4,500–11,000); hemoglobin, 13.3 g/dL (normal 12–16); platelets, 179,000/mm^3 (normal 150,000–400,000); BUN, 23 mg/dL (normal 7–20); creatinine, 0.4 mg/dL (normal 0.5–1); alanine aminotransferase, 28 U/L (normal <31); aspartate transaminase, 18 U/L (normal <31); albumin, 1.7 g/dL (normal 3.4–4.8); D-dimer, 3,516 ng/mL (normal <500); fibrinogen, 933 mg/dL (normal 200–400). The urine DPL was 10.3 g. Immunological studies were as follows: positive LA; aCL-IgG, 55 U/mL (normal <15); aCL-IgM, 19.6 U/mL (normal <15); anti-dsDNA, 394 IU/mL; C3, 48.8 mg/dL (normal 90–180); C4, 16.8 mg/dL (normal 10–40), and the serological test for syphilis was negative. Antithrombin III was 59% (normal 70–120). Multidetector-row computed tomography (MDCT) demonstrated a wedge-shaped infarction involving the right kidney (Figure 1), as well as segmental thrombus in the inferior vena cava (IVC) and main portal vein (Figure 2). Initially, the patient was managed with anticoagulants (low-molecular-weight heparin) and intravenous methylprednisolone 250 mg daily for three days. However, right lower quadrant abdominal pain with acute renal failure (serum creatinine: 2.5 mg/dL) progressed. Elevation of anti-dsDNA (412 IU/mL) and reduction of C3 and C4 (40 and 9 mg/dL) were also found from following laboratory data. Acute SLE flare with acute renal failure and multiple thrombus events was impressed. Due to poor response for anticoagulant and methylprednisolone therapy, plasma exchange was carried out 5 times by using fresh frozen plasma as the replacement fluid, followed by corticosteroids pulse therapy (1,000 mg intravenous methylprednisolone for 3 days). After therapy, she recovered and was discharged on the 14th hospital day with normal D-dimer and a targeted international normalized ratio (INR) of 2.5. The patient's renal functions were within normal range. Decreased serum levels of anti-dsDNA, and increased C3 and C4 was also found. The patient had no recurrent symptoms of thrombus or emboli in the following three months. Until now, she visited outpatient department regularly and received medication including prednisolone, hydroxychloroquine, and azathioprine.

3. Discussion

APS is an autoimmune disorder defined as the presence of antiphospholipid antibodies (aPLs) with arterial or venous thrombosis, recurrent spontaneous abortions, and thrombocytopenia. aPLs include aCL, LA, and anti-β2GPI, but small number is seronegative APS [2]. Approximately, half of the primary APS cases and one third of the secondary APS cases are associated with SLE. Other conditions that are associated with secondary APS include lupus-like syndrome, primary Sjogren's syndrome, rheumatoid arthritis, systemic sclerosis, systemic vasculitis, and dermatomyositis [1]. Most cases of APS present peripheral or pulmonary thrombosis and neurological manifestations, whereas intra-abdominal involvement is uncommon. Hepatic involvement is the most common abdominal manifestation in APS [1, 3, 4]. Intestinal infarction due to thrombosis of mesenteric vessels or IVC is infrequently reported.

Catastrophic APS (CAPS) is a variant form of APS and predominantly a small vessel occlusive disease mainly affecting parenchymal organs resulting in multiple organ failure, and its prevalence is less than 1% [5]. CAPS has a high mortality rate in the absence of aggressive and emergency therapy. Our patient had coexisting acute renal infarction and thrombosis of IVC and portal vein. Multiple large vessel involvement is different from the classical manifestation of

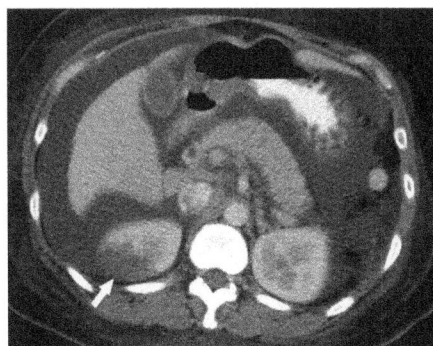

FIGURE 1: The axial contrast-enhanced CT image showing a wedge-shaped infarction (arrow) involving the right kidney.

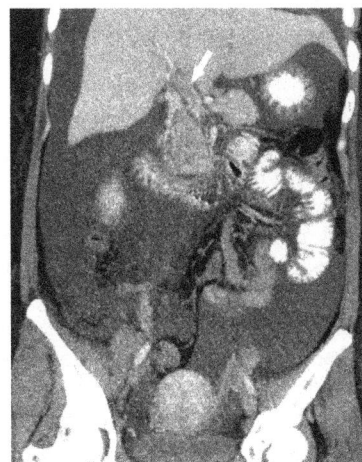

(a)

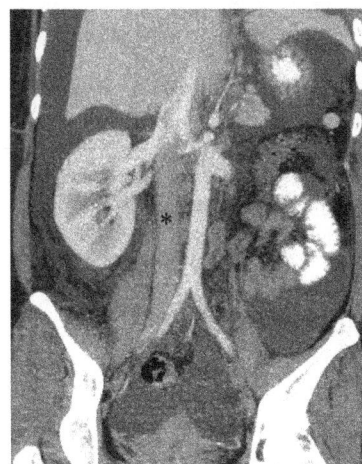

(b)

FIGURE 2: The reformatted coronal CT image showing (a) thrombosis of the main portal vein (arrow), and (b) a long segmental thrombus in the inferior vena cava (*).

CAPS which consists of multiple thromboses of medium and small vessels. However, multiple organ involvement including that of the liver, kidney, and intestine was observed in this case. The patient had membranous type of lupus nephritis with severe proteinuria. High incidence of thromboembolic complications is observed in patients with nephrotic syndrome, and most cases have venous events including renal, pulmonary, and deep-vein thromboses [6, 7]; however, arterial thrombosis-associated nephrotic syndrome is uncommon. The pathogenesis of thrombotic abnormalities in the nephritic syndrome includes increased platelet hyperaggregability, hyperfibrinogenemia, and decreased antithrombin III [6, 7]. From the laboratory data, our patient had significantly reduction of antithrombin III levels and elevation of fibrinogen levels. Therefore, the presentation of severe nephrotic syndrome may be one of the risk factors to develop IVC thrombosis in this case.

Most patients who undergo splenectomy are at an increased risk of developing portal system thrombosis within 1 month after the operation, but a few cases have late presentation (13–46 months postoperatively) [8]. Portal system thrombosis may be asymptomatic. Our patient received splenectomy 10 months ago, and we considered that her portal vein thrombosis may be associated with the operation of splenectomy. In this case, multiple factors were found to trigger thromboembolic complications including APS, poor control of nephrotic syndrome, and splenectomy.

Current therapies for APS include heparin (low-molecular-weight and unfractionated heparin), warfarin, antiplatelet agent (aspirin and clopidogrel), and hydroxychloroquine. The target INR of 2 to 3 is suggested for APS patients [9]. High dose methylprednisolone pulse therapy or plasma exchange is indicated in acute life-threatening manifestations of SLE [10]. We treated our patient by the combination of plasma exchange, corticosteroids pulse therapy, and anticoagulant therapy, and the condition was improved after medication.

In conclusion, early diagnosis and adequate treatment are important to prevent multiple organ failures in SLE patients with secondary APS or severe nephritic-syndrome-related thromboembolic events. Thrombotic microangiopathy, including thrombotic thrombocytopenic purpura, hemolytic uremic syndrome, HELLP (hemolysis, elevated liver enzymes, low platelets) syndrome, and CAPS, should be considered. Higher mortality rate can be found in the patients with thrombotic microangiopathy. Aggressive treatment by anticoagulation, plasma exchange with fresh frozen plasma replacement combined with glucocorticoid pulse therapy should be performed in SLE patients with multiple venous and arterial thromboses.

References

[1] R. Cervera, J. C. Piette, J. Font et al., "Antiphospholipid syndrome: clinical and immunologic manifestations and patterns of disease expression in a cohort of 1,000 patients," *Arthritis and Rheumatism*, vol. 46, no. 4, pp. 1019–1027, 2002.

[2] M. L. Bertolaccini and M. A. Khamashta, "Laboratory diagnosis and management challenges in the antiphospholipid syndrome," *Lupus*, vol. 15, no. 3, pp. 172–178, 2006.

[3] I. Uthman and M. Khamashta, "The abdominal manifestations of the antiphospholipid syndrome," *Rheumatology*, vol. 46, no. 11, pp. 1641–1647, 2007.

[4] S. Kaushik, M. P. Federle, P. H. Schur, M. Krishnan, S. G. Silverman, and P. R. Ros, "Abdominal thrombotic and ischemic manifestations of the antiphospholipid antibody syndrome: CT findings in 42 patients," *Radiology*, vol. 218, no. 3, pp. 768–771, 2001.

[5] R. A. Asherson, "Multiorgan failure and antiphospholipid antibodies: the catastrophic antiphospholipid (Asherson's) syndrome," *Immunobiology*, vol. 210, no. 10, pp. 727–733, 2005.

[6] T. J. Rabelink, J. J. Zwaginga, H. A. Koomans, and J. J. Sixma, "Thrombosis and hemostasis in renal disease," *Kidney International*, vol. 46, no. 2, pp. 287–296, 1994.

[7] F. Llach, "Hypercoagulability, renal vein thrombosis, and other thrombotic complications of nephrotic syndrome," *Kidney International*, vol. 28, no. 3, pp. 429–439, 1985.

[8] K. M. Stamou, K. G. Toutouzas, P. B. Kekis et al., "Prospective study of the incidence and risk factors of postsplenectomy thrombosis of the portal, mesenteric, and splenic veins," *Archives of Surgery*, vol. 141, no. 7, pp. 663–669, 2006.

[9] M. A. Crowther, J. S. Ginsberg, J. Julian et al., "A comparison of two intensities of warfarin for the prevention of recurrent thrombosis in patients with the antiphospholipid antibody syndrome," *The New England Journal of Medicine*, vol. 349, no. 12, pp. 1133–1138, 2003.

[10] C. Pagnoux, J. M. Korach, and L. Guillevin, "Indications for plasma exchange in systemic lupus erythematosus in 2005," *Lupus*, vol. 14, no. 11, pp. 871–877, 2005.

40

Life Threatening Idiopathic Recurrent Angioedema Responding to Cannabis

Amit Frenkel,[1] **Aviel Roy-Shapira,**[1] **Brotfain Evgeni,**[1] **Koyfman Leonid,**[1] **Abraham Borer,**[2] **and Moti Klein**[1]

[1]*General Intensive Care Unit, Soroka University Medical Center and the Faculty of Health Sciences,*
Ben-Gurion University of the Negev, 84101 Beersheba, Israel
[2]*Infection Control and Hospital Epidemiology Unit, Soroka University Medical Center and the Faculty of Health Sciences,*
Ben-Gurion University of the Negev, 84101 Beersheba, Israel

Correspondence should be addressed to Amit Frenkel; frenkela@prognosa.co.il

Academic Editor: Takahisa Gono

We present a case of a 27-year-old man with recurrent episodes of angioedema since he was 19, who responded well to treatment with medical grade cannabis. Initially, he responded to steroids and antihistamines, but several attempts to withdraw treatment resulted in recurrence. In the last few months before prescribing cannabis, the frequency and severity of the attacks worsened and included several presyncope events, associated with scrotal and neck swelling. No predisposing factors were identified, and extensive workup was negative. The patient reported that he was periodically using cannabis socially and that during these periods he was free of attacks. Recent data suggest that cannabis derivatives are involved in the control of mast cell activation. Consequently, we decided to try a course of inhaled cannabis as modulators of immune cell functions. The use of inhaled cannabis resulted in a complete response, and he has been free of symptoms for 2 years. An attempt to withhold the inhaled cannabis led to a recurrent attack within a week, and resuming cannabis maintained the remission, suggesting a cause and effect relationship.

1. Introduction

Angioedema is a potentially life threatening condition which has numerous hereditary, acquired, and iatrogenic causes. Although most patients present with urticaria [1], severe attacks may lead to airway obstruction and even death [2]. There are two main types of angioedema: histaminergic angioedema versus nonhistaminergic angioedema. Both types are equally dangerous and require an aggressive approach to diagnosis and treatment [2].

In most cases of angioedema, careful workup usually identifies the etiology of the attacks and allows appropriate preventive measures. According to guidelines published by The World Allergy Organization (WAO) [3], the workup of patients presenting with signs and symptoms of angioedema (urticaria, flushing, generalized pruritus, bronchospasm, throat tightness, and/or hypotension) includes detailed history of exposure to potential allergens, such as particular food items, drugs, inhaled materials, latex, and stinging insect.

In patients with recurrent episodes, further workup may require additional workup, such as immune components level, thyroid function and antibodies, chest and abdominal imaging, skin and gastrointestinal biopsies, stool examination for parasites, and bone marrow aspiration. The value of aeroallergen screening for patients with angioedema is limited [3].

Idiopathic angioedema (IAE) is defined as recurrent episodes of angioedema without urticaria for which no explanation can be found after full evaluation [4]. Currently recommended therapy is largely empiric. Available treatment modalities include a trial of nonsedating antihistamines, combination of nonsedating antihistamines with a leukotriene receptor antagonist, systemic corticosteroids, and immunosuppressant therapies. Plasmapheresis or intravenous immunoglobulin has also been used [5]. None of these treatments is universally successful.

Recent studies have demonstrated that cannabis has an important role in modulating the immune response [6].

There are at least two types of cannabinoid receptors, CB1 (CNR1) and CB2 (CNR2), both coupled to G proteins. CB2 receptors, the nonpsychoactive cannabinoid receptors, are present mainly on immune cells [7], suggesting that cannabinoids may have an important role in the regulation of the inflammatory response. This suggestion is supported by the observation that cannabinoids effectively suppress immunologic and inflammatory functions of leukocytes in vitro [8] and the reported effect of cannabis in modulating a variety of immune cell functions such as T helper cell development, chemotaxis, and tumor development [9].

Consequently, we hypothesized that the use of cannabis may be effective in the management of patients with refractory IAE.

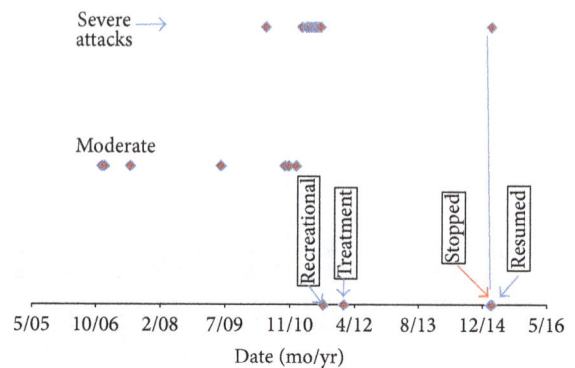

FIGURE 1: Attack severity by date.

2. Case Presentation

The patient was a 27-year-old man with a history of recurrent episodes of angioedema. The episodes begun when he was 19 years old, and their frequency and severity had been rising over the previous six months. There was a history of urticaria following penicillin administration in early childhood, but there were no other known allergies.

Initially, the episodes were manifested by mild urticaria which resolved spontaneously. But the severity and frequency of attacks increased over the years. In the last few months, the attacks became more frequent, at least twice a month, and included autonomic dysfunction: one episode of syncope and a few presyncopal episodes associated with scrotal and neck swelling and abdominal pain. Two of the episodes were considered "life threatening" due to imminent airway obstruction and were treated with subcutaneous epinephrine and intravenous steroids, which were tapered down gradually after each episode. Due to the severity of the episodes, the patient was instructed to carry epinephrine 0.3 mg autoinjector (EpiPen) at all times.

Extensive search for possible etiology was carried out. Ancillary studies were nonproductive. Blood tests included a complete blood count, full chemistry panel, serum levels of thyroid stimulating hormone, antinuclear antibodies, rheumatoid factor, antineutrophil cytoplasmic antibodies, C-1 inhibitor activity, tryptase, and chromogranin. Urinary vanillylmandelic acid and 5-hydroxyindoleacetic acid were also negative, as were urine and stool tests for OVA and parasites. Imaging studies (chest roentgenograms, abdominal ultrasound) did not show evidence of echinococcal infection, and endoscopically obtained biopsies from the GI tract did not show eosinophils or mast cells. Skin biopsy was negative for C-KIT, and bone marrow aspiration showed no evidence of increased mast cell count and was negative for tryptase and C-KIT. While the workup was in progress, the patient was placed on prophylactic antihistamines, using several preparations, but the attacks persisted, and periodically supplemental steroids were necessary.

The patient disclosed that from time to time he was using marijuana socially and that it seemed to him that the attacks were less frequent when he did. The patient declared that he did not prepare the cigarette himself, so we presumed he did not have a significant skin contact with cannabis. The history was consistent with the known effect of cannabis on the immune system as described in the introduction, so we conjectured that marijuana may have had a modulatory effect facing failure of other treatment modalities. We suggested that the patient should try medical grade marijuana inhalations (cannabis products for medical indications may be legally used in Israel, but authorization by the Ministry of Health is required for each individual patient and prescription must be renewed monthly). The patient was informed that there was no supporting evidence in the medical literature for this treatment in his condition but that the potential risk for side effects was minimal and he consented to try. He was instructed not to drive or engage in other potentially risky activities during treatment.

We prescribe a total of 20 grams of medical grade marijuana per month, inhaled two to three times a week, which in Israel is the minimal accepted dosage for medical indications. The patient stayed on this dose for two years during which the patient did not have a single attack and no adverse effects were observed. After two years, the patient tried to stop treatment, on his own initiative, but developed a recurrent severe attack a week later. After resuming the treatment no further attacks were observed over the next 4 months of close followup (the regulations for legal use of medical marijuana stipulate that the prescription must be renewed monthly). The timeline of the course of the disease is depicted in Figure 1.

3. Discussion

This is the first report in which a cannabis product for the treatment of refractory idiopathic angioedema was associated with an excellent clinical response. The rate of attacks dropped from at least twice a month to nil, appeared again a week after cessation, and disappeared again when treatment was restarted. This course is consistent with Koch's postulates for establishing causality: frequent attacks before treatment, no attacks during treatment, and recurrence after temporarily stopping treatment.

The exact mechanism by which the drug worked is not clear. Measuring IgE against LPTs (e.g., Pru p3) [7] may have shed some light on the mechanism because cross reactivity with cannabis has been described, but this test is not currently available in our institute.

In this case, the patient smoked medical grade marijuana, which affects both the CB1 and CB2 receptors. The CB2 cannabinoid receptors are present mainly in immune cells [6]. It is possible that using CB1 antagonists would allow elimination of potentially undesirable psychotropic effects [10].

While in this case it is hard to dispute the beneficial effect of inhaled marijuana at the prescribed dosage, it is possible that the effect would not last or that there would be a need to escalate the dosage. Therefore, this case report does not establish that the beneficial effects we observed would be maintained in the long run. However, the decrease of the number of potentially life threatening attacks from at least twice a month to nil and the effect of the drug on the patient's quality of life are encouraging.

More research into the exact mechanism of action of cannabis products in cases of idiopathic angioedema and on the modulation of the immune response in general is indicated.

Conflict of Interests

The authors declare that there is no conflict of interests regarding the publication of this paper.

References

[1] R. H. Champion, S. O. Roberts, R. G. Carpenter, and J. H. Roger, "Urticaria and angio-oedema. A review of 554 patients," *British Journal of Dermatology*, vol. 81, no. 8, pp. 588–597, 1969.

[2] M. Bas, V. Adams, T. Suvorava, T. Niehues, T. K. Hoffmann, and G. Kojda, "Nonallergic angioedema: role of bradykinin," *Allergy*, vol. 62, no. 8, pp. 842–856, 2007.

[3] M. Sánchez-Borges, R. Asero, I. J. Ansotegui et al., "Diagnosis and treatment of urticaria and angioedema: a worldwide perspective," *World Allergy Organization Journal*, vol. 5, no. 11, pp. 125–147, 2012.

[4] L. C. Zingale, L. Beltrami, A. Zanichelli et al., "Angioedema without urticaria: a large clinical survey," *CMAJ*, vol. 175, no. 9, pp. 1065–1070, 2006.

[5] A. P. Kaplan and M. W. Greaves, "Angioedema," *Journal of the American Academy of Dermatology*, vol. 53, no. 3, pp. 373–392, 2005.

[6] E. J. Downer, "Cannabinoids and innate immunity: taking a toll on neuroinflammation," *The Scientific World Journal*, vol. 11, pp. 855–865, 2011.

[7] S. Rom and Y. Persidsky, "Cannabinoid receptor 2: potential role in immunomodulation and neuroinflammation," *Journal of Neuroimmune Pharmacology*, vol. 8, no. 3, pp. 608–620, 2013.

[8] J. C. Ashton, "Cannabinoids for the treatment of inflammation," *Current Opinion in Investigational Drugs*, vol. 8, no. 5, pp. 373–384, 2007.

[9] T. W. Klein, C. Newton, K. Larsen et al., "The cannabinoid system and immune modulation," *Journal of Leukocyte Biology*, vol. 74, no. 4, pp. 486–496, 2003.

[10] M. A. Huestis, D. A. Gorelick, S. J. Heishman et al., "Blockade of effects of smoked marijuana by the CB1-selective cannabinoid receptor antagonist SR141716," *Archives of General Psychiatry*, vol. 58, no. 4, pp. 322–328, 2001.

41

Nocardia Brain Abscess and CD4$^+$ Lymphocytopenia in a Previously Healthy Individual

Norair Adjamian,[1] **Adeline Kikam,**[2] **Kathryn Ruda Wessell,**[3] **Jason Casselman,**[3]
Erin Toller-Artis,[3] **Olapeju Olasokan,**[3] **and Robert W. Hostoffer**[3]

[1]*Kansas City University of Medicine & Biosciences, Kansas City, MO 1750, USA*
[2]*Firelands Regional Medical Center, Sandusky, OH 1111, USA*
[3]*University Hospitals Richmond Medical Center, Richmond Heights, OH 27100, USA*

Correspondence should be addressed to Norair Adjamian; nadjamian@gmail.com

Academic Editor: Elena Bozzola

Nocardia brain abscesses are a known occurrence in patients with immunocompromised conditions. Nocardial infection is commonly an unfortunate sequela to other complications which these patients are being followed up and treated for. The incidence of nocardial brain abscess in an otherwise healthy patient is extremely rare. We present a case of *Nocardia* brain abscess in a previously healthy individual, who, upon workup for vision and gait abnormalities, was shown to have multiple brain abscesses and a decreased absolute CD4$^+$ lymphocyte count. Adding to the rarity of our case, the finding of lymphocytopenia in our patient was unrelated to any known predisposing condition or infectious state.

1. Introduction

Patients with deficiencies in cell-mediated immunity are at high risk of infection with opportunistic pathogens such as *Nocardia* [1]. Among these individuals are those with lymphoma, various malignancies, and human immunodeficiency virus (HIV), organ or hematopoietic stem-cell transplant recipients, and those receiving long term treatment of medications that suppress the immune system [1]. Of other known described conditions, Idiopathic CD4$^+$ Lymphocytopenia (ICL) was first defined in 1992 by the US Centers for Disease Control and Prevention (CDC) as

> ... a documented absolute CD4 T-lymphocyte count of <300 cells/mm3 or <20% of total T-cells on two separate time points at least six weeks apart, without evidence of infection of HIV-1 or HIV-2 testing, and without immunodeficiency or therapy related to decrease of CD4 T-cells... [2].

We report the case of a patient with depressed CD4$^+$ counts, unrelated to HIV infection or other immunocompromising conditions, presenting with *Nocardia* brain abscess. Her CD4 T-lymphocyte count, although not to the strict definition of <300 cells/mm^3, was clearly depressed from the normal value range and idiopathic in nature.

2. Case Presentation

At the age of 70, our patient presented to the Emergency Department (ED) with slurred speech, left peripheral visual field deficits, left sided weakness, and unsteady gate. Her past medical history includes asthma, allergic rhinitis, arthritis, and hypotension. Computed Tomography (CT) of the brain revealed large, low-density areas in the right temporal, occipital, and parietal regions, primarily involving the white matter. Magnetic Resonance Imaging (MRI) showed multiple ring enhancing lesions within the right hemisphere, with the dominant lesion found in the posterior parietal-occipital region, measuring 3.2 × 2.4 cm. Chest X-ray revealed mild left lower lobe density indicative of subsegmental atelectasis, but otherwise the lungs appeared clear. She underwent a right craniotomy with excision of the right occipital mass that confirmed abscess formation, culture positive for *Nocardia farcinica*. The patient was placed on intravenous (IV) antibiotics consisting of trimethoprim/sulfamethoxazole (TMP/SMX) and linezolid for two months following her diagnosis and then transitioned to oral TMP/SMX. She remains on TMP/SMX for prophylactic therapy. HIV-1 and HIV-2 antibodies were nonreactive 2 months after surgery. CD4$^+$ counts acquired 6 months and 11 months after surgery revealed depletion of CD4$^+$ T cells with a declining pattern. The values were 398 cells/uL and 343 cells/uL, respectively. The remainder of her immunodeficiency workup was negative, including no demonstrable Cluster Differentiation (CD) markers that revealed an additional underlying immunodeficiency. Malignancy workup was also negative.

3. Discussion

Nocardia is described as an opportunistic bacteria, most commonly infecting immunocompromised patients but not uncommon in immunocompetent individuals as well [1]. Those at particularly high risk are patients with deficiencies in cell-mediated immunity [1]. The most common anatomic site for nocardial infection is pulmonary due to inhalation being the primary route of exposure [1]. Classic pulmonary symptoms include cough, shortness of breath, chest pain, hemoptysis, fever, night sweats, and fatigue. Pulmonary nocardiosis is associated with patients with underlying pulmonary diseases including asthma, chronic sarcoidosis, emphysema, and chronic bronchitis, who have been treated with long term, high dose of corticosteroid therapy [3]. Observed sites for extrapulmonary nocardiosis include the central nervous system and skin [3]. CNS manifestations include multiple brain abscesses, which can present with headaches, nausea, vomiting, seizures, or other neurological symptoms [3]. Cutaneous nocardiosis may lead to superficial abscesses or localized cellulitis [3].

Similar to our reported case, patients with Idiopathic CD4$^+$ Lymphocytopenia (ICL) go undiagnosed until they develop symptoms suggestive of opportunistic infections [4]. Ahmad et al. found 258 diagnosed cases of ICL in 143 published papers [4]. This study was able to determine the ten most common opportunistic organisms to infect these patients: *Clostridium neoformans* (26.6%), *Mycobacterium* spp. (17%), *Candida* spp. (16.20%), Varicella Zoster Virus (13.10%), Human Papilloma Virus (11.60%), Herpes Simplex Virus (8.10%), *Pneumocystis carinii* pneumonia (7.70%), Cytomegalovirus (5.80%), John Cunningham Virus (3.90%), and *Toxoplasma* (3.10%) [4]. Among the unusual bacterial infections noted, there were only two nocardiosis cases. One, similar to our patient, was associated with *N. farcinica* brain abscesses, and the second nocardiosis case was disseminated *N. asteroides* without brain abscesses [5]. The patient with the *Nocardia* brain abscesses was a 19-year-old heterosexual male

who had accompanying epidermodysplasia verruciformis-like skin eruptions with dysplasia by HPV-16, along with pulmonary tuberculosis [5]. The patient died of respiratory failure during treatment [5]. After a thorough review of the literature, the case of *N. farcinica* brain abscess of the 19-year-old male was the only case of *Nocardia* brain abscesses reported in a patient with Idiopathic CD4$^+$ Lymphocytopenia [5].

We present, to our knowledge, the second reported case of *Nocardia* brain abscess in a patient with depressed absolute CD4$^+$ counts, unrelated to HIV or other conditions depleting cell mediated immunity. In contrast to the first ICL *Nocardia* brain abscess case, our patient had no underlying pulmonary comorbid disease besides her mild, well-controlled asthma. The 19-year-old male with the first reported *Nocardia* brain abscess case with ICL had underlying pulmonary tuberculosis. Our patient's CD4 T-lymphocyte count, although not to the strict definition of <300 cells/mm^3, was clearly depressed (down to 343 cells/uL) from the normal value range. Prior to her presentation at the Emergency Department, our patient had no major illnesses, and her comorbid conditions of asthma, allergic rhinitis, arthritis, and hypotension were all easily managed, and without complications. Similar to other reported cases of CD4$^+$ T-lymphopenia, her indolent condition went unrecognized until the *Nocardia* brain abscess manifested as acute neurologic symptoms.

4. Conclusion

Nocardia is a rare opportunistic pathogen found in immunocompromised patients. Nocardial brain abscesses in patients with idiopathic CD4$^+$ lymphopenia are exceedingly rare in the literature. To our knowledge, we present the first case of a nocardial brain abscess in an otherwise healthy patient with depressed CD4$^+$ counts idiopathic in nature. She did not present with other coinfections, displayed symptomatology limited to neurologic manifestations, demonstrated infection clearance with abscess resection and antibiotic therapy, and has remained infection-free since TMP/SMX prophylaxis was initiated.

Conflict of Interests

The authors declare that there is no conflict of interests regarding the publication of this paper.

References

[1] J. W. Wilson, "Nocardiosis: updates and clinical overview," *Mayo Clinic Proceedings*, vol. 87, no. 4, pp. 403–407, 2012.

[2] A. Régent, B. Autran, G. Carcelain et al., "Idiopathic CD4 lymphocytopenia: clinical and immunologic characteristics and follow-up of 40 patients," *Medicine*, vol. 93, no. 2, pp. 61–72, 2014.

[3] B. A. Brown-Elliott, J. M. Brown, P. S. Conville, and R. J. Wallace Jr., "Clinical and laboratory features of the *Nocardia* spp. based on current molecular taxonomy," *Clinical Microbiology Reviews*, vol. 19, no. 2, pp. 259–282, 2006.

[4] D. S. Ahmad, M. Esmadi, and W. C. Steinmann, "Idiopathic CD4 lymphocytopenia: spectrum of opportunistic infections,

malignancies, and autoimmune diseases," *Avicenna Journal of Medicine*, vol. 3, no. 2, pp. 37–47, 2013.

[5] F. Göktay, A. T. Mansur, M. Erşahin, R. Adaleti, and P. Güneş, "Idiopathic CD4+ T lymphocytopenia with epidermodysplasia verruciformis-like skin eruption, Nocardia farcinica brain abscesses and pulmonary tuberculosis: a case report with fatal outcome," *The Journal of Dermatology*, vol. 38, no. 9, pp. 930–933, 2011.

42

Intrapleural Bortezomib for the Therapy of Myelomatous Pleural Effusion: A Case Report

Magdalena Klanova,[1,2] **Pavel Klener,**[1,2] **Marek Trneny,**[1,3] **Jan Straub,**[1] **and Ivan Spicka**[1]

[1] *1st Department of Medicine and Clinical Department of Hematology, the General Teaching Hospital, Charles University in Prague, Prague, Czech Republic*
[2] *Institute of Pathological Physiology, First Faculty of Medicine, Charles University in Prague, Prague, Czech Republic*
[3] *Institute of Hematology and Blood Transfusion, Prague, Czech Republic*

Correspondence should be addressed to Ivan Spicka, spicka@cesnet.cz

Academic Editors: N. Martinez-Quiles, H. Narimatsu, M. M. Nogueras, and H. L. Trivedi

Myelomatous pleural effusion (MPE) is an extremely rare manifestation of multiple myeloma (MM). We present a case of MPE in a patient with IgG-κ MM treated with intrapleural bortezomib with systemic bortezomib-based therapy. Although we observed good local response, the patient succumbed due to systemic myeloma progression.

1. Introduction

Myelomatous pleural effusion is an extremely rare manifestation of multiple myeloma and only a few cases have been reported to date [1]. MPE in patients with MM is often associated with high-risk disease and poor prognosis despite aggressive treatment. There is no standard treatment strategy for MPE and the majority of cases of MM presenting with MPE were associated with resistance to therapy [2]. Bortezomib (the dipeptidylboronic acid analogue, proteasome inhibitor) belongs now to backbone antimyeloma drugs. The data concerning intrapleural administration of bortezomib is scarce. We present a case of MPE in a patient with IgG-κ MM treated with intrapleural bortezomib and concomitantly with systemic bortezomib-based-combined therapy.

2. Case History

A 43-year-old female initially presented to the hospital in November 2009 with a dry cough, dyspnea, and left chest pain. The chest X-ray showed bilateral pneumonia. The computer tomography demonstrated a massive tumor involving the left breast and chest cavity, a tumor in the uterus and right ovary, multiple osteolytic lesions in the skull and ribs, and bilateral axillar lymphadenopathy. Immunohistochemical analysis of the breast tumor biopsy revealed plasmacytoma/multiple myeloma. Bone marrow examination by trephine biopsy revealed 30% infiltration with atypical plasma cells. Cytogenetic studies including FISH showed a deletion of chromosome 13 and amplification of 1q21 and 1q26 genomic regions. On admission the total plasma protein was 106 g/L, albumin 40 g/L, urea 5.7 mmol/L, creatinine 74 umol/L, calcium 2.12 mmol/L, LDH 3.7 ukat/L (normal values 2,2–3,75 ukat/L), and β-2 microglobulin 3.0 mg/L (normal values 1.0–2,4 mg/L). The international staging system (ISS) score was 1. Serum protein electrophoresis with immunofixation confirmed monoclonal gammopathy IgG-κ 44 g/L. Initially, the patient was treated with cyclophosphamide, thalidomide, and dexamethasone (CTD), but achieved no objective response (stable disease). In the second line therapy bortezomib (Velcade) was added (VTD combination) but due to side effects (severe myopathy) dexamethasone had to be shortly discontinued.

In July 2010, after 2 VT cycles, the CT scan showed a progression of extranodal masses with massive left pleural effusion (Figure 1(a)). The flow-cytometry analysis of pleural

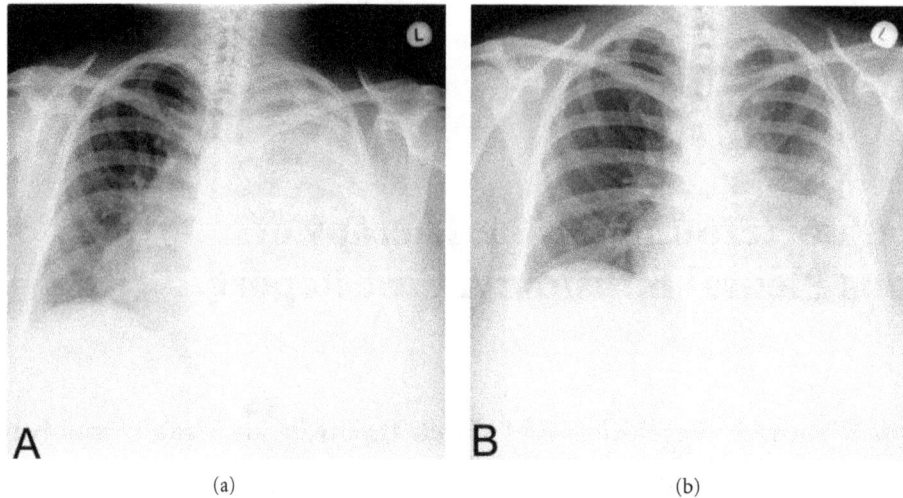

FIGURE 1: (a) Chest X-ray of patient showing massive left pleural effusion and (b) reduction of the pleural effusion after two doses of intrapleural bortezomib.

effusion demonstrated infiltration with atypical plasma cells thereby confirming the diagnosis of MPE. Repeated evacuations of the pleural fluid resulted only in short alleviations followed by rapid replenishment of the MPE. The patient was indicated to third-line therapy and received 1 modified cycle of bortezomib, doxorubicin, and dexamethasone (PAD), in which, on days 8 and 11, one-half of the bortezomib dose (i.e., $0.75 \, \text{mg/m}^2$) was administered intrapleurally and the other half (i.e., $0.75 \, \text{mg/m}^2$) intravenously. The patient thus received two doses of intrapleural bortezomib ($0.75 \, \text{mg/m}^2$) three days apart, namely, in an attempt to mitigate the symptoms associated with pleural effusion refractory to repeated thoracocenteses. After the intrapleural administration of bortezomib the patient became thoracocentesis-independent, and in a two-week period the CT scan confirmed significant regression of pleural effusion (Figure 1(b)). Subsequently, the patient received four cycles of fourth-line therapy—PAD with lenalidomide (added to combination due to the progression of extramedullary disease) but still with no effect on extramedullary tumors. Due to the progression of the disease and poor tolerance of previous therapy (hypotension after bortezomib, cytopenia) immediate high-dose melphalan therapy with stem cell support was planned; however, the patient eventually succumbed in November 2010 due to infectious complications just before the start of stem cell mobilization. The autopsy was not performed at the request of the family.

3. Discussion

Multiple myeloma is the second most common hematologic malignancy after non-Hodgkin's lymphoma and is responsible for 2% of cancer deaths [3]. The plasma cell disorder is characterized by the proliferation of malignant plasmocytes accumulating mainly in the bone marrow and by the production of monoclonal immunoglobulin [4]. Apart from this characteristic features the clinical manifestations of disease could be variable. Pleural effusion is an untypical finding in myeloma patients affecting approximately 6% of the cases [1]. The pathogenesis most frequently involves congestive heart failure due to amyloidosis and cardiac disease in the older myeloma population [5, 6]. MPE itself due to involvement of the pleura is extremely rare and only a few cases have been reported to date. Kintzer et al. reported 0.8% cases of MPE from 958 patients with MM [1]. MPE usually occurs as a late complication of MM in the course of the disease progression and is associated with very poor prognosis. A survival rate of less than 4 months has been reported in the few cases of MPE despite aggressive treatment [6].

There is no standard therapy for MPE. Various anti-myeloma agents in combination with local treatment approaches targeted at pleural effusion, for example, pleurodesis, were tested without significant effect. High-dose chemotherapy with peripheral blood stem cell support for MPE did not confer clear survival advantage [7]. The intrapleural administration of α-interferon [8] or doxorubicin [9] has been tested in an attempt to increase concentrations of the drugs in the pleural cavity. The data concerning intrapleural administration of bortezomib remains scarce. Iannitto et al. published a case report of intrapleurally administered bortezomib in a patient with refractory MM, in whom MPE occurred late in the course of the disease. Their patient first received two cycles of i.v. bortezomib, dexamethasone, and pegylated liposomal doxorubicin without any impact on the formation of pleural effusion. Thus, the therapy was modified and in the third cycle half of the bortezomib dose was administered intrapleurally (for the total of 4 injections). After completion of the single-modified cycle of bortezomib, MPE disappeared [10]. Similarly, in our patient only as few as two intrapleural administrations of bortezomib ($0.75 \, \text{mg/m}^2$ each) resulted in a rapid improvement of clinical symptoms, followed by a gradual disappearance of MPE. We assume that increased intrapleural concentration of bortezomib as a result of local administration might represent a major factor responsible for the rapid remission of MPE. In conclusion, intrapleural administration of bortezomib appears safe and efficacious treatment approach targeted at MPE and MPE-related clinical symptoms.

Conflict of Interests

None of the authors of the paper has declared any conflict of interests.

Acknowledgment

This work is supported by Grant nos. IGA MZ CR NT12215-4/2011, IGA MZ NS/10287-3, PRVOUK-P24/LF1/3, and GA-UK 44621.

References

[1] J. S. Kintzer, E. C. Rosenow, and R. A. Kyle, "Thoracic and pulmonary abnormalities in multiple myeloma. A review of 958 cases," *Archives of Internal Medicine*, vol. 138, no. 5, pp. 727–730, 1978.

[2] Y. M. Kim, K. K. Lee, H. S. Oh et al., "Myelomatous effusion with poor response to chemotherapy," *Journal of Korean Medical Science*, vol. 15, no. 2, pp. 243–246, 2000.

[3] R. A. Kyle and S. V. Rajkumar, "Multiple myeloma," *Blood*, vol. 111, no. 6, pp. 2962–2972, 2008.

[4] R. Bataille and J. L. Harousseau, "Multiple myeloma," *New England Journal of Medicine*, vol. 336, no. 23, pp. 1657–1665, 1997.

[5] J. N. Rodriguez, A. Pereira, J. C. Martinez, J. Conde, and E. Pujol, "Pleural effusion in multiple myeloma," *Chest*, vol. 105, no. 2, pp. 622–624, 1994.

[6] J. C. Hughes and M. L. Votaw, "Pleural effusion in multiple myeloma," *Cancer*, vol. 44, no. 3, pp. 1150–1154, 1979.

[7] R. Kamble, C. S. Wilson, A. Fassas et al., "Malignant pleural effusion of multiple myeloma: prognostic factors and outcome," *Leukemia and Lymphoma*, vol. 46, no. 8, pp. 1137–1142, 2005.

[8] S. Makino, S. Yamahara, Y. Nagake, and J. Kamura, "Bence-Jones myeloma with pleural effusion: response to α-interferon and combined chemotherapy," *Internal Medicine*, vol. 31, no. 5, pp. 617–621, 1992.

[9] E. Iannitto, R. Scaglione, M. Musso, V. Abbadessa, and G. Licata, "Intrapleural adriamycin in treatment of myelomatous pleural effusion: a case report," *Haematologica*, vol. 73, no. 4, pp. 325–326, 1988.

[10] E. Iannitto, V. Minardi, and C. Tripodo, "Use of intrapleural bortezomib in myelomatous pleural effusion," *British Journal of Haematology*, vol. 139, no. 4, pp. 621–622, 2007.

43

Cephazolin-Induced Toxic Epidermal Necrolysis Treated with Intravenous Immunoglobulin and N-Acetylcysteine

Carlos Saavedra, Paola Cárdenas, Héctor Castellanos, Kateir Contreras, and J. R. Castro

Units of Infectology and Dermatology, Department of Internal Medicine, National University of Colombia, 111321 Bogotá, Colombia

Correspondence should be addressed to Paola Cárdenas, paolajimena@gmail.com

Academic Editors: N. Kutukculer and A. Plebani

Toxic epidermal necrolysis is the most severe form of drug-induced skin reaction and includes denudation of >30% of total body surface area. The mechanism of disease is not completely understood, but immunologic mechanisms, cytotoxic reactions, and delayed hypersensitivity seem to be involved. We report a case of cephazolin-induced toxic epidermal necrolysis treated with intravenous immunoglobulin and N-acetylcysteine with excellent response.

1. Introduction

Drug-induced toxic epidermal necrolysis (TEN), also known as Lyell's syndrome, remains one of the most dramatic dermatological emergencies characterized by extensive destruction of the epidermis and mucosal epithelia that often can be caused by drugs [1]. TEN affects between 0.4 and 1.5 cases per million people every year [1, 2] with a mortality rate from 15% to 40%, with a large portion of patients dying from infections or multiorgan failure [3, 4].

The pathogenesis of drug-induced TEN is unknown, although several theories have been developed. Recent discoveries have shown that keratinocytes in TEN undergo apoptosis, not simply necrosis [5, 6]. Further research has elucidated that this apoptosis can be induced by interactions between cell surface death receptor Fas and its ligand, FasL or CD95L.

The management of these patients is primarily supportive, although use of corticosteroids and intravenous immunoglobulin (IVIG) therapy has been widely used with controversy.

We report a case of Cephazolin-induced toxic epidermal necrolysis with excellent response to N-acetylcysteine. Immunopathogenesis and current imputability of antibiotics in TEN will be discussed together with a review of the literature.

2. Case Report

A 38-year-old woman with a long history of type I diabetes was hospitalized in our institution for an acute episode of complicated urinary tract infection. She reported no history of allergy to antibiotics. Upon admission, physical examination revealed a temperature of 38°C, a pulse of 120 beats/min, and a blood pressure of 85/50. The patient developed septic and hypovolemic shock requiring aggressive fluid resuscitation and dopamine. Laboratory findings were white blood cells, 24 900/mm^3 (85.8% segmented, 7.6% lymphocyte, 5.7% monocyte, 0.4% eosinophil, and 0.5% basophil); red blood cells, 435 × 10^4/mm^3; hemoglobin, 14.0 g/dL; platelets, 23.2 × 10^4/mm^3. Blood chemistry documented: glucose level, 305 mg/dL; blood urea nitrogen (BUN), 27 mg/dL; creatinine, 1.6 mg/dL; C-reactive protein, 70 mg/dL; IgG, 1050 mg/dL; IgA, 290 mg/dL; IgM, 132 mg/dL.

She was first administered cephazolin intravenously. Three days later, she developed an erythematous rash and flaccid blisters mainly on her back and arm (Figure 1).

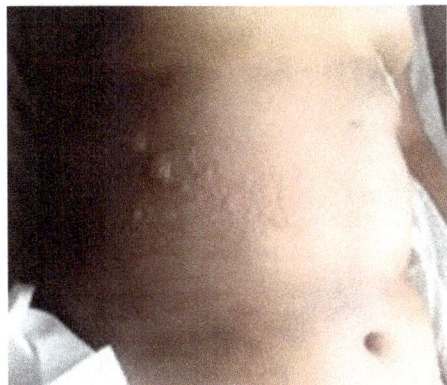

FIGURE 1

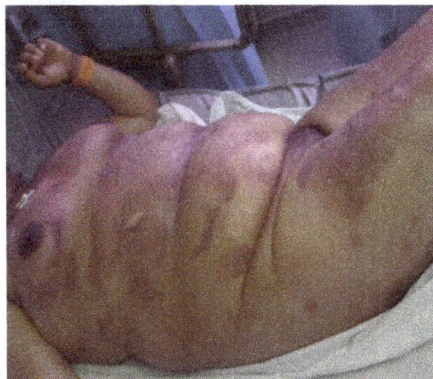

FIGURE 2

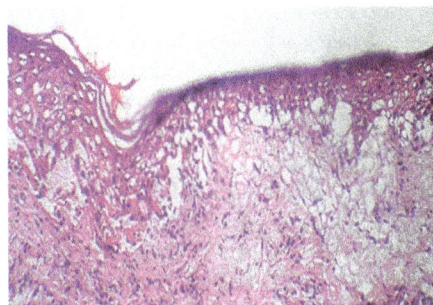

FIGURE 3

The administration of the antibiotic was stopped and was shifted to tigecycline according to the uroculture results. The cutaneous rash progressed onto the trunk, face, and limbs, reaching almost 52% of the body surface; blisters appeared progressively on the erythematous areas during the following 2 days (Figure 2).

A calculated SCORTEN value of 3 predicted a 35.8% mortality rate. Bilateral conjunctivitis and erosions of the genital and oral mucosae also developed. The diagnosis of TEN was confirmed by a skin biopsy, showing a subepidermal blister with presence of rare mononuclear cells scattered between confluent necrotic keratinocytes (Figure 3).

The patient was placed on a fluidized bed and benefited from supportive and antiseptic measures, including daily baths. No systemic corticosteroids were given. Massive rehydration was undertaken. In addition, intravenous immunoglobulins were administered on a daily dosage of 1 g/kg body weight for three consecutive days. On completion of the immunoglobulin perfusions, the clinical examination revealed that progression to 75% BSA epidermal detachment occurred over the next 48 hours (Figure 4). The Nikolsky sign was positive. In the context of a septic patient we decided to administrate N-acetylcysteine 600 mg every 8 hours intravenously; two days later the erosive lesions of the skin and mucosae had dried and eyes were cured. She was discharged after 16 days, with complete reepithelialization.

3. Discussion

The Stevens-Johnson syndrome (SJS) and toxic epidermal necrolysis (TEN) represent different degrees of a severe, acute mucocutaneous reaction that often can be caused by drugs [1].

TEN is most commonly characterized by skin changes (scattered 2-ring target-like lesions with a dark-red center and lighter red halo and red macules with central blistering that can coalesce to larger areas of denuded skin), hemorrhagic mucositis (mouth, eyes, genitals, and respiratory tract), and systemic symptoms (fever, malaise, and possible internal organ involvement) [3].

SCORTEN, a TEN-specific severity of illness scale, has been proven to be an accurate predictor of mortality in patients with TEN by evaluating 7 independent risk factors (age, presence of malignancy, body surface area involved, serum urea nitrogen level, glucose level, bicarbonate level and heart rate) [7]. The main factors associated with TEN mortality are the occurrence of sepsis at the time of hospitalization (odds ratio [OR] 3.04), age (OR 1.11 per year of age), and total body surface area involved (OR 1.03 per percent of body surface area involved) [8].

In 74%–94% of cases, TEN is triggered either by preceding medication or by an infection of the upper respiratory tract. More than 100 different drugs are considered as having caused TEN. Among them, antibiotics represent one of the most common class of culprit drugs [2].

The prevalence of antibiotics being responsible for TEN ranges from 29% to 42% [2]. Almost all antibiotics have been implicated, but the beta-lactam compounds and the sulfonamide antibiotics exhibit the largest risk group. The relative risk of using aminopenicillins and cephalosporins (relative risk, 6.7 and 14, resp., IC 95%) is much lower than that of sulfonamide antibiotics (relative risk, 172 IC 95%) [9]. Cephalosporins that belong to the beta-lactam antibiotics group are indeed well-known inducers of TEN. However, cephazolin itself has never been reported to be responsible for TEN.

As sepsis is the most dreadful complication, antibiotics are commonly administered to TEN patients. The medication necessary to treat the TEN complications may be in some instances related to the drug that initiated the process, leading to the risk of cross-reactions. In our patient the

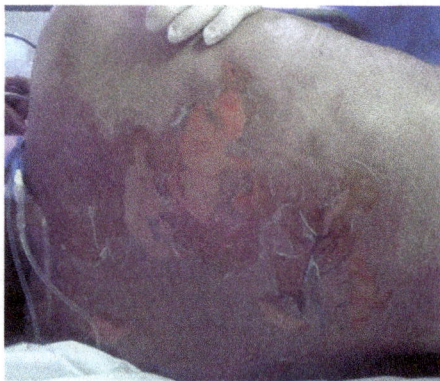

FIGURE 4

treatment for urinary sepsis was responsible for the TEN leading to the risk of cross-reactions as well.

Recent discoveries in the immunopathogenesis of TEN have shown that keratinocytes undergo apoptosis, not simply necrosis, following different phases [10, 11]. Phase I is determined by the immunogenic impact of xenobiotics. It involves a lack of balance between activation and detoxification processes in keratinocytes. Phase II corresponds to early apoptosis. Generation of strongly electrophilic metabolites in TEN keratinocytes is thought to lead to disruption of the electron transfer chain in the mitochondria. In TEN keratinocytes it is likely that reactive oxygen species (ROS), acting as second messengers, increase gene transcription of the TNF-a and CD95 proapoptotic systems. [11] In late apoptosis (phase III) the proinflammatory cytokine TNF-a is believed to act as an autocrine/paracrine factor on neighbouring keratinocytes, thus spreading epidermal destruction. In phase IV, cells with ruptured mitochondria are at risk of death through a slow nonapoptotic mechanism resembling necrosis [12].

There is currently no specific treatment for TEN. Discontinuation of the suspected drug with supportive care (e.g., wound care, hydration, and nutritional support) forms the basis of treatment [4].

Intravenous immunoglobulin therapy (IVIG) is considered by many clinicians as a treatment option, blocking the binding of CD95L [13]. An updated review stratified results according to TEN and SJS, and 14 studies in patients with TEN were evaluated. The majority of studies reported positive results, while three cohort studies did not observe statistically significant improvement with IVIG administration [14]. In a subanalysis of these controlled trials, mortality rate for patients receiving IVIG was 27% compared with 30% for the predicted/control group. Because of the heterogeneity of the studies, a meta-analysis could not be conducted for IVIG in TEN or SJS.

N-acetylcysteine (NAC) is a cysteine derivative precursor of GSH. Abnormal inherited metabolic pathways are presumed in some cases, which could lead to a diminished detoxifying capacity. Administration of N-acetylcysteine enhances the oxidant buffering capacity of glutathione and inhibits nuclear factor kappa B, a transcription factor induced by tumor necrosis factor alpha and interleukin-6. Few patients have been successfully treated with high-dose intravenous NAC in open-label studies [15, 16]. Further studies are required to confirm the beneficial therapeutic effect of NAC in TEN.

Our patient was treated with IVIG with no response. A good response was achieved with N-acetylcysteine, showing the potential benefit of this drug in the TEN treatment.

Different studies had used thalidomide, cyclosporine, infliximab, azathioprine, methotrexate, cyclophosphamide, and plasmapheresis but were limited data to be recommended as first-line treatment [17, 18].

In conclusion, TEN is a complex pathology; although the incidence is relatively low, it is important to identify patients at risk to avoid delaying therapy. We suggest that several molecular targets that block different apoptosis/necrosis pathways should be attacked simultaneously in order to achieve optimal efficacy in the treatment of TEN. We consider that N-acetylcysteine is a good alternative to patients who did not respond to IVIG, especially in septic patients.

To the best of our knowledge, this is the first report of a cephazolin-induced toxic epidermal necrolysis.

References

[1] J. Revuz, "Alan Lyell and Lyell's syndrome," *Journal of the European Academy of Dermatology and Venereology*, vol. 22, no. 8, pp. 1001–1002, 2008.

[2] E. Schöpf, A. Stuhmer, B. Rzany, N. Victor, R. Zentgraf, and J. F. Kapp, "Toxic epidermal necrolysis and Stevens-Johnson syndrome: an epidemiologic study from West Germany," *Archives of Dermatology*, vol. 127, no. 6, pp. 839–842, 1991.

[3] J. Revuz, D. Penso, and J. C. Roujeau, "Toxic epidermal necrolysis: clinical findings and prognosis factors in 87 patients," *Archives of Dermatology*, vol. 123, no. 9, pp. 1160–1165, 1987.

[4] I. Garcia-Doval, L. LeCleach, H. Bocquet, X. L. Otero, and J. C. Roujeau, "Toxic epidermal necrolysis and Stevens-Johnson syndrome: does early withdrawal of causative drugs decrease the risk of death?" *Archives of Dermatology*, vol. 136, no. 3, pp. 323–327, 2000.

[5] C. Paul, P. Wolkenstein, H. Adle et al., "Apoptosis as a mechanism of keratinocyte death in toxic epidermal necrolysis," *British Journal of Dermatology*, vol. 134, no. 4, pp. 710–714, 1996.

[6] I. Viard, P. Wehrli, R. Bullani et al., "Inhibition of toxic epidermal necrolysis by blockade of CD95 with human intravenous immunoglobulin," *Science*, vol. 282, no. 5388, pp. 490–493, 1998.

[7] S. Bastuji-Garin, N. Fouchard, M. Bertocchi, J. C. Roujeau, J. Revuz, and P. Wolkenstein, "Scorten: a severity-of-illness score for toxic epidermal necrolysis," *Journal of Investigative Dermatology*, vol. 115, no. 2, pp. 149–153, 2000.

[8] I. Ducic, A. Shalom, W. Rising, K. Nagamoto, and A. M. Munster, "Outcome of patients with toxic epidermal necrolysis syndrome revisited," *Plastic and Reconstructive Surgery*, vol. 110, no. 3, pp. 768–773, 2002.

[9] M. Mockenhaupt, C. Viboud, A. Dunant et al., "Stevens-Johnson syndrome and toxic epidermal necrolysis: assessment of medication risks with emphasis on recently marketed drugs.

The EuroSCAR-study," *Journal of Investigative Dermatology*, vol. 128, no. 1, pp. 35–44, 2008.

[10] C. Paul, P. Wolkenstein, H. Adle et al., "Apoptosis as a mechanism of keratinocyte death in toxic epidermal necrolysis," *British Journal of Dermatology*, vol. 134, no. 4, pp. 710–714, 1996.

[11] I. Viard, P. Wehrli, R. Bullani et al., "Inhibition of toxic epidermal necrolysis by blockade of CD95 with human intravenous immunoglobulin," *Science*, vol. 282, no. 5388, pp. 490–493, 1998.

[12] D. R. Green and J. C. Reed, "Mitochondria and apoptosis," *Science*, vol. 281, no. 5381, pp. 1309–1312, 1998.

[13] K. Ito, H. Hara, T. Okada, H. Shimojima, and H. Suzuki, "Toxic epidermal necrolysis treated with low-dose intravenous immunoglobulin: immunohistochemical study of Fas and Fas-ligand expression," *Clinical and Experimental Dermatology*, vol. 29, no. 6, pp. 679–680, 2004.

[14] N. Mittmann, B. Chan, S. Knowles, L. Cosentino, and N. Shear, "Intravenous immunoglobulin use in patients with toxic epidermal necrolysis and Stevens-Johnson syndrome," *American Journal of Clinical Dermatology*, vol. 7, no. 6, pp. 359–368, 2006.

[15] A. Velez and J. C. Moreno, "Toxic epidermai necrolysis treated with N-acctylcysteine," *Journal of the American Academy of Dermatology*, vol. 46, pp. 469–470, 2002.

[16] P. Redondo, I. De Felipe, A. De La Pena, J. M. Aramendia, and V. Vanaclocha, "Drug-induced hypersensitivity syndrome and toxic epidermal necrolysis. Treatment with N-acetylcysteine," *British Journal of Dermatology*, vol. 136, no. 4, pp. 645–646, 1997.

[17] R. Gerull, M. Nelle, and T. Schaible, "Toxic epidermal necrolysis and Stevens-Johnson syndrome: a review," *Critical Care Medicine*, vol. 39, pp. 1521–1532, 2011.

[18] T. Harr and L. E. French, "Toxic epidermal necrolysis and Stevens-Johnson syndrome," *Orphanet Journal of Rare Diseases*, vol. 5, pp. 39–50, 2010.

The Efficacy of Mizoribine (Inosine Monophosphate Dehydrogenase Inhibitor) for ANCA-Associated Vasculitis with Hepatitis B Virus Carrier

Jun Muratsu,[1] Atsuyuki Morishima,[1] Masayoshi Kukida,[1] Anzu Tanaka,[1] Shigeki Fujita,[2] and Katsuhiko Sakaguchi[1]

[1] *Department of Nephrology and Hypertension, Sumitomo Hospital, 5-3-20 Kitaku Nakanoshima, Osaka 530-0005, Japan*
[2] *Department of Pathology, Sumitomo Hospital, 5-3-20 Kitaku Nakanoshima, Osaka 530-0005, Japan*

Correspondence should be addressed to Jun Muratsu, jm27252725@yahoo.co.jp

Academic Editors: M. Hummel, A. M. Mansour, M. M. Nogueras, Y. Nozaki, M. T. Perez-Gracia, A. E. Tebo, and A. Vojdani

A 42-year-old female who was an asymptomatic carrier of hepatitis B virus (HBV) was diagnosed with antineutrophil cytoplasm antibody- (ANCA-) associated vasculitis and was induced to remission with 30 mg/day prednisolone nine years ago. Four years ago, she suffered recurrence of ANCA-associated vasculitis and with 30 mg/day prednisolone was induced to remission. This time, laboratory data showed 3-fold increase in myeloperoxidase antineutrophil cytoplasmic antibody (MPO-ANCA) levels. Administration of 30 mg/day prednisolone was started. Three days later, she was admitted to our hospital suffering from fatigue. After admission, urinalysis showed glomerular hematuria. Despite administration of 30 mg/day prednisolone, MPO-ANCA titer had been of high level, ranging from 42 to 83 EU for 2.5 months. Furthermore, the adverse effects of steroid were seen. We decided the tapering of prednisolone (25 mg/day) and the start of mizoribine (4-carbamoyl-1-β-D-ribofuranosyl imidazolium-5-olate) administration. After mizoribine treatment, MPO-ANCA titer was decreased without any mizoribine-related adverse effects. Six months later, MPO-ANCA titer was decreased to normal levels and she was induced to clinical remission without reactivation of HBV. We describe the effectiveness of mizoribine for the ANCA-associated vasculitis complicated with HBV-carrier.

1. Introduction

The common treatment for antineutrophil cytoplasm antibody- (ANCA-) associated vasculitis is oral cyclophosphamide-corticosteroid combination therapy. However, there are some reports that cyclophosphamide-corticosteroid combination therapy has serious complications such as increased risk of infection, leucopenia, osteoporosis, diabetes, and sterility and malignancy [1–4]. Reactivation of hepatitis B virus (HBV) replication is one of complications in patients with chronic HBV infection who receive immunosuppressive therapy [5].

Mizoribine (4-carbamoyl-1-β-D-ribofuranosyl imidazololium-5-olate), a purine synthesis inhibitor, has an immunosuppressive effect equivalent to that of azathioprine, but with less hepatic toxicity and myelosuppression [6].

Mizoribine and mycophenolic acid inhibit the rate-limiting enzyme inosine monophosphate dehydrogenase (IMPDH) in the *de novo* pathway of purine biosynthesis. It was reported that IMPDH inhibitors have potential antiviral effect *in vitro* and inhibited HBV replication with cultures of primary human hepatocytes, HepG2 2.2.15 cells [7–12].

There have been some reports that mizoribine is useful not only as a preemptive treatment to prevent relapse, but as also an aggressive strategy to induce the remission of relapsed ANCA-associated renal vasculitis [13, 14]. However, there have not been any reports about the effectiveness of mizoribine in ANCA-associated renal vasculitis with HBV carrier. Herein, we describe the successful treatment with mizoribine for the case of the ANCA-associated renal vasculitis complicated with HBV carrier who was induced to remission without reactivation of HBV.

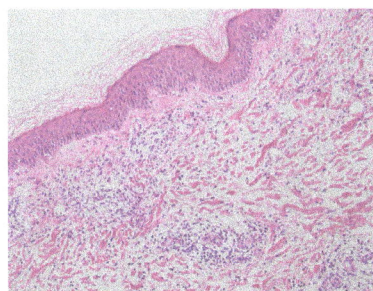

(a)

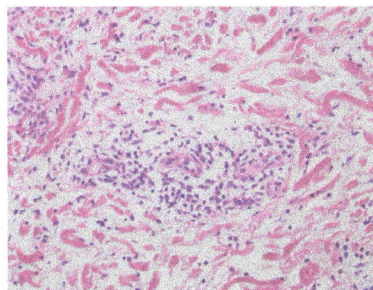

(b)

FIGURE 1: Skin biopsy showed findings of leukocytoclastic vasculitis (A, B H&E stain; A × 20; B × 40).

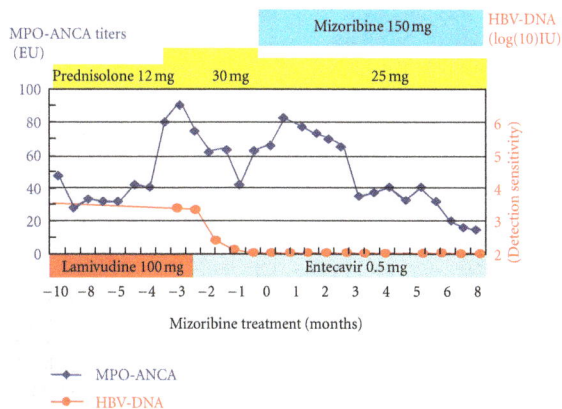

FIGURE 2: Time course plots of the MPO-ANCA levels and HBV-DNA. *MPO-ANCA*: myeloperoxidase antineutrophil cytoplasmic antibody; *HBV-DNA*: Hepatitis B Virus-DNA.

2. Case Presentation

A 42-year-old Japanese female experienced glomerular hematuria, bilateral pedal purpura, and arthralgia nine years ago. Elevation of MPO-ANCA titer and serum creatinine levels was shown. Percutaneous renal biopsy was performed. Nine glomeruli were observed by light microscopy. Five of them were totally obsolescent, and the rest were also collapsing to some extent. Two glomerulus showed cellular crescentic glomerulonephritis. Glomerular deposition of IgA, IgM, IgG, C1q, C3, and C4 was negative. In addition, skin biopsy was performed, which showed leukocytoclastic vasculitis (Figures 1(a) and 1(b)). Thus, she was diagnosed with antineutrophil cytoplasm antibody- (ANCA-) associated vasculitis. Her past medical histories included asymptomatic carrier of hepatitis B virus (HBV) in childhood. Administration of lamivudine was started. She was induced to remission with 30 mg/day prednisolone. Prednisolone had been gradually tapered to 5 mg. Elevation of aspartate aminotransferase and alanine aminotransferase had not been seen. Four years ago, the ANCA-associated vasculitis relapsed and was induced to remission 30 mg/day prednisolone. Prednisolone had been gradually tapered to 12 mg. HBV-DNA had been from 3.4 to 4.5 log(10)IU. Elevation of aspartate aminotransferase and alanine aminotransferase was not seen.

This time, laboratory data showed normal serum creatinine levels and, however, 3-fold increase in myeloperoxidase antineutrophil cytoplasmic antibody (MPO-ANCA) levels (82 EU). We speculated recurrence of the ANCA-associated vasculitis. Administration of 30 mg/day prednisolone was started. Three days later, she was admitted to our hospital suffering from fatigue. On admission, her pulse rate was 76/min regular, blood pressure was 130/84 mmHg, and body temperature was 36.2°C. Her consciousness was clear. Her bulbar conjunctiva was not icteric, and the palpebral conjunctiva was not pale. On auscultation, her lungs and heart were normal. Cough, pulmonary alveolar hemorrhage, and gastrointestinal bleeding were not observed. On palpation, hepatosplenomegaly and ascites were not observed. She did not have any neurological abnormalities. In addition, purpura, rash, arthralgia, myalgia, edema, or oral and genital ulceration were not found. Table 1 shows laboratory data at the admission. Laboratory data showed myeloperoxidase antineutrophil cytoplasmic antibody (MPO-ANCA) levels and showed 3-fold increase, 93 EU. HBs antigen was positive, and HBV-DNA level was 3.4 log(10)IU. Her chest X-ray and echocardiography were normal and electrocardiography had no problem. Abdominal ultrasonography showed that liver was not atrophy. After admission, a urinalysis indicated +/− proteinuria and a 3+ occult blood reaction with 21–50 red blood cells per high-power field. Her 24-hour urinary protein excretion was 0.03 g. Her urine volume was 2300 mL/day. Figure 2 shows time course plots of the MPO-ANCA levels and HBV-DNA. Despite administration of 30 mg/day prednisolone for 2.5 months, MPO-ANCA titers increased and hematuria had been seen without elevation of serum creatinine levels. Furthermore, the adverse effects of steroid, such as moon face, insomnia, and femur head necrosis, were seen. Because she strongly desired pregnancy in the future, we did not start cyclophosphamide. We decided tapering of prednisolone (25 mg/day) and start of mizoribine (4-carbamoyl-1-β-D-ribofuranosyl imidazololium-5-olate) (150 mg/day) administration. Before the start of mizoribine, HBV-DNA was 2.5 log(10)IU and elevation of aspartate aminotransferase and alanine aminotransferase was not seen. Because HBV-DNA was detectable and longer duration (>12 months) of treatment for HBV and ANCA-associated renal vasculitis is anticipated, we changed lamivudine to entecavir before the start of mizoribine administration. We monitored serum concentration of mizoribine (Figure 3). Trough level of mizoribine was 0 μg/mL, after 2 hours

TABLE 1: Laboratory data on admission.

Complete blood count	
White blood cell count	12100/μL
Red blood cell count	$354 \times 10^4/\mu$L
Hemoglobin	11.9 g/dL
Hematocrit	35.8%
Platelets	$33.1 \times 10^4/\mu$L
Blood chemical	
Aspartate aminotransferase	23 IU/L
Alanine aminotransferase	12 IU/L
Alkaline phosphatase	117 IU/L
Lactate dehydrogenase	202 IU/L
γ-GTP	24 IU/L
Total bilirubin	0.7 mg/dL
Creatine phosphokinase	77 IU/L
Total cholesterol	312 mg/dL
Triglyceride	69 mg/dL
Sodium	136 mEq/L
Chloride	99 mEq/L
Potassium	4.5 mEq/L
Uric acid	4.2 mg/dL
Blood urea nitrogen	13 mg/dL
Creatinine	0.56 mg/dL
Total protein	6.7 g/dL
Albumin	4.6 g/dL
C-reactive protein	0.04 mg/dL
Fasting plasma glucose	79 mg/dL
Hemoglobin A1c	5.0%
KL-6	151 U/mL
Immunology	
Immunoglobulin G	782 mg/dL
Immunoglobulin A	145 mg/dL
Immunoglobulin M	48 mg/dL
Complement titer (CH50)	36.9 U/mL
Complement C3	84 mg/dL
Complement C4	18 mg/dL
Antinuclear antibody	<40
HBs antigen	(+)
HBe antigen	(−)
HBe antibody	(+)
HBV-DNA	3.4 log (10) IU
HCV-antibody	(−)
Coagulation	
APTT	25.1 second
PT-INR	0.80
<ELISA>	
MPO-ANCA	93 EU
PR3-ANCA	<10 EU
Urinalysis	
pH	7.0
Specific gravity	1.010
Glucose	(−)
Protein	(−)

TABLE 1: Continued.

Cast	Hyaline cast (+)
Erythrocytes	1–5/HPF
Leukocytes	1–5/HPF

γ-GTP: gamma-glutamyl transpeptidase, PR3-ANCA: proteinase-3 anti-neutrophil cytoplasmic antibody, MPO-ANCA: myeloperoxidase anti-neutrophil cytoplasmic antibody, APTT: activated partial thromboplastin time, PT-INR: prothrombin time-international normalized ratio.

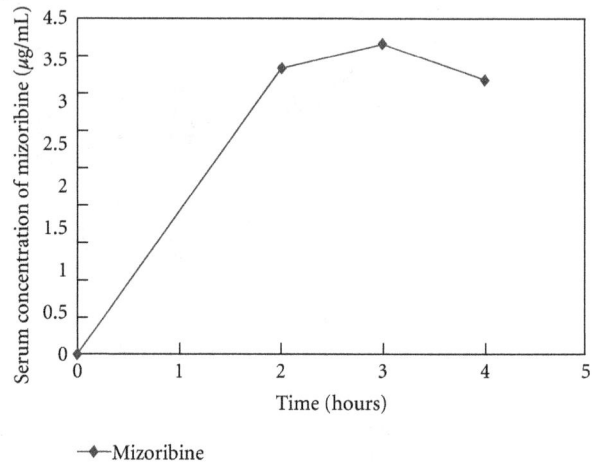

FIGURE 3: Serum concentration-time curve of mizoribine in this case.

the level was 3.82 μg/mL, after 3 hours the level (peak level of mizoribine) was 4.17 μg/mL, and after 4 hours the level was 3.67 μg/mL. After mizoribine treatment, MPO-ANCA titer was decreased without any mizoribine-related adverse effects. Six months later, hematuria and fatigue had not been shown. She was induced to clinical remission without reactivation of HBV. Elevation of MPO-ANCA titers has not been presented for one year.

3. Discussion

We describe a case of the ANCA-associated vasculitis with HBV carrier who was induced remission with mizoribine without reactivation of HBV.

In general, the treatment of relapsed ANCA-associated vasculitis is based on cyclophosphamide and high-dose corticosteroids. However, high-dose corticosteroids are of high risk for HBV replication because HBV-DNA contains a glucocorticoid responsive element [15]. Reactivation of hepatitis B virus (HBV) replication is a well-recognized complication in patients with chronic HBV infection who receive immunosuppressive therapy [5]. However, it was reported that corticosteroid is relatively safe under administration of entecavir [16]. No reports have been described if mizoribine caused HBV replication and fulminant hepatitis.

Mizoribine has an immunosuppressive effect equivalent to that of azathioprine; however, it shows less hepatic toxicity and myelosuppression [6]. Mizoribine has recently been proved clinically effective and relatively safe for the treatment of nephritic syndrome, lupus nephritis, IgA nephropathy, and ANCA-associated renal vasculitis [14, 17–19]. The administration should also only be done in facilities where the blood level of mizoribine can be monitored. It is important to monitor serum concentration of mizoribine because mizoribine is excreted through kidney. There have been some reports that more than $5\,\mu g/mL$ of mizoribine trough level induce hepatic dysfunction [6]. Mizoribine showed an inhibition of 50% on human mixed-lymphocyte reaction at a concentration of about $1\,\mu g/mL$.

Mizoribine and mycophenolic acid inhibit the rate-limiting enzyme inosine monophosphate dehydrogenase (IMPDH) in the de novo pathway of purine biosynthesis. It has been reported that mycophenolic acid inhibits the replication of human immunodeficiency virus (HIV) *in vitro* by depletion of the deoxynucleoside triphosphate substrate of the reverse transcriptase, thus blocking formation of the viral DNA [7]. It was reported that *in vitro* mycophenolic acid inhibited HBV replication. Experiments were performed using cultures of primary human hepatocytes, HepG2 2.2.15 cells in the report [8]. Inhibition of IMPDH reduces the level of intracellular guanine nucleotides required for adequate RNA and DNA synthesis. Therefore, IMPDH inhibitors have potential antiviral effect [9–12]. In addition, it was reported that mizoribine was able to suppress cytomegalovirus plaque formation dose dependently [20]. Thus, we speculate that mizoribine would inhibit HBV replication. However, there was no evidence that mizoribine inhibited HBV replication *in vivo*. Entecavir may suppress HBV replication in this case. This case revealed that mizoribine is safe for ANCA-associated renal vasculitis complicated with HBV carrier under administration of entecavir. It is important to consider mizoribine administration for ANCA-associated renal vasculitis with HBV carrier. However, we must take care of reactivation of HBV replication and monitor HBV-DNA.

In conclusion, mizoribine may be useful and safe for ANCA-associated vasculitis with HBV carrier. There is the possibility that mizoribine is one of the choices for the treatment of ANCA-associated renal vasculitis complicated with HBV carrier. Further experience is needed to confirm our conclusions.

Conflict of Interests

The authors have declared that no conflict of interests exists.

References

[1] J. Turnbull and L. Harper, "Adverse effects of therapy for ANCA-associated vasculitis," *Best Practice and Research: Clinical Rheumatology*, vol. 23, no. 3, pp. 391–401, 2009.

[2] H. Nawata, S. Soen, R. Takayanagi et al., "Guidelines on the management and treatment of glucocorticoid-induced osteoporosis of the Japanese Society for Bone and Mineral Research (2004)," *Journal of Bone and Mineral Metabolism*, vol. 23, no. 2, pp. 105–109, 2005.

[3] M. C. Park, Y. B. Park, S. Y. Jung, I. H. Chung, K. H. Choi, and S. K. Lee, "Risk of ovarian failure and pregnancy outcome in patients with lupus nephritis treated with intravenous cyclophosphamide pulse therapy," *Lupus*, vol. 13, no. 8, pp. 569–574, 2004.

[4] J. E. Hader, L. Marzella, R. A. M. Myers, S. C. Jacobs, and M. J. Naslund, "Hyperbaric oxygen treatment for experimental cyclophosphamide-induced hemorrhagic cystitis," *Journal of Urology*, vol. 149, no. 6, pp. 1617–1621, 1993.

[5] A. S. F. Lok, R. H. S. Liang, E. K. W. Chiu, K. L. Wong, T. K. Chan, and D. Todd, "Reactivation of hepatitis B virus replication in patients receiving cytotoxic therapy: report of a prospective study," *Gastroenterology*, vol. 100, no. 1, pp. 182–188, 1991.

[6] K. Sonda, K. Takahashi, K. Tanabe et al., "Clinical pharmacokinetic study of mizoribine in renal transplantation patients," *Transplantation Proceedings*, vol. 28, no. 6, pp. 3643–3648, 1996.

[7] H. Ichimura and J. A. Levy, "Polymerase substrate depletion: a novel strategy for inhibiting the replication of the human immunodeficiency virus," *Virology*, vol. 211, no. 2, pp. 554–560, 1995.

[8] Z. J. Gong, S. De Meyer, C. Clarysse et al., "Mycophenolic acid, an immunosuppressive agent, inhibits HBV replication in vitro," *Journal of Viral Hepatitis*, vol. 6, no. 3, pp. 229–236, 1999.

[9] P. Franchetti and M. Grifantini, "Nucleoside and non-nucleoside IMP dehydrogenase inhibitors as antitumor and antiviral agents," *Current Medicinal Chemistry*, vol. 6, no. 7, pp. 599–614, 1999.

[10] E. Padalko, E. Verbeken, P. Matthys, J. L. Aerts, E. De Clercq, and J. Neyts, "Mycophenolate mofetil inhibits the development of Coxsackie B3-virus-induced myocarditis in mice," *BMC Microbiology*, vol. 3, article 25, 2003.

[11] M. C. Livonesi, R. L. Moro De Sousa, and L. T. Moraes Figueiredo, "In vitro study of antiviral activity of mycophenolic acid on Brazilian orthobunyaviruses," *Intervirology*, vol. 50, no. 3, pp. 204–208, 2007.

[12] W. Markland, T. J. Mcquaid, J. Jain, and A. D. Kwong, "Broad-spectrum antiviral activity of the IMP dehydrogenase inhibitor VX-497: a comparison with ribavirin and demonstration of antiviral additivity with alpha interferon," *Antimicrobial Agents and Chemotherapy*, vol. 44, no. 4, pp. 859–866, 2000.

[13] K. Hirayama, M. Kobayashi, Y. Hashimoto et al., "Treatment with the purine synthesis inhibitor mizoribine for ANCA-associated renal vasculitis," *American Journal of Kidney Diseases*, vol. 44, no. 1, pp. 57–63, 2004.

[14] Y. Nishioka, Y. Horita, M. Tadokoro et al., "Mizoribine induces remission of relapsed ANCA-associated renal vasculitis," *Nephrology Dialysis Transplantation*, vol. 21, no. 4, pp. 1087–1088, 2006.

[15] A. L. Cheng, C. A. Hsiung, I. J. Su et al., "Steroid-free chemotherapy decreases risk of hepatitis B virus (HBV) reactivation in HBV-carriers with lymphoma," *Hepatology*, vol. 37, no. 6, pp. 1320–1328, 2003.

[16] A. S. F. Lok and B. J. McMahon, "Chronic hepatitis B," *Hepatology*, vol. 45, no. 2, pp. 507–539, 2007.

[17] K. Yoshioka, Y. Ohashi, T. Sakai et al., "A multicenter trial of mizoribine compared with placebo in children with frequently relapsing nephrotic syndrome," *Kidney International*, vol. 58, no. 1, pp. 317–324, 2000.

[18] K. Kaneko, "Mizoribine for childhood IgA nephropathy," *Nephron*, vol. 83, no. 4, pp. 376–377, 1999.

[19] K. Hirayama, M. Kobayashi, Y. Hashimoto et al., "Treatment with the purine synthesis inhibitor mizoribine for ANCA-associated renal vasculitis," *American Journal of Kidney Diseases*, vol. 44, no. 1, pp. 57–63, 2004.

[20] T. Kuramoto, T. Daikoku, Y. Yoshida et al., "Novel anticytomegalovirus activity of immunosuppressant mizoribine and its synergism with ganciclovir," *Journal of Pharmacology and Experimental Therapeutics*, vol. 333, no. 3, pp. 816–821, 2010.

Permissions

List of Contributors

Chad J. Cooper, Sarmad Said and German T. Hernandez
Department of Internal Medicine, Texas Tech University Health Sciences Center, 4800 Alberta Avenue, El Paso, TX 79905, USA

Benjamin Smith and Matthew B. Carroll
81st Medical Group Hospital, 301 Fisher Street, Keesler Air Force Base, MS 39534, USA

Vasantha Nagendran and Amolak S. Bansal
Epsom and St Helier University Hospitals NHS Trust, Carshalton, Surrey SM5 1AA, UK

Vasantha Nagendran
St Georges University of London, London SW17 0RE, UK

Noel Emmanuel
St George's University Hospitals NHS Foundation Trust, Tooting, London SW17 0QT, UK

Sajal Ajmani, Durga Prasanna Misra and Vikas Agarwal
Department of Clinical Immunology, Sanjay Gandhi Postgraduate Institute of Medical Sciences, Lucknow 226014, India

Deep Chandh Raja
Department of Cardiology, Sanjay Gandhi Postgraduate Institute of Medical Sciences, Lucknow 226014, India

Namita Mohindra
Department of Radiodiagnosis, Sanjay Gandhi Postgraduate Institute of Medical Sciences, Lucknow 226014, India

J. Campbell, R. Kee and A. Fulton
Department of Neurology, Royal Victoria Hospital, Belfast BT12 6BA, UK

D. Bhattacharya and P. Flynn
Department of Neuroradiology, Royal Victoria Hospital, Belfast BT12 6BA, UK

M. McCarron
Neurology Centre, Altnagelvin Area Hospital, Londonderry BT47 6SB, UK
Pinar Ataca, Erden Atilla and Muhit Ozcan
Department of Hematology, Ankara University, Cebeci, 06590 Ankara, Turkey

Resat Kendir and Sevim Bavbek
Department of Pulmonary Medicine, Immunology and Allergy Clinic, Ankara University, Cebeci, 06590 Ankara, Turkey

Piyush Ranjan and Manish Soneja
Department of Medicine, All India Institute of Medical Sciences, New Delhi 110029, India

Nellai Krishnan Subramonian, Vivek Kumar and Shuvadeep Ganguly
All India Institute of Medical Sciences, New Delhi 110029, India

Tarun Kumar and Geetika Singh
Department of Pathology, All India Institute of Medical Sciences, New Delhi 110029, India

Luigi Nespoli, Silvia Tajè, Francesco Paolo Pellegrini and Maddalena Marinoni
Pediatrics Unit, Department of Clinical and Experimental Medicine, University of Insubria, 21100 Varese, Italy

Annapia Verri
Neurological Institute C. Mondino Foundation IRCCS, 27100 Pavia, Italy

Durga Prasanna Misra, Jyoti Ranjan Parida, Abhra Chandra Chowdhury and Vikas Agarwal
Department of Clinical Immunology, Sanjay Gandhi Postgraduate Institute of Medical Sciences, Lucknow 226014, India

Krushna Chandra Pani, Niraj Kumari and Narendra Krishnani
Department of Pathology, Sanjay Gandhi Postgraduate Institute of Medical Sciences, Lucknow 226014, India

Wolfgang Hartung and Martin Fleck
Department of Rheumatology and Clinical Immunology, Asklepios Clinic, 93077 Bad Abbach, Germany

Judith Maier and Martin Fleck
Department of Internal Medicine I, University of Regensburg, 93042 Regensburg, Germany

Michael Pfeifer
Department of Pulmonology and Internal Medicine II, University of Regensburg, 93042 Regensburg, Germany

Saliha Esenboga, Deniz Çagdas Ayvaz, Ozden Sanal and Ilhan Tezcan
Division of Immunology, Department of Pediatrics, Hacettepe University Faculty of Medicine, 06100 Ankara, Turkey

Arzu Saglam Ayhan
Department of Pathology, Hacettepe University Faculty of Medicine, 06100 Ankara, Turkey

Banu Peynircioglu
Department of Medical Biology and Genetics, Hacettepe University Faculty of Medicine, 06100 Ankara, Turkey

Ian A. Myles
Bacterial Pathogenesis Unit, Laboratory of Clinical Infectious Diseases, National Institute of Allergy and Infectious Diseases, National Institutes of Health, 9000 Rockville Pike, Building 33, Room 2W10A, Bethesda, MD20892,USA

Satyen Gada
Allergy/Immunology/Immunization Service, Department of Medicine, Walter Reed National Military Medical Center, 8901Wisconsin Avenue, Bethesda, MD 20889, USA

Teresa Urraro, Laura Gragnani, Alessia Piluso, Alessio Fabbrizzi, Monica Monti, Elisa Fognani, Barbara Boldrini, Jessica Ranieri and Anna Linda Zignego
Center for Systemic Manifestations of Hepatitis Viruses (MASVE), Department of Experimental and Clinical Medicine, University of Florence, Lagro Brambilla 3, 50134 Florence, Italy

Jelena Paovic and Predrag Paovic
University Eye Clinic, Clinical Center of Serbia, Pasterova 2, 11000 Belgrade, Serbia

Vojislav Sredovic
Primary Health Care Center, Jove Negusevica 5, 22140 Pecinci, Serbia

M. M. G. Vollebregt and A. Malfroot
Department of Pediatrics, University Hospital Brussels, 1090 Brussels, Belgium

M. De Raedemaecker
Department of Genetics, University Hospital Brussels, 1090 Brussels, Belgium
M. van der Burg
Department of Immunology, Erasmus MC, 3015 CN Rotterdam, Netherlands

J. E. van der Werff ten Bosch
Department of Pediatric Hematology, Oncology and Immunology, University Hospital Brussels, 1090 Brussels, Belgium

Maria Giovanna Danieli and Ramona Morariu
Clinica Medica, Dipartimento di Scienze Cliniche e Molecolari, Universitá Politecnica delle Marche & Ospedali Riuniti, Via Tronto 10, 60126 Ancona, Italy

Lucia Pettinari
U.O. di Medicina-LPA, Presidio di Loreto, 66025 Loreto, Italy

Fernando Monteforte
U.O. di Radiodiagnostica, Ospedale di Casarano, 73042 Lecce, Italy

Francesco Logullo
Clinica Neurologica, Dipartimento di Medicina Sperimentale e Clinica, Polo Didattico Scientifico, Universita Politecnica delle Marche & Azienda Ospedali Riuniti, Via Tronto 10, 60126 Ancona, Italy

Saul Oswaldo Lugo Reyes and Lizbeth Blancas Galicia
Immunodeficiencies Research Unit, National Institute of Pediatrics, Coyoacan, 04530 Mexico City, DF, Mexico

Saul Oswaldo Lugo Reyes, Lizbeth Blancas Galicia, Marjorie Hubeau, Capucine Picard, Jean-Laurent Casanova, and Jacinta Bustamante
Laboratory of Human Genetics of Infectious Diseases, INSERM U980, University Paris Descartes, Paris Sorbonne Cite, 75014 Paris, France

Capucine Picard, Jacinta Bustamante and Nizar Mahlaoui
French Reference Center for Primary Immune Deficiencies (CEREDIH), Necker-Enfants Malades University Hospital, AP-HP, 75015 Paris, France

Capucine Picard, Stéphane Blanche, Jean-Laurent Casanova and Nizar Mahlaoui
Pediatric Immunology-Hematology Unit, Necker-Enfants Malades University Hospital, AP-HP, 75015 Paris, France

Carolina Prando and Jean-Laurent Casanova
St. Giles Laboratory of Human Genetics of Infectious Diseases, Rockefeller University, New York, NY 10065, USA

Carolina Prando
Bioinformatics Laboratory, Pele Pequeno Principe Research Institute, 80250-060 Curitiba, PR, Brazil

Santiago Bernal-Macías, Laura-Marcela Fino-Velásquez, Benjamín Reyes-Beltrán and Adriana Rojas-Villarraga
Center for Autoimmune Diseases Research (CREA), School of Medicine and Health Sciences, Universidad del Rosario, Bogota, Colombia

Felipe E. Vargas-Barato
Surgery Department, School of Medicine and Health Sciences, Universidad del Rosario, Bogota, Colombia
Surgery Department, Hospital Universitario Mayor-Mederi (HUM), Bogota, Colombia

Lucio Guerra-Galue
Gynaecology Department, Hospital Universitario Mayor-Mederi (HUM), Bogota, Colombia

Anju Bharti
Department of Pathology, King George Medical University, Lucknow 226003, India

Lalit Prashant Meena
Department of General Medicine, Institute of Medical Sciences, Banaras Hindu University, Varanasi 221005, India

Eli Magen and Hadari Israel
Leumit Health Services, Ashkelon, Israel

Eli Magen and Mishal Joseph
Medicine B Department, Barzilai Medical Center, 78306 Ashkelon, Israel

Eli Magen
Allergy and Clinical Immunology Unit, Barzilai Medical Center, Barzilai Hospital, Ben Gurion University of Negev, Ashkelon, Israel

Viktor Feldman
Orthopedic Department, Meir Medical Center, Kfar Saba, Israel

Pietro Sartorelli, Riccardo Romeo, Giuseppina Coppola, Roberta Nuti and Valentina Paolucci
Unit of Occupational Medicine and Toxicology, University of Siena, 16 Bracci Avenue, 53100 Siena, Italy

Soheyla Alyasin, Reza Amin and Hamidreza Houshmand
Department of Pediatrics, Division of Immunology and Allergy, Allergic Research Center, Shiraz University of Medical Science, Shiraz 7134845794, Iran

Alireza Teymoori
School of Medicine, Department of Neurosurgery, Ahvaz Jundishapur University of Medical Sciences, Ahvaz 6135715794, Iran

Gholamreza Houshmand
Department of Pharmacology and Toxicology, Pharmacy School, Ahvaz Jundishapur University of Medical Sciences, Ahvaz 6135715794, Iran

Mohammad Bahadoram
Medical Student Research Committee and Social Determinant of Health Research Center, Ahvaz Jundishapur University of Medical Sciences, Ahvaz 6135715794, Iran

Moushumi Lodh
Department of Biochemistry, The Mission Hospital, Durgapur, West Bengal 713212, India

Debkant Pradhan
Department of Microbiology, The Mission Hospital, Durgapur, West Bengal 713212, India

Ashok Parida
Department of Cardiology, The Mission Hospital, Durgapur, West Bengal 713212, India

James B. Geake
Department of Respiratory and Sleep Medicine, Monash Medical Centre, Melbourne, VIC 3206, Australia

Graeme Maguire
Cairns Clinical School, School of Medicine and Dentistry, Faculty of Medicine, Health and Molecular Sciences, James Cook University, P.O. Box 902, Cairns, QLD 4870, Australia

Baker IDI Central Australia, P.O. Box 1294, Alice Springs, NT 0870, Australia

Raheleh Assari and Mohammad-Hassan Moradinejad
Division of Pediatric Rheumatology, Children's Medical Center, Pediatrics Center of Excellence, Tehran 14194, Iran

Vahid Ziaee
Pediatric Rheumatology Research Group, Rheumatology Research Center, Tehran University of Medical Sciences, Tehran, Iran

Nima Parvaneh, Mohammad-Hassan Moradinejad and Vahid Ziaee
Department of Pediatrics, Tehran University of Medical Sciences, Tehran, Iran

Nima Parvaneh
Research Center for Immunodeficiencies, Tehran University of Medical Sciences, Tehran, Iran

J. F. Moreau
School of Medicine, University of Pittsburgh, Pittsburgh, PA 15261, USA

John A. Ozolek
Division of Pathology, Children's Hospital of Pittsburgh of UPMC, One Children's Hospital Drive, 4401 Penn Avenue, Pittsburgh, PA 15224, USA

P. Ling Lin
Division of Infectious Disease, Children's Hospital of Pittsburgh of UPMC, One Children's Hospital Drive, 4401 Penn Avenue, Pittsburgh, PA 15224, USA

Todd D. Green
Division of Pulmonary Medicine, Allergy and Immunology, Children's Hospital of Pittsburgh of UPMC, One Children's Hospital Drive, 4401 Penn Avenue, Pittsburgh, PA 15224, USA

Elaine A. Cassidy
Division of Rheumatology, Children's Hospital of Pittsburgh of UPMC, One Children's Hospital Drive, 4401 Penn Avenue, Pittsburgh, PA 15224, USA

Veena L. Venkat
Division of Gastroenterology, Children's Hospital of Pittsburgh of UPMC, One Children's Hospital Drive, 4401 Penn Avenue, Pittsburgh, PA 15224, USA

Andrew R. Buchert
The Paul C. Gaffney Diagnostic Referral Service, Children's Hospital of Pittsburgh of UPMC, One Children's Hospital Drive, 4401 Penn Avenue, Pittsburgh, PA 15224, USA

Avni Y. Joshi
Division of Pediatric and Adult Allergy and Immunology, Department of Pediatric and Adolescent Medicine, Mayo Clinic, Rochester, MN 55905, USA

Avni Y. Joshi and Erin K. Ham
Department of Internal Medicine, Mayo Clinic, Rochester, MN 55905, USA

Neel B. Shah
Department of Medical Genetics, Mayo Clinic, Rochester, MN 55905, USA

Xiangyang Dong and Roshini S. Abraham
Department of Laboratory Medicine and Pathology, Mayo Clinic, Rochester, MN 55905, USA

Shakila P. Khan
5Division of Pediatric Hematology and Oncology, Department of Pediatric and Adolescent Medicine, Mayo Clinic, Rochester, MN 55905, USA

Jocelyn R. Farmer
Department of Medicine, Massachusetts General Hospital, Harvard Medical School, Boston, MA 02114, USA

Caroline L. Sokol and Mandakolathur R. Murali
Division of Allergy & Immunology, Massachusetts General Hospital, Harvard Medical School, Boston, MA 02114, USA

Francisco A. Bonilla
Division of Allergy & Immunology, Boston Children's Hospital, Harvard Medical School, Boston, MA 02115, USA

Richard L. Kradin
Department of Pathology, Massachusetts General Hospital, Harvard Medical School, Boston, MA 02114, USA

Todd L. Astor
Division of Pulmonary & Critical Care Medicine, Massachusetts General Hospital, Harvard Medical School, Boston, MA 02114, USA

Jolan E. Walter
Pediatric Allergy & Immunology and the Center for Immunology and Inflammatory Diseases, Massachusetts General Hospital, Harvard Medical School, Boston, MA 02114,USA

Napoleon Patel, Lisbet D. Suarez and Sakshi Kapur
Department of Internal Medicine, Atlantic Health System, Overlook Medical Center, 99 Beauvoir Avenue, Summit, NJ 07902, USA
Leonard Bielory Division of Allergy and Immunology, Rutgers University RobertWood Johnson University Hospital, New Brunswick, NJ 07103, USA

Marjolein A. C. Mattheij, Ellen J. H. Schatorjé and Esther de Vries
Department of Pediatrics, Jeroen Bosch Hospital, P.O. Box 90153, 5200 ME's-Hertogenbosch, The Netherlands

Marjolein A. C. Mattheij
University Medical Centre Antwerp, Antwerp, Belgium

Ellen J. H. Schatorjé
Radboud University Medical Centre Nijmegen, Nijmegen, The Netherlands

Eugenie F. A. Gemen
Laboratory for Clinical Chemistry and Hematology, Jeroen Bosch Hospital, P.O. Box 90153, 5200 ME's-Hertogenbosch, The Netherlands

Lisette van de Corput
Department of Medical Immunology, University Medical Center Utrecht, P.O. Box 85500, Utrecht, The Netherlands

Peet T. G. A. Nooijen
Department of Pathology, Jeroen Bosch Hospital, P.O. Box 90153, 5200 ME's-Hertogenbosch, The Netherlands

Mirjam van der Burg
Department of Immunology, Erasmus Medical Center, P.O. Box 2040, 3000 CA Rotterdam, The Netherlands

Masayuki Ishida, Hiroaki Fushiki and Yukio Watanabe
Department of Otolaryngology, Head & Neck Surgery, University of Toyama, Toyama 930-0194, Japan

Romina Pace
Department of Medicine, McGill University Health Centre, Montreal, QC, Canada H3G 1A4

Donald C. Vinh
Division of Infectious Diseases, Division of Allergy & Clinical Immunology (Department of Medicine), Department of Medical Microbiology, Department of Human Genetics, McGill University Health Centre, Montreal General Hospital, 1650 Cedar Avenue, Rm A5-156, Montreal, QC, Canada H3G 1A4

Joselyn Rojas, Marjorie Villalobos, María Sofía Martínez, Mervin Chávez-Castillo, Wheeler Torres, José Carlos Mejías, Edgar Miquilena and Valmore Bermúdez
Endocrine and Metabolic Diseases Research Center, School of MedicineThe University of Zulia, Maracaibo 4004, Venezuela

Joselyn Rojas and Marjorie Villalobos
Endocrinology Department, Maracaibo University Hospital (SAHUM), Maracaibo 4004, Venezuela

Aristo Vojdani
Deptartment of Immunology, Immunosciences Lab., Inc., Los Angeles, CA 90035, USA
Cyrex Laboratories, Phoenix, AZ 85015, USA

David Perlmutter
Perlmutter Health Center, Naples, FL 34102, USA

Oswald Moling, Raffaella Binazzi, Lathá Gandini, Giovanni Rimenti and Peter Mian
Division of Infectious Diseases, Ospedale Generale, 39100 Bolzano, Italy

Alfonsina Di Summa and Loredana Capone
Division of Neurology, Ospedale Generale, 39100 Bolzano, Italy

Josef Stuefer
Radiology, Ospedale Generale, 39100 Bolzano, Italy

Andrea Piccin
Division of Hematology, Ospedale Generale, 39100 Bolzano, Italy

Alessandra Porzia, Antonella Capozzi and Maurizio Sorice
Department of Experimental Medicine, Sapienza University, 00161 Rome, Italy

Carolina Mejia-Otero and Shelley Singh
Internal Medicine Department, Mount Sinai Medical Center, Miami, FL 33140, USA

Luis Arias Urdaneta and Carlos Sesin
Division of Rheumatology, Internal Medicine Department, Mount Sinai Medical Center, Miami, FL, USA

Anindita Chakrabarti
Department of Infectious Disease, University of Miami Miller School of Medicine, Miami, FL 33136, USA

Nanci Mae Miller
Department of Pathology, Mount Sinai Medical Center, Miami, FL, USA

Claudio Tuda
Division of Infectious Disease, Internal Medicine Department, Mount Sinai Medical Center, Miami, FL, USA

Stalin Viswanathan and Kandan Balamurugesan
Indira Gandhi Medical College, Kadhiramam, Pondicherry 605009, India

Sunny Garg, Mousumi Kundu, Lalit Prashant Meena, Neeraj Varyani, Asif Iqbal and Kamlakar Tripathi
Department of General Medicine, Institute of Medical Sciences, Banaras Hindu University, Varanasi 221005, India

Amit Nandan Dhar Dwivedi
Department of Radiology, Institute of Medical Sciences, Banaras Hindu University, Varanasi 221005, India

Deng-Ho Yang
Division of Rheumatology/Immunology/Allergy, Department of Internal Medicine, Armed-Forces Taichung General Hospital, Number 348, Section 2, Chung Shan Road, Taiping District, Taichung City 411, Taiwan

Institute of Medicine, Chung Shan Medical University, Taichung city, Taiwan

Amit Frenkel, Aviel Roy-Shapira, Brotfain Evgeni, Koyfman Leonid and Moti Klein
General Intensive Care Unit, Soroka University Medical Center and the Faculty of Health Sciences, Ben-Gurion University of the Negev, 84101 Beersheba, Israel

Abraham Borer
Infection Control and Hospital Epidemiology Unit, Soroka University Medical Center and the Faculty of Health Sciences, Ben-Gurion University of the Negev, 84101 Beersheba, Israel

Norair Adjamian
Kansas City University of Medicine & Biosciences, Kansas City, MO 1750, USA

Adeline Kikam
Firelands Regional Medical Center, Sandusky, OH 1111, USA

Kathryn Ruda Wessell, Jason Casselman, Erin Toller-Artis, Olapeju Olasokan and Robert W. Hostoffer
University Hospitals Richmond Medical Center, Richmond Heights, OH 27100, USA

Magdalena Klanova, Pavel Klener, Marek Trneny, Jan Straub and Ivan Spicka
1st Department of Medicine and Clinical Department of Hematology, the General Teaching Hospital, Charles University in Prague, Prague, Czech Republic

Magdalena Klanova and Pavel Klener
Institute of Pathological Physiology, First Faculty of Medicine, Charles University in Prague, Prague, Czech Republic

Marek Trneny
Institute of Hematology and Blood Transfusion, Prague, Czech Republic

Carlos Saavedra, Paola Cárdenas, Héctor Castellanos, Kateir Contreras, and J. R. Castro
Units of Infectology and Dermatology, Department of Internal Medicine, National University of Colombia, 111321 Bogotá, Colombia

JunMuratsu, Atsuyuki Morishima, Masayoshi Kukida, Anzu Tanaka, and Katsuhiko Sakaguchi
Department of Nephrology and Hypertension, Sumitomo Hospital, 5-3-20 Kitaku Nakanoshima, Osaka 530-0005, Japan

Shigeki Fujita
Department of Pathology, Sumitomo Hospital, 5-3-20 Kitaku Nakanoshima, Osaka 530-0005,Japan